A GUIDE TO THE
MRCP PART 2
WRITTEN PAPER

'Fully updated in line with new MRCP exam format'

A GUIDE TO THE MRCP PART 2 WRITTEN PAPER

Second edition

Dr Anthony N. Warrens DM PhD FRCP

MRC Clinician Scientist Fellow and Honorary Senior Registrar, Renal
Unit, Royal Postgraduate Medical School, Hammersmith Hospital,
London, UK

Dr Malcolm Persey MD FRCP

Consultant Rheumatologist, Barnet & Chase Farm Hospitals NHS
Trust, London, UK

Dr Michael Fertleman MRCP Of Gray's Inn, Barrister

Specialist Registrar, General and Geriatric Medicine, Northwick Park
Hospital, London, UK

Professor Stephen H. Powis BSc BM BCh PhD FRCP

Professor of Renal Medicine, Royal Free and University College
Medical School, University College London, London, UK

Professor Alimuddin Zumla PhD FRCP

Director, Division of Infectious Diseases, Department of Medicine,
University College Medical School, London, UK

Hodder Arnold

A MEMBER OF THE HODDER HEADLINE GROUP

First published in Great Britain in 1998 by Hodder Arnold
This second edition published in 2005 by
Hodder Arnold, an imprint of Hodder Education and a member of the
Hodder Headline Group,
338 Euston Road, London NW1 3BH

http://www.hoddereducation.com

Distributed in the United States of America by
Oxford University Press Inc.,
198 Madison Avenue, New York, NY10016
Oxford is a registered trademark of Oxford University Press

Whilst the advice and information in this book are believed to be true and
accurate at the date of going to press, neither the author[s] nor the publisher
can accept any legal responsibility or liability for any errors or omissions that
may be made. In particular (but without limiting the generality of the preceding
disclaimer) every effort has been made to check drug dosages; however it is still
possible that errors have been missed. Furthermore, dosage schedules are
constantly being revised and new side-effects recognized. For these reasons the
reader is strongly urged to consult the drug companies' printed instructions
before administering any of the drugs recommended in this book.

British Library Cataloguing in Publication Data
A catalogue record for this book is available from the British Library

Library of Congress Cataloging-in-Publication Data
A catalog record for this book is available from the Library of Congress

ISBN-10   0 340 80658 3
ISBN-13   978 0 340 806 58 6

1 2 3 4 5 6 7 8 9 10

Commissioning Editor: Joanna Koster
Project Editor: Heather Fyfe
Production Controller: Lindsay Smith
Cover Designer: Amina Dudhia

Typeset in 10 on 12pt Sabon by Phoenix Photosetting, Chatham, Kent
Printed and bound in Italy

What do you think about this book? Or any other Hodder Arnold title?
Please send your comments to www.hoddereducation.com

Contents

Preface

It is 11 years since the publication of the first edition of this book. There have been many changes in medicine over that period; new evidence, new technologies and even one or two new diseases. With time it has become clear that the favourable reception accorded the first edition would not be sustained by further reprints without adapting to these changing circumstances. With the encouragement of the staff at the publishers, Hodder Arnold, we have therefore, not always willingly, laboured to produce a second edition.

In that time there have also been many changes in the approach of the Royal Colleges to examining those applying for their seal of approval, but the importance of that approval remains undiminished. We have therefore also had to adapt, for better or for worse, to the new (and ever-changing) examinations format, while trying to update the questions to more closely reflect the practice of medicine more than a decade on.

Progression through most careers involves crossing the thresholds of examinations set by professional associations. The further you get, the more important it becomes not just to have 'the knowledge', but also the technique.

As in the previous edition we have attempted to distil our own experiences with advice and feedback we have received to present a medical textbook for MRCP in the context of typical questions and answers, with advice about how to approach the questions. Recognizing that to cover the full range of subjects would be impossible we have tried to emphasize those areas often poorly understood by candidates.

We have co-opted a further author (MF), who is still young enough to sympathize with those of you about to pass through the trauma of the MRCP Examination, while some of the original authors have moved on to senior posts, including an examiner or two!

We hope this double authorial perspective will enhance the book and help to make it worthy of its titular claims to be a true aid to the MRCP written papers.

Acknowledgements

First and foremost we must acknowledge that the tradition of thanking families for support in preparation of a book is no mere formality and, in this case at least, truly reflects how difficult such an undertaking would be without their encouragement and patience.

We are grateful to our publishers, and in particular, Jo Koster, Dan Edwards and more recently Heather Fyfe, for not only their practical help but for making sure that we did get on with the job.

A number of colleagues, senior and junior, have contributed material and comments, as well as reviewing the papers. Their contributions have been invaluable, and in particular we would like to thank the following:

Dr A. Ansari, Dr J. Ball, Dr C. Baynes, Dr E. Beck, Dr R. Behrens, Dr J. Chambers, Dr P. Chiodini, Dr E. Choi, Mr J. Conway, Dr F. Flinter, Dr M. Friston, Miss J.M. Heaton, Prof D. Isenberg, Dr Murali Kotechwara, Dr G. Llewelyn, Dr A.Lulat, Prof K.P.W.J. McAdam, Dr D. McEnirey, Dr Shaun McGee, Dr T. McKay, Dr Tom Maher, Dr S. Makinole, Dr P.D. Mason, Dr M. Medlock, Dr P. Nunn, Dr W. Rakowicz, Dr B. Ramsey, Dr Jeremy Rees, Dr W. Rosenberg, Dr N. J. Simmonds, Dr A.K.L. So, Dr Campbell Tait, Dr S.M. Tighe, Dr Enric Vilar, Dr W.R.C. Weir, Dr P.R. Wilkinson, Dr Steve Williams, Dr M.K.B. Whyte, Dr P. Wong.

Introduction

Times have changed and modern education reflects technological advance and an emphasis on equality and fair assessment, no less at MRCP level than elsewhere.

The examination

The old MRCP written examination with separate grey, data interpretation and pictorial cases, followed by a lunchtime analysis in the nearest pub, is now a distant and perhaps unpleasant memory for those already at consultant level. It has been replaced by a day and a half marathon of three 3-hour papers, each containing between 80 and 100 questions. The questions usually contain a combination of at least two and sometimes all three of history, data or photographic components. The question will ask the candidate to select one of the 'best of five' given options, or occasionally 'two from ten'. Each candidate is given a question booklet, an answer sheet and a 'brochure' of images, photographs and ECGs.

It is all computer marked and candidates should expect to see an answer grid similar to that met in Part I. Education research has shown that negative marking discriminates unfairly against some candidates and therefore there are no deductions for an incorrect answer and nothing is lost by guessing. Blank and wrong answers alike earn no points.

The book

Candidates fail because they lack the degree of knowledge required or their examination technique is poor. Despite the syllabus, it is hard to know how much should be covered and in what depth. This book contains many examples of questions we think might come up, but we could never hope to cover all possibilities. This is where good examination technique becomes indispensable.

Knowing all there is to know about medicine does not necessarily guarantee success in the MRCP – although of course it would be a great asset – rather like the losing football manager who knows everything about the game, but fails to study the tactics of the opposing team. Likewise, you must have a plan before going into the examination. It is no good memorizing the contents of numerous textbooks without having ever tried a specimen question. Quite simply, approach the exam as if you were going into battle with the College – not such an inappropriate analogy. You must develop an examination technique that will allow you to make the best use of your knowledge on the day. We have deliberately structured our book to help you achieve this.

The book is divided into 3 exam papers of 100 questions. Some of these contain a subset of several questions – unlikely in the examination itself, but allowing us to show you how the same information can lead to a variety of questions. If you chose to use the book as 3 mock examinations you should answer 100 questions in 3 hours or 50 questions in 1½ hours before looking at the answers. Alternatively you could use the book as textbook, going through the questions by subject. An appendix indexes the 12 subject areas covered in the book (Cardiology, Dermatology, Endocrinology, Gastroenterology, Haematology, Infectious Diseases, Nephrology, Neurology, Respiratory, Rheumatology, Therapeutics & Others) across all three exams.

Whichever way you choose, write down your answers, as otherwise you will tend to credit your-self with an answer that passed through your mind, even if you rejected it. If you have written evidence of your conclusions, your impression of your performance will be similar to that of your examiners.

Tackling questions

Read the question stem with its possible answers first. This will give you an idea as to what is required. Differentiate between the 'hard data' and the 'soft data'. By 'hard data' we mean unequivocal abnormalities, usually physical signs or abnormal laboratory results. The history can provide hard data but remember that as in real clinical practice, what the patients say might not mean what you think it means, and something important may be withheld. You may assume that physical signs have been correctly elicited and reported and also that the examiner is not withholding from you a relevant physical sign which you would expect to find on thorough routine examination.

Try constructing a mental differential diagnosis around a piece of hard laboratory data such as eosinophilia or hypercalaemia, or from a feature of the physical examination such as splenomegaly. Choose the most unusual of the given observations.

As regards laboratory and radiological data you can expect that common investigations such as an ECG will be difficult to interpret whereas the less common cardiac pressure data will be easier to interpret.

For the more common investigations practice a logical and reproducible approach to the data which will help you arrive at the correct diagnosis – much as you are taught to examine the various components of the ECG one at a time.

For the less common investigations try to construct short lists of the conditions likely to be represented. In the examination, if you are having difficulty reaching an answer, run through your list to see which fits best. It may trigger in your mind what is the appropriate answer to the question. In this book, we shall try to provide you with a list of the most likely diagnoses for most of these specialist investigations.

We demonstrate how pictorial material can be integrated into questions in a variety of ways. Almost anything can be shown and breadth of knowledge from the widely available books of pictures is recommended. However, like the laboratory data it is impossible to predict the range of what will be shown. Common investigations like chest x-rays and CT scans are favourites. Prior to the examination you should prepare lists of the more common conditions likely to be presented. Practice logical methods of looking at pictures for use when an abnormality is not immediately present. We will suggest these for certain classes of picture – for example the mnemonic for looking at an apparently normal chest x-ray.

If you are having difficulty with a question, move on and come back to it later. Time is limited and there is nothing more soul-destroying that running out of time because you have spent too long on a question that you could not do. Many candidates report rushing through the last 10 questions.

Using the answers

Take time over going through the answers. You will find detailed descriptions of how to approach the particular type of question. Extra information is provided in 2 types of boxes. In the shaded boxes we present generalised tips on technique. In the unshaded boxes we present information that you may find particularly useful in tackling the examination. In subsequent papers, you will encounter similar types of question. If you have read and understood the discussion provided with the first example, then these should become progressively easier to tackle.

We have attempted to be as comprehensive as possible, but there will clearly be important gaps. There is also occasional repetition. This is deliberate as it reinforces the message that the same information can be presented in a variety of ways. We have always put in what we feel to be the best answer. Others will fit, but not as well as ours. This reflects what you will find in the examination.

All we can say is that we have done our best. Like its predecessor this edition has been reviewed and re-reviewed not only by candidates sitting the examination but also by expert colleagues, who are, after all, the people who set the questions.

Please feel free to write to us (c/o Hodder Arnold) with other areas of discussion that you feel should have been included as well as criticism of what is here.

Examination A

Questions

Question 1

A 32-year-old renal transplant recipient presents with dyspnoea 6 weeks after transplantation. She had required transplantation after a rapid and irreversible deterioration in renal function due to type I diabetes mellitus. She had had one episode of acute rejection 10 days after transplantation which had been reversed with high-dose corticosteroids. She was discharged 3 weeks after transplantation on prednisolone, azathioprine and cyclosporin A with a plasma creatinine of 119 µmol/L. She had failed to present for regular review for 2 weeks before the present assessment.

On examination, she was afebrile and clinically well. Palpation of the graft was unremarkable. Results of investigations were as follows:

Plasma sodium	144 mmol/L
Plasma potassium	4.9 mmol/L
Plasma urea	20.2 mmol/L
Plasma creatinine	343 µmol/L
Urgent urine microscopy	normal
Urgent ultrasound of renal tract	no evidence of obstruction

1   Which of the following would be your next two investigations?
    (a) Graft renal artery angiogram
    (b) Renal transplant biopsy
    (c) Urine microscopy and culture
    (d) Serum cyclosporin A levels
    (e) Blood cultures
    (f) Ultrasound of renal tract
    (g) Glycosylated haemoglobin level
    (h) Cytomegalovirus serology
    (i) Blood film examination
    (j) Chest x-ray

Question 2

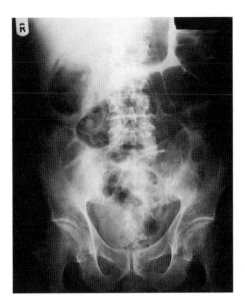

1   What is the diagnosis in this diabetic woman?
    (a) Toxic megacolon
    (b) Emphysematous cholecystitis
    (c) Ileus
    (d) Diverticular disease
    (e) Volvulus

Question 3

A 30-year-old male suffers from Crohn's disease and epilepsy. The inflammatory bowel disease proved very difficult to control over the years, requiring frequent courses of steroids. At initial presentation he was still having frequent episodes of loose, but relatively inoffensive, stool, but was otherwise generally well with no symptoms outside the gastrointestinal system.

He was taking phenytoin and prednisolone 10 mg/day. He has been a vegetarian since the onset of his bowel disease and has never smoked.

He was referred for evaluation of frequent episodes of cramp in his hand. At initial presentation, examination was normal apart from his being thin with ankle oedema.

Results of investigations performed were as follows:

Plasma calcium	1.95 mmol/L
Plasma phosphate	1.1 mmol/L
Plasma alkaline phosphatase	90 IU/L *(normal range 30–100)*
Hb	10.6 g/dL

1   What single investigation is most likely to explain his cramps?
     (a) Parathyroid hormone levels
     (b) Serum albumin
     (c) 24-hour urine calcium collection
     (d) Vitamin D level
     (e) Serum magnesium

Some years later he was referred again, this time because of deterioration in his gait. His Crohn's disease was now quiescent with improved overall well-being and a weight gain of almost 10 kg and resolution of the oedema. However, he had severe proximal myopathy and had fallen several times, most recently down the stairs outside the clinic.
     Results of investigations performed were as follows:

Plasma calcium	2.14 mmol/L
Plasma phosphate	1.35 mmol/L
Serum albumin	38 g/dL
Plasma alkaline phosphatase	1600 IU/L *(normal range 30–100)*
Hb	13.5 g/dL
Serum vitamin D level	36 pmol/L *(normal range 38–101)*

2   What is the most useful test?
     (a) Bone density scan
     (b) Bone biopsy
     (c) CT scanning of parathyroid glands for parathyroid adenoma
     (d) Subtraction radioisotope scan of thyroid and parathyroid glands
     (e) Creatine kinase

Question 4

A 25-year-old mechanic presents with apathy and tremor. Urinalysis shows glycosuria. The blood chemistry showed:

Plasma sodium	140 mmol/L
Plasma potassium	3.0 mmol/L
Plasma glucose	4.8 mmol/L
Plasma bicarbonate	14 mmol/L
Plasma aspartate aminotransferase	55 IU/L *(normal range 5–35)*
Plasma bilirubin	31 µmol/L

1   The two most useful investigations to confirm the diagnosis would be:
    (a) Glucose tolerance test
    (b) Urinary analysis for lead
    (c) Liver biopsy
    (d) Plasma γ-gluconeryltransferase level
    (e) Autoimmune screen
    (f) Serum caeruloplasmin level
    (g) HLA typing
    (h) Blood alcohol level
    (i) Bone marrow biopsy
    (j) Blood film

Question 5

A 53-year-old woman was investigated for a 6-month history of low back pain. Investigations showed:

Plasma sodium	136 mmol/L
Plasma potassium	4.2 mmol/L
Plasma urea	5.7 mmol/L
Plasma creatinine	98 μmol/L
Serum bilirubin	36 μmol/L
Serum albumin	42 g/L
Plasma aspartate aminotransferase	16 IU/L *(normal range 5–35)*
Plasma alkaline phosphatase	78 IU/L *(normal range 30–100)*
Serum IgG	28.5 g/L *(normal range 7.2–19)*
Serum IgA	2.3 g/L *(normal range 0.85–5)*
Serum IgM	2.0 g/L *(normal range 0.5–2)*
Hb	13.5 g/dL
WBC	5.9×10^9/L
Platelets	187×10^9/L
ESR	49 mm in the first hour
Serum electrophoresis	IgG A paraprotein band paraprotein concentration 18 g/L
Urine electrophoresis	no protein
Skeletal survey	no abnormality

1   The response to initial management in this condition is best measured through regular assessment of which of the following:
    (a) ESR
    (b) Protein electrophoresis
    (c) Serum creatinine
    (d) Serum calcium
    (e) Bone scan

Question 6

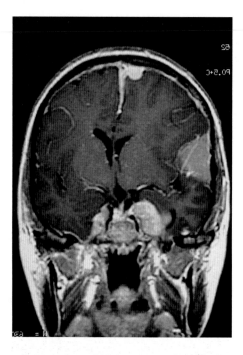

1   This patient with a hereditary disease was losing hearing. What is the underlying diagnosis?
    (a) Tuberous sclerosis
    (b) Multiple gliomata
    (c) Neurofibromatosis type I
    (d) Acoustic neuroma
    (e) Neurofibromatosis type II

Question 7

A 23-year-old male presented to A and E because he had become breathless during the course of the day. He was a non-smoker with no past history of disease.

On examination, he is dyspnoeic on moderate exertion with a respiratory rate of 20/min and a regular pulse of 100/min. His first and second heart sounds are normal, but there is an added systolic click.

1   What is the likely diagnosis?
    (a) Pneumothorax
    (b) Tension pneumothorax
    (c) Mitral valve prolapse
    (d) Pulmonary embolism
    (e) Lobar pneumonia

2   He has a normal chest x-ray; which single investigation do you arrange next?
    (a) Pulmonary angiogram
    (b) VQ scan
    (c) Echocardiogram
    (d) Chest x-ray in expiration
    (e) Pulmonary function tests

Hint
If you cannot decide which of the possible answers is right, ask yourself which would be the most dangerous to get wrong.

Question 8

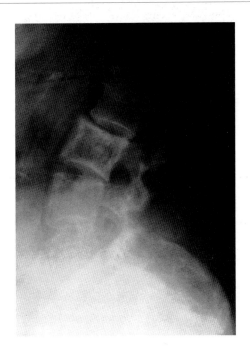

1   What are the two possible diagnoses?
    (a) Paget's disease
    (b) Metastasis from breast primary
    (c) Lymphoma
    (d) Osteoporotic collapse
    (e) Haemangioma
    (f) Acromegaly
    (g) Ankylosing spondylitis
    (h) Metastasis from lung primary
    (i) Osteomyelitis

Question 9

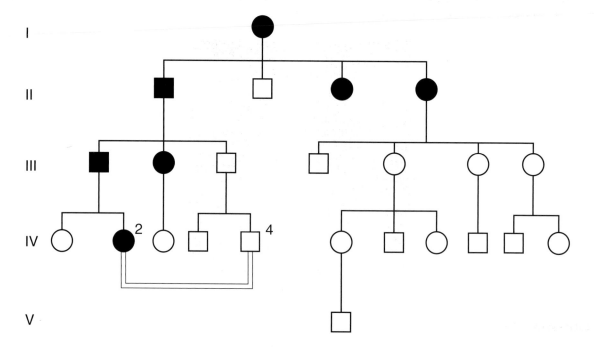

1   What is the mode of inheritance illustrated in this pedigree?
(a) Autosomal recessive
(b) Autosomal recessive with incomplete penetrance
(c) Autosomal dominant
(d) Autosomal dominant with incomplete penetrance
(e) X-linked

2   What is the probability of an affected offspring resulting from the marriage of IV^2 and IV^4?
(a) 1:1
(b) 1:2
(c) 1:3
(d) 1:4
(e) 1:8

Question 10

1   The pacemaker is likely to have been inserted:
(a) To treat hypertrophic cardiomyopathy
(b) To treat congenital heart block

(c) To treat acquired heart block
(d) To treat an arrhythmia following withdrawal of amiodarone
(e) To treat an arrhythmia following myocardial infarction

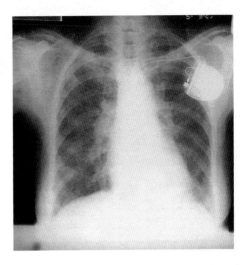

Question 11

A 21-year-old remains breathless after successful treatment of an apparently spontaneous pneumothorax. He mentions having to pass urine frequently. The chest x-ray report reads: 'Resolution of pneumothorax. Diffuse honeycomb appearance. Would be interested to know pathological diagnosis.'

Respiratory function tests show the following:

Test	Predicted	Actual
FEV (L)	4.00	1.43
FVC (L)	4.93	2.93
FEV$_1$/FVC		48 per cent
TLC (L)	5.95	6.30
TLCO (mmol/min/kPa)	10.64	5.1
KCO (mmol/min(kPa/L)	1.90	1.4

1 Suggest the likely diagnosis for the radiologist:
(a) Histiocytosis X
(b) Hand–Schuller–Christian disease
(c) Eosinophilic granuloma
(d) Neurofibromatosis
(e) Lymphangio(leio)myomatosis

Question 12

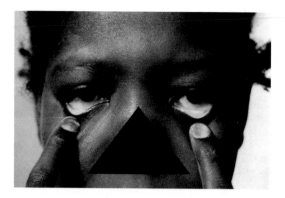

1 What is the likely diagnosis?
   (a) Megaloblastic anaemia
   (b) Iron-deficiency anaemia
   (c) Sideroblastic anaemia
   (d) Anaemia of chronic disease
   (e) Chronic liver disease

Question 13

1 What is the most appropriate treatment for stress polycythaemia?
   (a) Venesection
   (b) Heparin therapy
   (c) Warfarin therapy
   (d) Angiotensin-converting enzyme therapy
   (e) It does not need treatment

Question 14

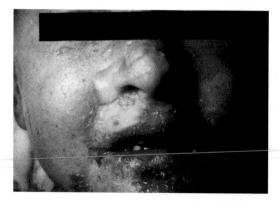

1   What is this lesion?
    (a) Erysipelas
    (b) Herpes simplex
    (c) Herpes zoster
    (d) Impetigo
    (e) Stevens–Johnson syndrome

Question 15

A 36-year-old woman presents with a 2-week history of haemoptysis and a 5-day history of haematuria. In the last 24 hours she has become increasingly dyspnoeic and oliguric.
    Investigations show:

Plasma sodium	136 mmol/L
Plasma potassium	8.9 mmol/L
Plasma bicarbonate	14 mmol/L
Plasma urea	48 mmol/L
Plasma creatinine	987 μmol/L
Hb	10 g/dL
Chest x-ray	patchy interstitial infiltrate

1   Give two investigations which would confirm the most likely diagnosis:
    (a) 24-hour urine collection
    (b) Anti-double-stranded DNA antibodies
    (c) Anti-GBM antibodies
    (d) pANCA
    (e) cANCA
    (f) Renal biopsy
    (g) CT thorax
    (h) Bronchoscopy
    (i) Serum calcium and phosphate
    (j) Serum angiotensin-converting enzyme

Question 16

The man to whom this fundus belongs has always had difficulty finding shoes to fit, and is wheelchair-bound by the age of 25 years. There is a no family history.

1   What would you not expect to find on examination and investigation?
    (a) Brisk tendon reflexes
    (b) Peripheral neuropathy
    (c) Optic atrophy
    (d) Spastic limbs
    (e) Abnormal ECG

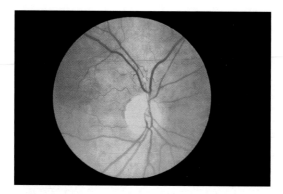

2   How do you make the diagnosis?
    (a) On the basis of history and clinical findings
    (b) Genetic test requesting triplet repeat analysis of DNA
    (c) Typical nerve conduction studies
    (d) Echocardiography
    (e) PCR to identify recessive mutation

Question 17

A 50-year-old former shipyard worker complained of breathlessness. Respiratory function tests were performed:

	Predicted	Actual
FEV (L)	4.1	3.9
FVC (L)	5.0	2.6
TLco (mmol/min/kPa)	10.2	6.6
Kco (mmol/min/kPa/L)	1.9	2.1

1   What is the probable diagnosis?
    (a) Emphysema
    (b) Pulmonary fibrosis
    (c) Mesothelioma
    (d) Asbestosis
    (e) Pleural thickening

Question 18

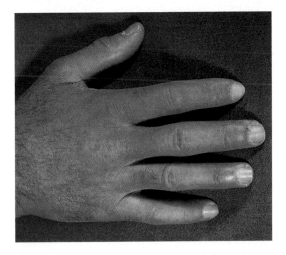

This patient complained of arthralgia and excessive post-prandial fullness.

1   What is the likely diagnosis?
(a) Bronchogenic carcinoma
(b) Systemic sclerosis
(c) Linitis plastica
(d) Osler–Weber–Rendu syndrome
(e) NSAID induced ulceration

Question 19

The following data were obtained at cardiac catheterization:

Site	Oxygen saturation (per cent)
Superior vena cava	72
Inferior vena cava	76
Right atrium	75
Right ventricle	84
Pulmonary artery	85
Left ventricle	98
Aorta	97

1   What is the diagnosis?
(a) Ostium primum atrial septal defect with right-to-left shunt
(b) Ostium primum atrial septal defect with left-to-right shunt

(c) Ostium secundum atrial septal defect with left-to-right shunt
(d) Ventricular septal defect with a left-to-right shunt
(e) Ventricular septal defect with a right-to-left shunt

Question 20

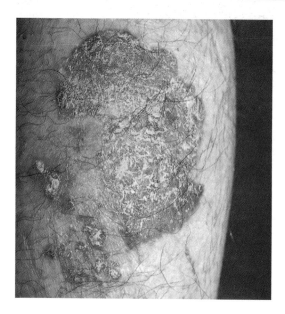

1   What is this isolated skin lesion?
    (a) Mycosis fungoides
    (b) Psoriasis
    (c) Arsenic poisoning
    (d) Dermatophyte infection
    (e) Bowen's disease

Question 21

You are asked to consent a 17-year-old girl for an HIV test following an admission after a violent sexual assault. Her parents have just left the hospital to go and pick up her younger sister from school. Whilst consenting her for the test she tells you that the assailant was her father, but she doesn't want you to tell anyone.

1   You should:
    (a) Tell no one
    (b) Inform the police
    (c) Inform the ward sister
    (d) Inform social services
    (e) Inform the mother

Question 22

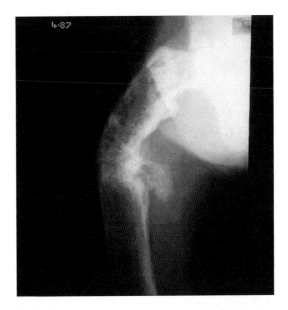

1   Give the diagnosis.
     (a) Rickets
     (b) Pathological fracture
     (c) Paget's disease
     (d) Metastatic disease
     (e) Osteoarthritis

Question 23

You are asked to see a 76-year-old-man who has been brought into A and E by his carer who helps him get dressed in the morning. She told the A and E receptionist that the patient was 'not quite himself' but gave no further information and left before being seen by a nurse or doctor. You are unable to find another informant. His old notes report several attendances to the rheumatology clinic because of degenerative joint disease.

The patient himself is inattentive and drowsy. He can give you no coherent history. On examination there are no other physical signs. Although he resists neurological examination, there is no obvious focal deficit.

The nurses tell you that his BM is 4.2 and his 12-lead ECG shows normal sinus rhythm. His FBC is normal.

1   What are the next two investigations that should be performed?
     (a) CT brain
     (b) Full blood count
     (c) Urea and electrolytes

(d) Laboratory glucose
(e) Chest x-ray
(f) Urine microscopy
(g) Blood cultures
(h) Troponin measurement
(i) Paracetamol and salicylate level
(j) Urine Dipstix

Question 24

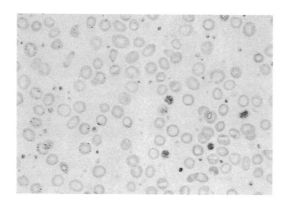

1   Suggest the underlying diagnosis.
   (a) *Helicobacter pylori* infection
   (b) Multiple myeloma
   (c) Alcoholism
   (d) Essential thrombocythaemia
   (e) Crohn's disease

Question 25

A 55-year-old greengrocer was referred with a history of several months of a hacking dry cough, particularly bad first thing in the morning. On direct questioning, it was clear that it had troubled him intermittently for at least 2 years. It was almost never productive. He also tended to be short of breath after walking only 100 metres on the flat, although this was rather variable.

He had never smoked. He had been prescribed salbutamol, ipratropium bromide, and beclomethasone inhalers variously for several years. Initially helpful, they had seemed to be much less useful over the past year or so. Two 1-week courses of oral prednisolone, starting at a dose of 30 mg, had brought no significant benefit.

On examination, he was dyspnoeic on mild exertion. His chest was hyperinflated. Otherwise there were occasional inspiratory and expiratory wheezes audible throughout the chest. His peak expiratory flow rate was 250 L/min. His JVP was not visible and the apex beat was not displaced. Cardiac auscultation was normal. The liver was palpable 2 cm below the right subcostal margin. By percussion, the upper border was in the seventh intercostal space. Urinalysis was normal.

Biochemistry and haematological studies were normal.

1   What is the likely diagnosis?
    (a) Extrinsic allergic alveolitis
    (b) Chronic asthma
    (c) Chronic obstructive airways disease
    (d) Primary pulmonary hypertension
    (e) Cardiac failure

2   Which single pulmonary function test would you use to confirm this?
    (a) Arterial blood gas analysis
    (b) Transfer factor (DLCO)
    (c) FEV_1/FVC before and after bronchodilators
    (d) Peak expiratory flow rate before and after bronchodilators
    (e) Flow–volume loops

Question 26

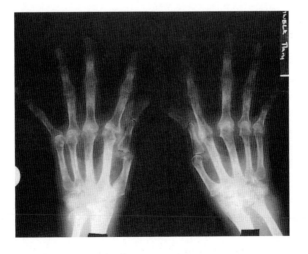

1   What is the diagnosis?
    (a) Gout
    (b) Osteoarthritis
    (c) Rheumatoid arthritis
    (d) Systemic sclerosis
    (e) Pseudogout

Question 27

A 30-year-old brittle diabetic presents with a grand mal fit. In A and E, her blood glucose is normal, having had no intervention.

1   The commonest cause of her fit would have been:
   (a) Hypoglycaemia
   (b) Hyperglycaemia
   (c) Acidosis
   (d) Space-occupying lesion
   (e) Head trauma

Question 28

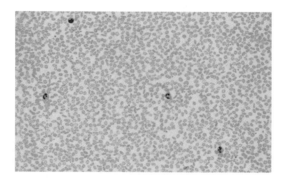

1   How is this condition inherited?
   (a) Autosomal recessive
   (b) Autosomal dominant
   (c) X-linked dominant
   (d) X-linked recessive
   (e) Mitochondrial disease inheritance pattern

Question 29

You are called to a cardiac arrest where you find that a 47-year-old man admitted earlier that week with a suspected myocardial infarct has collapsed in the corridor. You establish that the airway is patent but that he is not breathing spontaneously. You are unable to feel any pulsation in his carotid or femoral arteries. You instruct two colleagues to institute assisted cardiopulmonary resuscitation while you await an anaesthetist and equipment.

1   What ratio of rescue breathing to sternal massage do you request?
   (a) Non-synchronous with 100 compressions and 20 breaths per minute
   (b) 15:2

(c) 5:1
(d) 10:1
(e) Non-synchronous with 100 compressions and 10 breaths per minute

The patient is connected to a cardiac monitor and VF is noted. He is given two shocks though a monophasic defibrillator. Fifteen seconds following the second shock the monitor shows sinus rhythm. There is no pulse palpable.

2   The correct course of action is to:
(a) Continue basic CPR for another 45 seconds and reassess
(b) Continue basic CPR for another 165 seconds and reassess
(c) Give 1 mg of adrenaline and commence CPR for 3 minutes
(d) Give 1 mg of adrenaline and commence CPR for 1 minute
(e) Commence temporary pacing

Following the correct management in question 2, a weak pulse is detected. After 35 seconds VF again is seen on the monitor with no pulse detectable.

3   The correct management would be:
(a) Shock at 360 J
(b) Shock at 200 J
(c) 1 mg adrenaline
(d) 300 mg amiodarone
(e) Abandon resuscitation as futile

Question 30

An elderly lady presented with hyperosmolar non-ketotic diabetic coma.

1   Give three important steps in the management of this patient:
(a) Intravenous fluid replacement with twice normal saline
(b) Intravenous fluid replacement with normal saline
(c) Intravenous fluid replacement with hypotonic saline
(d) Intravenous fluid replacement with dextrose-saline
(e) Intravenous fluid replacement with 5 per cent dextrose
(f) Potassium replacement at rate of 40 mmol/h
(g) Potassium replacement at rate of 40 mmol/30 min
(h) Manage potassium abnormalities by coadministering dextrose and insulin
(i) Restoration of normoglycaemia with intravenous insulin
(j) Avoid administering insulin to prevent risk of hypoglycaemia
(k) Administer 8.4 per cent sodium bicarbonate via peripheral line
(l) Administer 8.4 per cent sodium bicarbonate via central line
(m) Anticoagulation with heparin
(n) Control anxiety with benzodiazepines
(o) Following resolution, change from insulin to biguanide therapy

Question 31

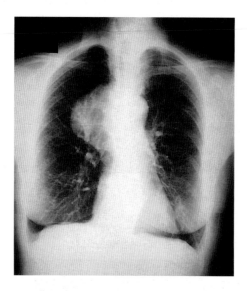

This is the chest x-ray of a patient complaining of weakness.

1 What is the diagnosis and why is she weak?
   (a) Dissecting aortic aneurysm with consequent vascular insufficiency
   (b) Paraspinal meningioma with cord compression
   (c) Carcinoma of lung with Eaton–Lambert syndrome
   (d) Rheumatoid arthritis with lung nodulosis and cervical myelopathy
   (e) Thymoma and myasthenia gravis

Question 32

A 40-year-old woman is investigated as part of a routine life assurance medical.

Plasma sodium	135 mmol/L
Plasma potassium	4.1 mmol/L
Plasma urea	2.3 mmol/L
Plasma creatinine	45 µmol/L
Plasma bicarbonate	19 mmol/L
Plasma calcium	2.3 mmol/L
Plasma phosphate	1.4 mmol/L
Plasma glucose	6 mmol/L
Plasma bilirubin	7 µmol/L
Plasma aspartate aminotransferase	14 IU/L *(normal range 5–35)*
Plasma alkaline phosphatase	42 IU/L *(normal range 30–100)*
Serum albumin	34 g/L

Serum urate	0.12 mmol/L
Serum thyroxine	170 nmol/L *(normal range 70–140)*
Hb	9.8 g/dL
WBC	5×10^9/L
Platelets	180×10^9/L
Urinalysis	glucose ++

1 How would you confirm the diagnosis?
   (a) Oral glucose tolerance test
   (b) Urine hormone evaluation
   (c) Thyroid uptake scan
   (d) Colonoscopy
   (e) Ultrasound abdomen

Question 33

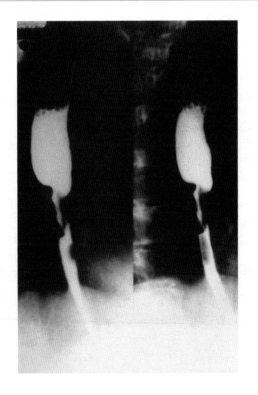

1 What is the diagnosis?
   (a) Achalasia
   (b) Oesophageal web
   (c) Scleroderma
   (d) Peptic stricture
   (e) Malignant stricture

Question 34

A 23-year-old man returns from a holiday in the USA with a skin rash. He complains of a drooping right eyelid.

CSF examination reveals clear fluid with an opening pressure of 16 cm. Fluid analysis:

Protein	1.5 g/L
White cells	56/mm^3 (80 per cent lymphocytes)
Glucose	2.0 mmol/L
Plasma glucose	5 mmol/L

1   What is the likely diagnosis?
   (a) Neurosyphilis
   (b) Neurosarcoidosis
   (c) Lyme disease
   (d) SLE
   (e) Fungal meningitis

Question 35

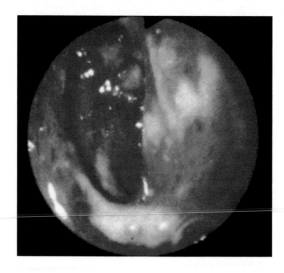

1   The pathology should initially be treated with:
   (a) Oral vancomycin
   (b) Oral metronidazole
   (c) Oral corticosteroids
   (d) Topical corticosteroids
   (e) Intravenous corticosteroids

Question 36

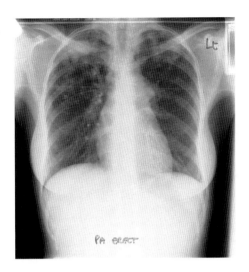

A 37-year-old presents with haemoptysis.

1   What are the radiological diagnoses?
   (a) Cryptogenic fibrosing alveolitis
   (b) Tuberculosis
   (c) Aspergillosis
   (d) Aspergilloma
   (e) Small cell carcinoma
   (f) Squamous cell carcinoma
   (g) Caplan's syndrome
   (h) Varicella pneumonia
   (i) Goodpasture's syndrome
   (j) Extrinsic allergic alveolitis

2   What tests would you do initially?
   (a) Aspergillosis precipitins
   (b) Skin tests for aspergilla sensitivity
   (c) Heaf test
   (d) Bronchoscopy
   (e) Sputum smear microscopy and culture
   (f) Serology for anti-BM antibodies
   (g) ANCA
   (h) Open lung biopsy
   (i) Rheumatoid factor and lupus serology
   (j) HIV test

Questions: Exam A

Question 37

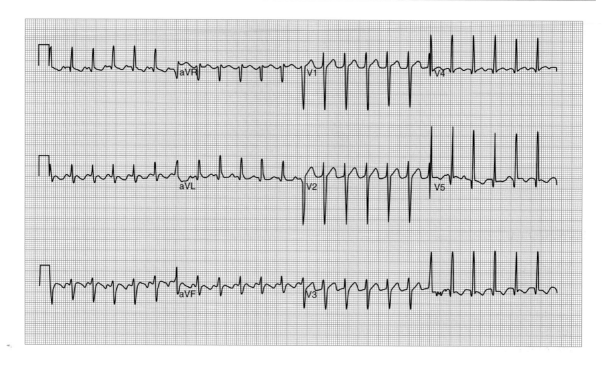

1   What is the most significant abnormality on this ECG?
    (a) Sinus tachycardia
    (b) Atrial fibrillation
    (c) Atrial flutter
    (d) Lateral ischaemia
    (e) Left axis deviation

2   How might you confirm this?
    (a) Intravenous adenosine
    (b) Carotid sinus massage
    (c) Intravenous amiodarone
    (d) Intravenous digoxin
    (e) Echocardiogram

Question 38

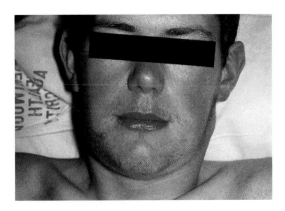

This patient has a sore throat and a fever.

1   What is the diagnosis?
  (a) Glandular fever
  (b) CMV infection
  (c) *Toxoplasma gondii* infection
  (d) *Streptococcus pyogenes* infection
  (e) Kawasaki's disease

Question 39

A 45-year-old man with a background history of diabetes and severe hypercholesterolaemia is seen in A and E feeling unwell. The following results were obtained:

Plasma sodium	133 mmol/L
Plasma potassium	6.9 mmol/L
Plasma urea	22 mmol/L
Plasma creatinine	2254 µmol/L
Plasma calcium	1.87 mmol/L
Plasma phosphate	1.99 mmol/L

1   What is the cause of his renal impairment?
  (a) Cholesterol emboli syndrome
  (b) Renal papillary necrosis
  (c) Renal artery stenosis
  (d) Diabetic nephropathy
  (e) Rhabdomyolysis

Question 40

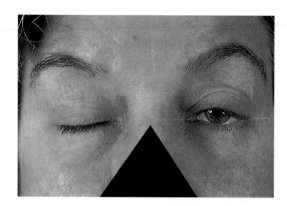

1   What is the likely diagnosis?
   - (a) Hypothyroidism
   - (b) Third cranial nerve palsy
   - (c) Horner's syndrome
   - (d) Myotonia dystrophica
   - (e) Myasthenia gravis

Question 41

A 28-year-old West Indian woman is 27 weeks into a second pregnancy. Her first, 10 years previously, had ended in a spontaneous abortion at 20 weeks. Following the abortion she had suffered breathlessness and chest pain and was anticoagulated for 6 months. During that pregnancy, in the West Indies, she had been told that she had rheumatoid arthritis but this had not concerned her since. Now the GP has admitted her to hospital with hypertension (BP 170/100 mmHg) and an active urinary sediment. A medical opinion is sought and you note a few splinter haemorrhages on each hand, a systolic cardiac murmur and no peripheral oedema.

1   Of the following which is the most likely diagnosis of the current problem?
   - (a) Rheumatoid vasculitis
   - (b) Pre-eclampsia
   - (c) Systemic lupus erythematosus
   - (d) Systemic sclerosis
   - (e) Subacute bacterial endocarditis

The initial investigations available to you are:

Hb   9.8 g/dL
WBC 3.8×10^9/L
Platelets 125×10^9/L
MCV 101 fL
Na   138 mmol/L
K   3.8 mmol/L
Creatinine   124 μmol/L
Blood culture   pending

2 What further two investigations would you order?
   (a) Erythrocyte sedimentation rate
   (b) SLE-serology (ANA and anti-DNA)
   (c) Transthoracic echocardiography
   (d) Anticardiolipin antibody
   (e) Chest x-ray
   (f) C-reactive protein
   (g) Further blood cultures
   (h) Electrocardiogram
   (i) Rheumatoid factor
   (j) Anti Scl-70

3 Other than appropriate blood pressure control, give two treatments you would consider for your first
   diagnosis:
   (a) Delivery of fetus
   (b) Warfarin
   (c) Heparin
   (d) Azathioprine
   (e) Cyclophosphamide
   (f) Magnesium
   (g) Methotrexate
   (h) Non-steroidal anti-inflammatory
   (i) Prednisolone
   (j) Vasodilators

Question 42

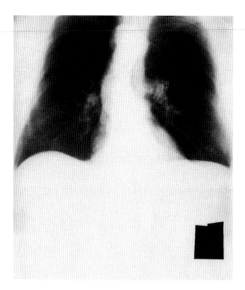

1   What is the abnormality?
    (a) Right-sided aortic arch
    (b) Mediastinal widening
    (c) Pleural thickening
    (d) Tumour in the left mid-zone
    (e) Elevated hemi-diaphragm

Question 43

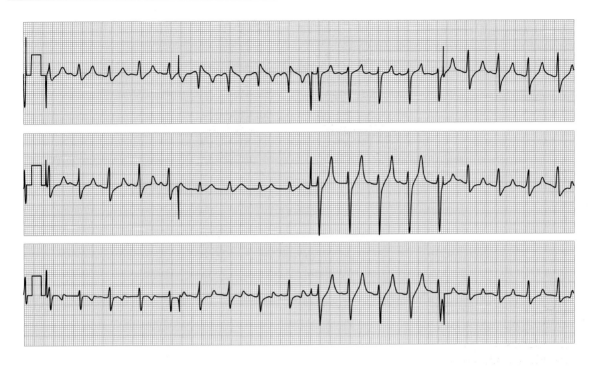

This is the ECG of a 45-year-old man who has been brought to A and E breathless.

1   What is the cause of the ECG abnormalities?
   (a) Anterolateral ischaemia
   (b) Pulmonary embolism
   (c) Hyperkalaemia
   (d) First-degree heart block
   (e) Hypothermia

Question 44

A 38-year-old City solicitor was admitted because of rapidly increasing jaundice immediately following her return from holiday in Ibiza. She had been entirely well prior to leaving the UK 2 weeks previously. Five days before her return she began to feel unwell and 2 days later she was first noted to have developed jaundice. She experienced mild epigastric fullness and discomfort, anorexia and nausea. She was now unable to keep any food down and still complained of abdominal fullness.

She had smoked 5–10 cigarettes/day for 20 years and drank three or four glasses of wine on social occasions, on average three times per week, although she had drunk 'rather more' on holiday. She denied intravenous or other drug abuse and had had no recent blood transfusions. She knew of no infectious contacts. She was married and had no other sexual partners.

On examination, she was jaundiced but afebrile. She was slightly drowsy and displayed a minor coarse tremor. There was some evidence of constructional apraxia. There were no stigmata of chronic liver disease. She was mildly tender in the epigastrium but there was no hepatic or splenic enlargement. There was no lymphadenopathy. Her blood pressure was 145/70 mmHg lying and 150/80 mmHg sitting. The rest of the examination was normal.

Her full blood count was normal. The results of further investigations were as follows:

Plasma sodium	132 mmol/L
Plasma potassium	3.9 mmol/L
Plasma urea	24.7 mmol/L
Plasma creatinine	198 µmol/L
Plasma aspartate aminotransferase	554 IU/L *(normal range 4–20)*
Plasma alkaline phosphatase	900 IU/L *(normal range 30–100)*
Hb	12.4 g/dL
WBC	8.2×10^9/L
Platelets	235×10^9/L
Prothrombin time	34 s (control 14 s)
Partial thromboplastin time	51 s (control 34 s)
Chest x-ray	no abnormalities
Plain abdominal radiograph	normal
HbsAb	positive
Urinalysis	no cells, protein, or glucose; specific gravity 1.030

1   What is the diagnosis?
(a) Acute hepatic failure due to alcohol abuse with the hepatorenal syndrome
(b) Idiopathic acute hepatic failure
(c) Acute hepatic failure due to hepatitis B virus
(d) Acute hepatic failure due to paracetamol overdose with the hepatorenal syndrome
(e) Acute hepatic failure due to leptospirosis

Question 45

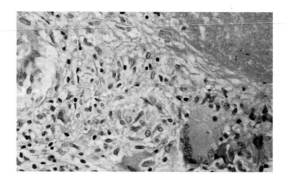

1   This lesion should be treated with:
(a) Oral antituberculous therapy

(b) Oral steroids
(c) Wide local excision
(d) Radiotherapy
(e) Oral antiretroviral therapy

Question 46

A GP asks for your advice. He has just received a copy of these investigations, performed in the outpatient department on a patient who had recently presented with hypertension and peripheral oedema.

Plasma sodium	137 mmol/L
Plasma potassium	8.9 mmol/L
Plasma urea	13.8 mmol/L
Plasma creatinine	210 μmol/L
Plasma calcium	2.1 mmol/L
Plasma phosphate	3.9 mmol/L
Plasma glucose	1.5 mmol/L

1   What is the cause of these abnormalities?
(a) Ectopic Cushing's syndrome
(b) Haemolysis
(c) Delayed sample analysis
(d) Type II renal acidosis
(e) Acute renal failure

Question 47

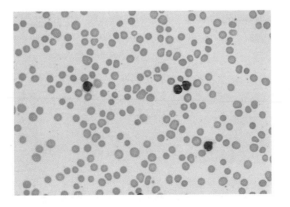

This is the peripheral blood film of a 69-year-old man who presented with herpes zoster. His blood count revealed a WBC count of 70×10^9/L.

1 What is the diagnosis?
   (a) Acute myeloblastic leukaemia
   (b) Chronic lymphocytic leukaemia
   (c) Acute lymphoblastic leukaemia
   (d) Chronic myeloid leukaemia
   (e) Erythroleucoplakia

Question 48

A 62-year-old man is referred to a renal physician for investigation of impaired renal function. He has lost 19 kg in weight over the previous 3 years, with intermittent episodes of nausea and vomiting.
Investigations show:

Plasma sodium	134 mmol/L
Plasma potassium	3.0 mmol/L
Plasma bicarbonate	40 mmol/L
Plasma chloride	83 mmol/L
Plasma urea	15.4 mmol/L
Plasma creatinine	201 μmol/L
Plasma calcium	2.59 mmol/L
Plasma phosphate	1.06 mmol/L
Plasma alkaline phosphatase	69 IU/L *(normal range 30–100)*
Serum albumin	41 g/L
Abdominal ultrasound	normal size kidneys; no evidence of obstruction; moderate enlargement of the prostate

1 How would you confirm the likely diagnosis?
   (a) Renal biopsy
   (b) Arterial pH
   (c) Gastroscopy
   (d) Renin and aldosterone levels
   (e) Drug history

Question 49

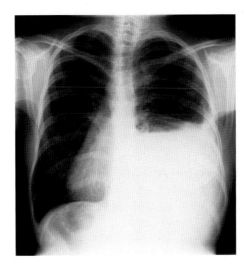

A woman in her thirties presents breathless; her chest x-ray is shown; her gas transfer is about 20 per cent expected and the pleural aspirate is milky.

1   Apart from dextrocardia, what is the diagnosis?
    (a) Carcinomatosis
    (b) Hypothyroidism
    (c) Adult respiratory distress syndrome
    (d) Thoracic duct rupture
    (e) Lymphangioleiomatosis

Question 50

A 60-year-old male presents with swelling and stiffness in his hands and shoulders of 6 months' duration. Some years ago he had required bilateral surgery for carpal tunnel syndrome; he was a little breathless on exertion, and admitted to impotence since his GP had prescribed diuretics for his dyspnoea, but otherwise his history was unremarkable.

On examination there was symmetrical swelling of the metacarpophalangeal joints of both hands, which were remarkably non-tender. There was bruising over the index finger of the right hand which he said had come on while turning a stiff key that morning. He felt dizzy when he stood up from the examination couch but recovered rapidly.

The GP had arranged some investigations:

Full blood count:
   Haemoglobin   12.5 g/dL
   White cell count 8×10^9/L
   Platelets 351×10^9/L
   ESR   87 mm/h

Urinalysis in clinic showed ++ proteinuria.

1   Which initial further investigation might most further your diagnosis?
   (a) CRP
   (b) Protein electrophoresis
   (c) Serum ANCA
   (d) Blood pressure measurement
   (e) Serum ACE

2   What is the diagnosis?
   (a) AL amyloidosis
   (b) Sarcoidosis
   (c) Wegener's granulomatosis
   (d) AA amyloidosis
   (e) Multiple myeloma

Question 51

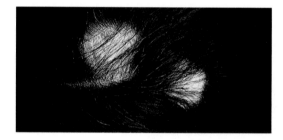

1   What is the diagnosis?
   (a) Discoid lupus
   (b) Tinea capitis
   (c) Alopecia areata
   (d) Previous evacuated subdural haematoma
   (e) En coup de sabre

Question 52

A 27-year-old Indian aeronautics engineer presented with a 2-week history of colicky abdominal pain, borborygmi, intermittent fever and diarrhoea of increasing frequency producing loose mucus-containing stool without blood. Over the past year he had noticed occasional loose stools and was feeling generally tired. He had lost 4 kg in weight recently and had developed low back pain. There was no history of travel abroad. He had received two courses of antibiotics during the past year for upper respiratory tract infections. He had a steady girlfriend.

On examination, he looked ill, was thin, pale and febrile (37.8°C). The abdomen was slightly distended, tender, and there was a diffuse mass in the right iliac fossa. The bowel sounds were increased in frequency. The remainder of the examination, including urinalysis, was normal.

The results of investigations performed were as follows:

Hb	10.8 g/dL
WBC	11.6×10^9/L
Neutrophils	69 per cent
Lymphocytes	29 per cent
Eosinophils	2 per cent
Platelets	352×10^9/L
ESR	56 mm in first hour
Plasma sodium	138 mmol/L
Plasma potassium	3.9 mmol/L
Plasma urea	4.9 mmol/L
Serum C-reactive protein	66 mg/L *(normal range <5 mg/L)*
Serum albumin	32 g/L
Plasma aspartate aminotransferase	38 IU/L *(normal range 4–20)*
Plasma alanine aminotransferase	90 IU/L *(normal range 2–17)*
Plasma bilirubin	7 µmol/L
Plasma alkaline phosphatase	82 IU/L
Plasma calcium	2.30 mmol/L
Plasma phosphate	0.80 mmol/L
Plasma thyroxine	104 nmol/L *(normal range 70–140)*
Faecal analysis	*Clostridium difficile* toxin not detected; no ova, cysts of parasites seen

1   What is the likely diagnosis?
   (a) Crohn's disease
   (b) Ileocaecal tuberculosis
   (c) Small bowel lymphoma
   (d) *Yersinia* enterocolitis
   (e) Chronic appendicitis

Question 53

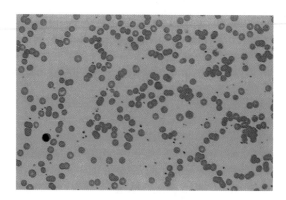

This is the peripheral blood film at 20°C of a woman who complains of recurrent abdominal pain and digital discoloration in the cold.

1   What is the diagnosis?
   (a) Raynaud's phenomenon
   (b) Sjögren's syndrome
   (c) Paroxysmal cold haemoglobinuria
   (d) Systemic lupus erythematosus
   (e) Polycythaemia rubra vera

Question 54

A 26-year-old intravenous drug abuser was brought as an emergency to A and E by his girlfriend. Four days prior to admission he had developed fever, non-productive cough and generalized muscle aches. Despite being prescribed amoxicillin by his GP, he had become worse and was now dyspnoeic. He had recently returned from a visit to Morocco. He drank heavily and smoked 30 cigarettes per day. He and his girlfriend had been treated for syphilis 3 months previously.

On examination he was acutely ill, centrally cyanosed with a temperature of 38.8°C, normotensive, and had a pulse of 100/min. He had mild jaundice, and tattoo marks on his right forearm. There were a few bilateral fine crackles on auscultation of the chest. His venepuncture sites were clean. There was no clinical evidence of deep vein thromboses of the calves.

The results of investigations were as follows:

Hb	12.8 g/dL
WBC	12×10^9/L
ESR	42 mm in first hour
Plasma sodium	136 mmol/L
Plasma potassium	3.5 mmol/L
Plasma urea	5.1 mmol/L

Plasma creatinine	98 μmol/L
Plasma bilirubin	90 μmol/L
Plasma aspartate aminotransferase	56 IU/L *(normal range 4–20)*
Plasma γ-glutamyltransferase	101 IU/L *(normal range 7–33)*
Plasma alkaline phosphatase	306 IU/L *(normal range 30–100)*
ECG	sinus tachycardia
Chest x-ray	upper and mid zone shadowing
Arterial blood gases	
pH	7.46 (on 30 per cent oxygen)
PaO_2	7.0 kPa
$PaCO_2$	3.8 kPa
Blood cultures	negative
Cold agglutinins	negative
Urinalysis	no abnormality

1   What is the likely diagnosis?
   (a) *Mycoplasma* pneumonia
   (b) *Pneumocystis carinii* pneumonia
   (c) Pulmonary tuberculosis
   (d) *Legionella* pneumonia
   (e) Amoxicillin-induced hepatitis

2   Which two investigations would you perform?
   (a) Bronchoscopy, lavage, and transbronchial biopsy
   (b) High-resolution CT chest
   (c) Pulmonary function tests with gas transfer
   (d) HIV test
   (e) Urinary *Legionella* antigen
   (f) Heaf test
   (g) Early morning gastric aspirate
   (h) Induced sputum
   (i) Clotting studies
   (j) Liver biopsy

3   Which two treatments would you prescribe?
   (a) Nebulized pentamidine
   (b) Antituberculous chemotherapy
   (c) Oral corticosteroids
   (d) Oral co-trimoxazole
   (e) Intravenous co-trimoxazole
   (f) Intravenous vitamin K
   (g) Triple therapy
   (h) Intravenous clarithromycin
   (i) Oral erythromycin
   (j) Intravenous amoxicillin

Question 55

A university science student doing his finals has become lethargic and irritable. Examination was unremarkable. The cerebrospinal fluid examination was clear with an opening pressure of 300 mm.

CSF:
White cells   3/mm^3
Protein   2.1 g/L
Glucose   4 mmo/L
Plasma glucose   6 mmol/L

1   What investigation would you order next?
     (a) PCR on CSF sample
     (b) EEG
     (c) CT brain
     (d) Blood film
     (e) Conduction studies

Question 56

An 18-year-old male was brought in to A and E by the police, having been found collapsed in the street. They had phoned his employers (whose name was written in his diary) who confirmed that he had been totally well at work 4 hours earlier. No other history was available.

He was cyanosed, had a temperature of 41.7°C and was generally floppy except around his mouth where he seemed to be chewing. His pulse was 165/min and his blood pressure 80/65. He had fixed dilated pupils. There was no neck stiffness or papilloedema and no focal neurological signs.

Results of investigations were as follows:

Plasma sodium   114 mmol/L
Plasma potassium   4.4 mmol/L
Plasma urea   5.5 mmol/L
Lumbar puncture   normal

1   What is the causative agent?
     (a) Cocaine
     (b) Ecstasy
     (c) Amphetamine
     (d) LSD
     (e) Selegiline

Question 57

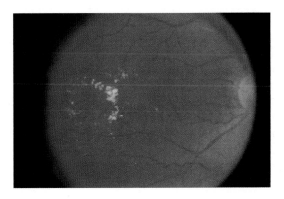

1   The diagnosis is:
    (a) Tay–Sachs disease
    (b) Background diabetic retinopathy
    (c) Grade II hypertensive retinopathy
    (d) Choroiditis
    (e) Retinal detachment

Question 58

A 59-year-old man with a history of angina is admitted to hospital for investigation of intermittent claudication. He has a history of hypertension for which he was initially prescribed a thiazide diuretic. Six months ago this was changed to a calcium antagonist. On the surgical ward his blood pressure is consistently around 200/110 mmHg. He has a trace of ankle oedema. Investigations show:

Plasma sodium	137 mmol/L
Plasma potassium	2.7 mmol/L
Plasma urea	8.9 mmol/L
Plasma creatinine	221 µmol/L
Hb	11.9 g/dL
WBC	8.9×10^9/L
Platelets	388×10^9/L

1   What is the most likely underlying diagnosis?
    (a) Renal artery stenosis
    (b) Conn's syndrome
    (c) Cushing's syndrome
    (d) Phaeochromocytoma
    (e) Essential hypertension

Question 59

A 37-year-old man has been on a hiking holiday with his partner in North Wales. He had been well until hours before his admission to a hospital near the camping site. He complained of general malaise and a productive cough, with no other specific symptoms.

He looked like a fit man with unremarkable observations including a heart rate of 60 and BP of 95/60. Examination of the chest and abdomen was normal apart from some faecal staining on his underpants. Neurological examination showed him to have fixed pupils and some diplopia on looking to the right. Otherwise his cranial nerve examination was normal. Examination of his limbs revealed mild reduced power in his arms and in his legs, with normal tone and reflexes. His plantars were downgoing.

Investigations:

FBC	normal
U + E	normal
LFT	normal
CSF	normal
CXR	normal
ECG	normal
Lung function tests:	
FEV_1	60 per cent
FVC	62 per cent
FEV_1/FVC	82 per cent
TL_{CO}	96 per cent
K_{CO}	102 per cent

1   What is the diagnosis?
(a) Viral gastroenteritis
(b) Botulism
(c) Guillain–Barré syndrome
(d) Organophosphate poisoning
(e) Myasthenia gravis

Question 60

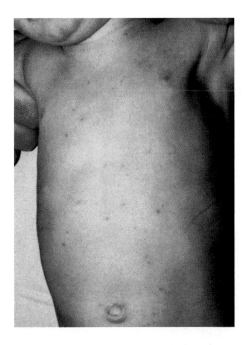

This child had a rising fever and constipation after a visit to India.

1   What is the diagnostic test of choice?
    (a) Stool culture
    (b) Blood culture
    (c) Serology
    (d) Clinical diagnosis
    (e) Culture of skin lesion

Question 61

A 26-year-old woman was admitted for an elective laparoscopic investigation of infertility. Unfortunately, the common iliac artery was torn during the procedure and an urgent laparotomy was required to staunch the haemorrhage. This proved difficult and she required two further urgent laparotomies in the next 24 hours. She required intubation and management on the Intensive Care Unit. Oliguria failed to respond to conservative measures and continuous venovenous haemofiltration was commenced through an indwelling double lumen femoral cannula, with total parenteral nutrition via an internal jugular cannula.

In the first 10 days of her illness she had a continuous pyrexia of 37.5–38.0°C despite ampicillin, flucloxacillin and metronidazole. The white cell count was 13–15×10^9/L and platelet count 60–80×10^9/L. On the eleventh day, the temperature rose to 38.5°C, white cell count to 20×10^9/L and the platelet count fell to 40×10^9/L. The antibiotics were changed to ceftazidime and metronidazole. Seventy-two hours later she was no better. There were no positive microbiological results from any stage in her illness.

1   What would be your first lines of management?
    (a) Change to intermittent haemodialysis
    (b) Stop all drugs
    (c) Repeat cultures after discontinuing antimicrobial therapy
    (d) Extend anti-staphylococcal cover with fusidic acid
    (e) Change and culture tips of IV cannulae and catheters and repeat blood cultures
    (f) Commence antifungal therapy
    (g) Platelet transfusion
    (h) Give hydrocortisone
    (i) Further laparotomy
    (j) Give fresh frozen plasma

Question 62

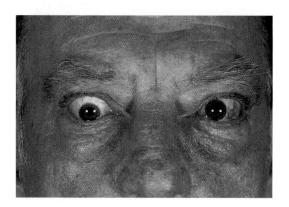

1   What is the likely diagnosis?
    (a) Retro-orbital tumour
    (b) Right IV nerve palsy
    (c) Graves' disease
    (d) Left Horner's syndrome
    (e) Left glass eye

(c) IgM fluorescent treponemal antibody test

(d) IgG fluorescent treponemal antibody test

(e) Serial antibody assays for rising titres of fluorescent treponemal antibody

Question 67

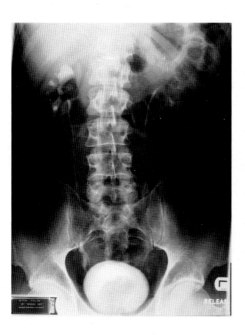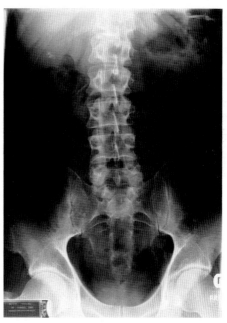

1   What prompted this investigation?
(a) Abnormal renal function
(b) Abdominal pain
(c) Sterile pyuria
(d) Red cell casts in urine
(e) Recurrent urinary tract infection

2   What is the diagnosis?
(a) Analgesic nephropathy
(b) Partially treated urinary tract infection
(c) Reflux nephropathy
(d) Schistosomiasis
(e) Tuberculosis

Question 68

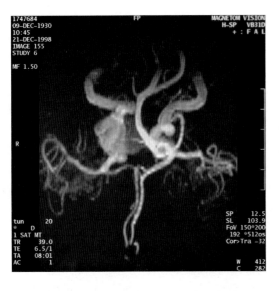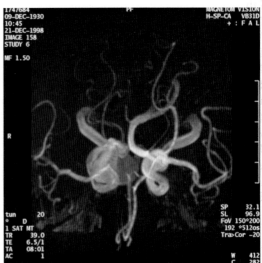

This man developed a sudden, severe headache.

1 What is the investigation?
   (a) Venous digital subtraction angiography
   (b) Arterial digital subtraction angiography
   (c) Cerebral angiography
   (d) CT angiography
   (e) MR angiography

2 What does it show?
   (a) Subarachnoid haemorrhage
   (b) Haemorrhage into cerebral tumour
   (c) Middle cerebral artery aneurysm
   (d) Posterior cerebral artery aneurysm
   (e) Dissection of internal carotid artery

Question 69

A 16-year-old girl is seen by her GP because of lethargy. She was often in the sick bay of her boarding school for the month of June and so missed many of her GCSEs. On one occasion she had a painful rash on her legs but this disappeared shortly after the end of term. She has had pain in her left ankle, although was still able to attend the leavers' ball. Since returning to her family home for the summer holidays she has become increasingly tired.

There is nothing abnormal to find on examination.

Blood tests reveal:

Hb	10.7 g/dL
MCV	78 fL
WBC	6.5×10^9/L
Platelets	527×10^9/L
Na	137 mmol/L
K	4.5 mmol/L
Urea	5.3 mmol/L
Creatinine	97 µmol/L
ALT	25 IU/L
Bilirubin	12 µmol/L
ALP	97 IU/L
Albumin	36 g/L
Pregnancy test	negative

1   The highest diagnostic yield will be by:
   (a) Referral to a psychiatrist
   (b) Colonoscopy
   (c) Autoimmune screen
   (d) Haemoglobin electrophoresis
   (e) Thyroid function tests

Question 70

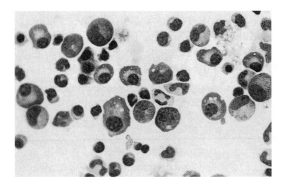

This is the bone marrow of a 49-year-old man.

1   What is the diagnosis?
   (a) Multiple myeloma
   (b) Chronic lymphocytic leukaemia
   (c) Infectious mononucleosis
   (d) Iron deficiency anaemia
   (e) Acute lymphoblastic leukaemia

Question 71

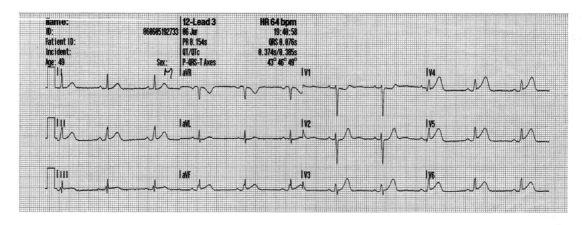

A 67-year-old Type II diabetic is seen in A and E following a road traffic accident. This is his ECG. He has been given aspirin, oxygen and diamorphine.

1   What is the next step ?
   (a) Thrombolysis with streptokinase
   (b) Thrombolysis with tPA
   (c) Echocardiogram
   (d) CT scan
   (e) Subcutaneous heparin

Question 72

A 35-year-old man was admitted for investigation of intermittent blurring of his vision. During these episodes his pupils would dilate, which caused him great anxiety. He also had problems with his balance, for which reason he walked with a stick. He had no other medical problems and was on no medication. On examination, there were no neurological signs. His gait was non-diagnostic and he did not really need the stick.

   While in hospital he suffered one of his attacks of blurred vision, during which it was confirmed that both pupils were widely dilated and totally unresponsive to light or accommodation.

1   What is the diagnosis?
   (a) Multiple sclerosis
   (b) Brain stem transient ischaemic attack
   (c) Clandestine self-medication with a mydriatic
   (d) Chronic subdural haematoma
   (e) Pancoast tumour

Question 73

A 28-year-old male presents with an itchy vesicular rash on his buttocks and a 4-month history of intermittent, foul-smelling, liquid stools and weight loss.
Investigations show:

Hb	7.9 g/dL
WBC	6×10^9/L
MCV	105 fL
MCHC	30 g/dL
ESR	14 mm in first hour
Blood film	macrocytosis and microcytosis
Serum iron	8 mmol/L *(normal range 13–22)*
Serum albumin	27 g/L
Serum globulin	40 g/L
Plasma aspartate aminotransferase	18 IU/L *(normal range 5–35)*
Plasma alkaline phosphatase	40 IU/L *(normal range 30–100)*

1   What single test would you request?
   (a) Skin biopsy
   (b) IgA anti-endomysial antibodies
   (c) Stool examination
   (d) Endoscopic duodenal biopsy before and after gluten-free diet
   (e) Sigmoidoscopy

Question 74

A 30-year-old woman presented to A and E as an emergency, having developed a widespread, symmetrically distributed, macular rash and ulceration of the mucous membranes of the mouth, eyes and vagina. She gave a 3-day history of a sore throat and 'flu-like illness' for which she was prescribed amoxicillin by her GP.

Her 6-year-old son had had chickenpox 2 weeks ago. She had never been abroad. She owned a budgie and an Alsatian dog. There was no history of allergies.

On examination, she was acutely ill and distressed with a temperature of 39.2°C but was normotensive. There was conjunctival injection and small beads of pus were seen at the inner canthus. There were painful ulcers in the mouth and in the genital tract. Erythematous macules of varying size were distributed all over the body including the palms and soles of her feet. There were some erythematous lesions and three bullous lesions on her thigh. Urinalysis was normal.

Investigations yielded the following results:

Hb	11.2 g/dL
WBC	10.8×10^9/L (65 per cent neutrophils)
ESR	36 mm in first hour
Chest x-ray	normal
VDRL	negative
Mycoplasma serology	negative
Throat swab	no growth

1 What is the diagnosis?
(a) *Mycoplasma* pneumonia
(b) *Legionella* pneumonia
(c) Stevens–Johnson syndrome
(d) Erythema multiforme
(e) Behçet's syndrome

Question 75

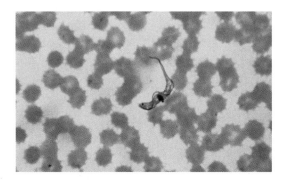

1 What is the diagnosis?
(a) Malaria
(b) Schistosomiasis
(c) Leishmaniasis
(d) Filariasis
(e) Trypanosomiasis

Question 76

A 39-year-old male with a history of rhinitis develops asthma and a purpuric rash. Results of investigations are as follows:

Hb	11.9 g/dL
MCV	93 fL
MCH	31 pg
WBC	10.0×10^9/L
Neutrophils	4.6×10^9/L
Eosinophils	1.9×10^9/L
Basophils	0.04×10^9/L
Monocytes	0.6×10^9/L
Lymphocytes	2.9×10^9/L
Platelets	239×10^9/L
ESR	45 mm in first hour

Plasma sodium	144 mmol/L
Plasma potassium	4.1 mmol/L
Plasma urea	5.1 mmol/L
Antineutrophil cytoplasmic antibody	detected perinuclear pattern of staining ethanol-fixed neutrophils
Anti-myeloperoxidase antibody	detected
Urinalysis	no abnormality detected
Chest x-ray	several patchy shadows in both lung fields

1   What is the diagnosis?
(a) Churg–Strauss syndrome
(b) Wegener's granulomatosis
(c) Classical polyarteritis nodosa
(d) Microscopic polyangiitis
(e) Systemic lupus erythematosus

Question 77

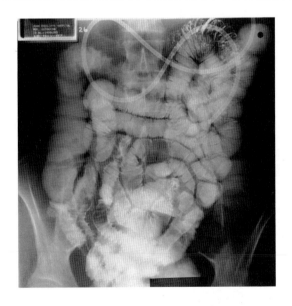

1   What is the diagnosis?
(a) Ulcerative colitis
(b) Ischaemic colitis
(c) Tuberculous enteritis
(d) Crohn's disease
(e) Coeliac disease

Question 78

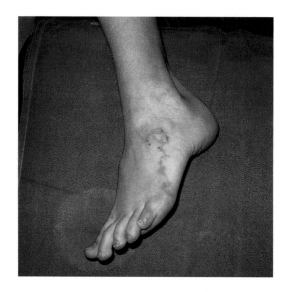

1   What is this abnormality?
    (a) Erythema marginatum
    (b) Scabies
    (c) Hookworm infestation
    (d) Eczema
    (e) Urticaria

Question 79

1   What two investigations would you perform to confirm a diagnosis of primary biliary cirrhosis?
    (a) Serum anti-mitochondrial antibody
    (b) Serum anti-smooth muscle antibody
    (c) Serum anti-gliadin antibody
    (d) Serum anti-endomysial antibody
    (e) Serum anti-liver/kidney microsomal antibody
    (f) Abdominal ultrasound
    (g) Liver biopsy
    (h) Endoscopic retrograde cholangiopancreaticogram (ERCP)
    (i) CT scan of upper abdomen
    (j) Mean corpuscular volume of erythrocytes

Question 80

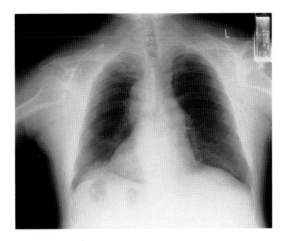

This is the routine chest x-ray of a man who is seeking health insurance.

1   The next investigation that you would advise his GP to arrange is:
   (a) Nothing
   (b) CT chest
   (c) Bronchoscopy
   (d) Echocardiogram
   (e) Lung function tests

Question 81

A 2-week-old baby presents with snuffles, skin rash and hepatomegaly. The VDRL is positive.
1   What is the most likely diagnosis?
   (a) Neonatal lupus
   (b) Congenital syphilis
   (c) Passive transfer of anti-Ro antibody from mother with lupus
   (d) Passive transfer of antibody from mother seropositive following syphilis exposure
   (e) Neonatal hepatitis

Question 82

A 35-year-old male complains of joint pains for many years and cold hands. He recalls an episode of a painful rash on his lower limbs some years ago. Otherwise the history is unrevealing.

Examination fails to show any evidence of an arthropathy. There is minor peripheral sensory loss and he wears dentures. There are a few fine basal inspiratory crepitations but otherwise normal findings.

Investigations:

Hb	13.5 g/dL
WCC	8.3×10^9/L
Platelets	433×10^9/L
ESR	79 mm in the first hour
U+E	normal
CRP	<1 mg/L
ANA	+ve 1/320
IgG	17 g/L *(6–13)*
IgA	6 g/L *(0.8–3)*
IgM	5 g/L *(0.8–2.5)*
CXR	normal

1   What two tests would you organize to confirm your clinical diagnosis?
   (a) Protein electrophoresis
   (b) Rheumatoid factor
   (c) Cryoglobulins
   (d) Autoimmune screen
   (e) Mycoplasma serology
   (f) Hepatitis serology
   (g) Differential white cell count
   (h) High resolution CT of the chest
   (i) Antibodies to double-stranded DNA
   (j) Antibodies to extractable nuclear antigens

Question 83

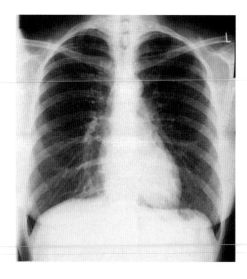

1   What is the abnormality?
   (a) Lytic lesion of the right clavicle
   (b) Chronic obstructive airways disease

(c) Cervical rib
(d) Osteoporosis
(e) Pulmonary hypertension

Question 84

The MN blood group is determined by three genotypes, L^ML^M, L^ML^N and L^NL^N at the L locus. The distribution of genotypes in a population of 1000 individuals is:

Blood group	Genotype	Number of individuals
M	L^ML^M	450
MN	L^ML^N	500
N	L^NL^N	50

1 Assuming random mating between members of the population and no selective pressure, what will the genotype frequencies be in the next generation?
  (a) $L^ML^M = 0.49$; $L^ML^N = 0.42$; $L^NL^N = 0.09$
  (b) $L^ML^M = 0.09$; $L^ML^N = 0.42$; $L^NL^N = 0.49$
  (c) $L^ML^M = 0.45$; $L^ML^N = 0.5$; $L^NL^N = 0.05$
  (d) $L^ML^M = 0.7$; $L^ML^N = 0$; $L^NL^N = 0.3$
  (e) $L^ML^M = 0.33$; $L^ML^N = 0.33$; $L^NL^N = 0.33$

Question 85

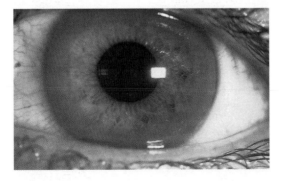

1 What is the diagnosis?
  (a) Primary hyperparathyroidism
  (b) Down's syndrome
  (c) Alport's syndrome
  (d) Wilson's disease
  (e) Horner's syndrome

Question 86

A 37-year-old woman presents with weight gain, amenorrhoea and hypertension. Investigations show:

Plasma sodium	138 mmol/L
Plasma potassium	2.7 mmol/L
Plasma cortisol at 9 a.m.	840 nmol/L
Plasma cortisol at 9 a.m. following 2 mg dexamethasone 6-hourly for 2 days	150 nmol/L *(normal range 280–700)*

1   What is the likely diagnosis?
(a) Cushing's syndrome
(b) Conn's syndrome
(c) Cushing's disease
(d) Polycystic ovaries syndrome
(e) Alcoholism

Question 87

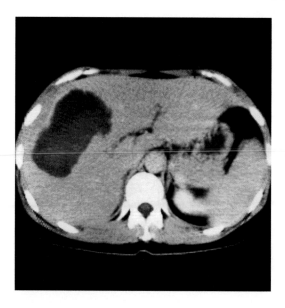

1   What is the likely radiological diagnosis?
(a) Pyogenic liver abscess
(b) Amoebic liver abscess
(c) Hepatoma
(d) Liver metastasis
(e) Hydatid cyst

Question 88

A 25-year-old woman presents with bruises and occasional nose bleeds over a period of 2 months. In the middle of that 2-month period the bruising seemed to be less of a problem. She is otherwise well. Specifically, she had had no shortness of breath or tiredness and had had no recent infections. She was rather a heavy drinker, consuming 2–3 gin and tonics a day.

On examination, she looked well and was not clinically anaemic. She had petechiae on the ulnar surfaces of both forearms. She had neither lymphadenopathy nor splenomegaly.

The results of investigations were as follows:

Hb	13.4 g/dL
WBC	9.8×10^9/L *(normal differential)*
Platelets	95×10^9/L
Blood film	normal
Prothrombin time	14 s *(normal range 11–15)*
Activated partial thromboplastin time	30 s *(normal range 25–34)*

1 What is the most likely cause of this woman's bleeding disorder?
   (a) Heterozygous factor X deficiency
   (b) Heterozygous factor IX deficiency
   (c) Fluctuating thrombocytopenia
   (d) Vitamin C deficiency
   (e) Acute myeloid leukaemia

Question 89

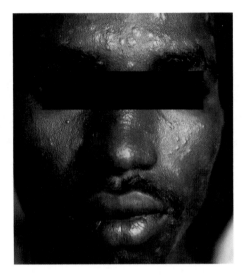

1   What is the likely diagnosis in this patient with lymphadenopathy and a non-itchy rash?
(a) Sarcoidosis
(b) Tertiary syphilis
(c) Secondary syphilis
(d) Staphylococcal septicaemia
(e) Sézary's syndrome

Question 90

A 26-year-old man is referred because of an episode of macroscopic haematuria that developed after a bout of tonsillitis. He had never previously been unwell.

1   The most likely diagnosis is:
(a) Post-streptococcal glomerulonephritis
(b) IgA nephropathy
(c) Acute leukaemia with leucopenia and thrombocytopenia
(d) Wegener's granulomatosis
(e) Benign bladder neoplasm

When he comes to your clinic he no longer has macroscopic haematuria.

2   The most likely combination of investigation results is:
(a) Normal urinalysis, normal serum creatinine
(b) Normal urinalysis, elevated creatinine
(c) Nephrotic-range proteinuria, normal serum creatinine
(d) Nephrotic-range proteinuria, elevated creatinine
(e) Oliguria, potassium 6.2 mmol/L and creatinine 667 μmol/L

Question 91

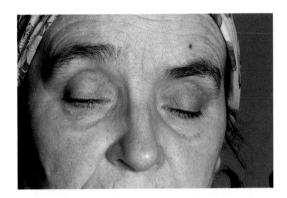

This woman is no longer able to open her eyes.

1   Which of the following would be the most appropriate first investigation?
    (a) CT brain scan
    (b) Muscle biopsy
    (c) Tensilon test
    (d) MR brain scan
    (e) CT thorax

Question 92

A 45-year-old farmer with a long history of hay fever developed an intermittent dry cough. Respiratory function tests results were as follows:

Predicted	Actual	After bronchodilators	
FEV$_1$ (L)	2.7	1.4	2.2
FVC (L)	3.6	2.6	3.2
FEV$_1$/FVC	75 per cent	54 per cent	
TL$_{CO}$ (mmol/min/kPa)	8.9	8.1	
K$_{CO}$ (mmol/min/kPa/L)	1.4	1.7	

1   What is the diagnosis?
    (a) Farmer's lung
    (b) Undefined restrictive lung disease
    (c) Pulmonary haemorrhage
    (d) Atopic asthma
    (e) Occupational asthma

Question 93

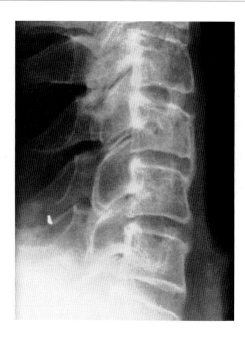

1 What is the likely diagnosis?
   (a) Diffuse idiopathic skeletal hyperostosis (DISH)
   (b) Vertebral spondylosis
   (c) Tuberculosis
   (d) Ankylosing spondylitis
   (e) Psoriatic arthritis

Question 94

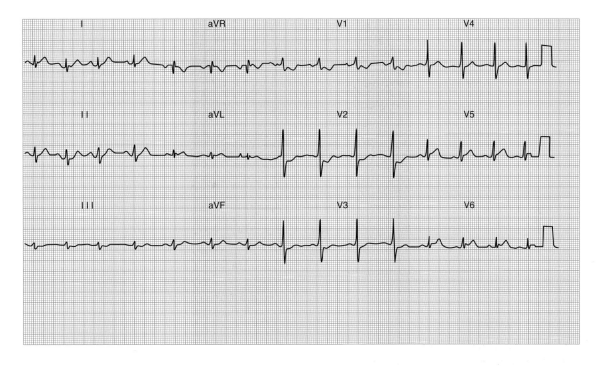

This is the ECG of a 60-year-old man who presents with chest pain.

1   What is the diagnosis?
    (a) Right ventricular myocardial infarction
    (b) Acute angina
    (c) Pericarditis
    (d) Posterior myocardial infarction
    (e) Dextrocardia

Question 95

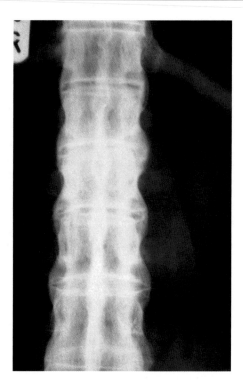

1 What is the diagnosis?
   (a) Diffuse idiopathic skeletal hyperostosis
   (b) Alkaptonuria
   (c) Spondylosis
   (d) Haemochromatosis
   (e) Ankylosing spondylitis

Question 96

You are called to a ward where a 17-year-old has been found unconscious. A note has been found by her bed to say that she doesn't want to be resuscitated should she be found alive. She has taken an overdose of tablets, but the note does not say which tablets have been taken. She is on the adolescent oncology ward and the nurses tell you that her proposed bone marrow transplant donor has withdrawn his consent.

1 What should you do?
   (a) Accept the suicide note as a valid advance directive
   (b) Commence treatment
   (c) Call her parents for further information
   (d) Call her consultant for further advice
   (e) Accept the suicide note as a valid contemporaneous refusal

Question 97

A 65-year-old man with lymphoma who is being treated with cytotoxic drugs and steroids presents with polyuria. He also has a history of manic-depressive illness. After normal baseline investigations, a water deprivation test was performed.

Date	Time	Urine osmolality (mOsm/kg)	Plasma osmolality (mOsm/kg)
25 August	1030	294	
	1130	243	
	1230	205	
	1300		289
	1330	203	
	1430	190	
	1600		299
	1630	250	
	1730	279	
	1730	DDAVP 2 mg given intramuscularly	
	1800	288	
	1830		289
	1830	276	
	1900	390	
	1930	411	
26 August	0030	486	
	0600	513	

1 What it the diagnosis?
   (a) Psychogenic polydipsia
   (b) Nephrogenic diabetes insipidus
   (c) Cranial diabetes insipidus
   (d) Syndrome of inappropriate antidiuretic hormone secretion
   (e) Diabetes mellitus

Question 98

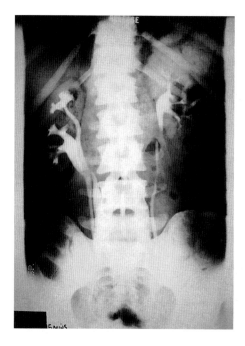

1   The abnormality shown predisposes to:
   (a) Vesicoureteric reflux
   (b) Renal cell carcinoma
   (c) Aortic regurgitation
   (d) Colovesical fistula
   (e) Lower limb ischaemia

Question 99

The following results were obtained from an apparently healthy 57-year-old man:

Hb	19.2 g/dL
PCV	54 per cent
RBC	6.6×10^9/L
MCV	83 fL
MCH	29 pg
MCHC	35 g/dL
WBC	8.5×10^9/L
Platelets	200×10^9/L

Further investigations showed:

Red cell mass	normal
Arterial blood gases	
PaO_2	10.9 kPa
$PaCO_2$	4.2 kPa

1   What is the most likely diagnosis?
   (a) Pseudopolycythaemia
   (b) Polycythaemia rubra vera
   (c) Chronic hypoxia
   (d) Asymptomatic unilateral hydronephrosis
   (e) Alpha thalassaemia trait

Question 100

A previously fit, sensible 70-year-old man was prescribed ibuprofen by his GP for osteoarthritis. He returned the following month complaining of breathlessness.

On examination, the only abnormalities found were changes of osteoarthritis. There were no physical signs in his respiratory system.

Respiratory function tests show his peak expiratory flow rate, FEV, and FVC to be within the predicted range.

1   For which of the following causes of his breathlessness is there NO support from the clinical information elicited above?
   (a) Asthma
   (b) Nephrotic syndrome
   (c) Anaemia
   (d) Pulmonary embolism
   (e) Acute renal failure due to interstitial nephritis

Answers

temic infection at this stage. For this reason blood cultures would not attract marks. The preferred initial investigations would be directed at the most likely diagnoses: acute rejection and cyclosporin A toxicity; infection and ureteric obstruction are unlikely given the normal microscopy and ultrasound.

Answer 1

1 (b), (d)

Essence

A renal transplant patient presents with a rise in creatinine shortly after transplantation.

Differential diagnosis

Investigations should be directed at revealing the cause of the graft failure, not excluding associated problems. Like all causes of renal failure, failure of a renal transplant may be classified as prerenal, renal and postrenal. It is reasonable to assume that the patient would have other prominent features of haemorrhage or hypotension; however, all anastomoses created at surgery (ureteric, arterial and venous) are subject to mechanical problems including dehiscence and stenosis. Renal artery pathology could cause prerenal uraemia.

The most likely intrinsic renal causes are cyclosporin A toxicity, rejection or infection. This early after transplantation, any rejection would be of the acute, potentially reversible type. After a few months, acute rejection episodes do not occur but the kidney becomes subject to chronic irreversible rejection. The other issue to consider is recurrence in the transplant of the original disease. Although diabetes may affect transplants, the only condition to recur early is focal and segmental glomerulosclerosis (FSGS). Postrenal causes of uraemia in transplants include ureteric obstruction and renal vein thrombosis.

Fever occurs both in acute rejection and infection. The lack of a fever excludes neither as the patient is immunosuppressed. However, it would be unusual for the patient to have no signs of sys-

Answer 2

1 (b)

The diagnosis here is emphysematous cholecystitis because air can be seen in the wall of the gallbladder. The condition, due to infection, most commonly occurs in elderly female diabetics and is usually caused by coliforms.

Causes of gas in the biliary tree

Within the bile ducts
- Incompetence of the sphincter of Oddi following sphincterotomy, passage of a gallstone or in the elderly ('patulous sphincter')
- Postoperative cholecystectomy or choledochoenterostomy
- Spontaneous biliary fistula due to passage of gallstone from gallbladder to bowel, duodenal ulcer perforating into common bile duct, tumour or malignancy

Within the gallbladder
- All of the above
- Emphysematous cholecystitis

Answer 3

1 (e)
2 (b)

Essence

A young man with Crohn's disease and epilepsy presenting initially with chronic diarrhoea, cramps in his hands and oedema has a low uncorrected calcium, with normal alkaline phosphatase. He later develops proximal myopathy and a raised alkaline phosphatase.

Differential diagnosis

We shall first address the initial part of the question, to which question 1 applies. Although this patient's total calcium is low, there are several reasons to suspect that the ionized calcium level is normal: the diarrhoea is not offensive, which argues against malabsorption, as does the normal haemoglobin; the oedema suggests significant hypoalbuminaemia, for which the calcium would have to be corrected; and, finally, significant hypocalcaemia would provoke a rise in the alkaline phosphatase provided the parathyroids are functioning (there is no reason to postulate that the hypocalcaemia is of such acute onset that it is too early to induce increased parathyroid hormone secretion). Each of these would be rather soft evidence in a real clinical situation but in the context of this examination they are significant. On the positive side, any prolonged diarrhoea is associated with low magnesium levels and possible tetany. In summary, you are given a reasonable amount of evidence that correcting his calcium is not going to provide you with an answer. For that reason, magnesium is a better answer than albumin.

In the second question, you have to appreciate the existence of a second pathology. The situation has changed, both clinically and biochemically. As always, ascribing the situation to a complicating problem is preferable to making an additional unrelated diagnosis. The most striking feature now is the raised alkaline phosphatase. This is most likely to be of bony origin in this case. Chronic phenytoin therapy is associated with osteomalacia, as is vegetarianism. Malabsorption may cause osteomalacia, but as discussed, this is a less likely cause here. Osteomalacia is associated with secondary hyperparathyroidism where the interplay of calcium homeostatic mechanisms is able to maintain serum calcium in the normal range, at the expense of bone resorption (hence the raised alkaline phosphatase). The low (corrected) serum calcium in this case should alert you to the fact that homeostasis is breaking down: vitamin D is necessary for parathormone to have its full effect. Finally, Crohn's disease may be associated with granulomatous infiltration of the liver or with malignancy, both of which can cause a raised alkaline phosphatase. However, that is unlikely to be the explanation here.

The fact that the vitamin D level is almost normal leaves the possibility that parathormone is elevated as a primary event: the chicken rather than the egg. This is less attractive since it is not linked to pre-existing pathology, but it cannot be excluded on the basis of the information provided. Steroid myopathy remains a possibility but would score low marks as the patient's steroid-dependent disease is quiescent and the steroids are presumably now only being given in low dose, if at all.

Causes of raised alkaline phosphatase
- Bone disease
- Osteomalacia
- Rickets
- Primary hyperparathyroidism (if bone disease)
- Paget's disease (very high levels)
- Secondary deposits
- Primary osteogenic sarcoma
- Liver disease
- Cholestasis
- Hepatitis
- Cirrhosis (but not always)
- Malignancy
- Granulomata
- Hepatic congestion
- Pregnancy (third trimester)
- Children until puberty

Muscle enzymes are of no help in establishing the cause of the myopathy, not least because he has just fallen down a flight of stairs. Bone biopsy will establish the presence of defective mineralization in osteomalacia, and will show the characteristic fibrosis of hyperparathyroidism if there is adequate vitamin D. Imaging of parathyroid adenomas is difficult, and in a simpler case, referral for surgery could be made even without visualizing an adenoma, because failure to image preoperatively does not exclude the presence of a tumour.

The nature of anticonvulsant osteomalacia is not clearly understood. It is simplest to presume that hepatic enzyme induction by anticonvulsants results in conversion of precursors to metabolites other than 25-hydroxycalciferol, but some patients have normal levels of 1,25-dihydroxycalciferol despite florid osteomalacia, suggesting a more complex mechanism.

Another moot point in this question is the nature of osteomalacia-related myopathy; muscle enzymes are often normal (unlike in the myopathy of hypothyroidism) and there is some evidence to suggest that high levels of parathormone themselves are associated with myopathy.

Answer 4

1   (c), (f)

Explanation

The combination of these observations should suggest Wilson's disease. This is a good Membership question because its multisystem features allow the same information to be presented in numerous ways. It is an autosomal recessive disorder characterized by an inability to excrete copper. It most commonly presents in the second or third decade, at which stage Kayser–Fleischer rings are invariably present, but the diagnosis cannot be excluded without slit-lamp examination. Any movement disorder may be present, including chorea, parkinsonism, spasticity or cerebellar ataxia. Patients with neurological disease invariably have liver disease that may have been 'silent'. However, liver disease may dominate the picture with acute hepatic failure, chronic active hepatitis and cirrhosis. Presentations involving other systems occur more rarely (except in MRCP papers!), but may be renal as in this case, with proximal renal tubular acidosis, renal glycosuria and bicarbonate wasting, or endocrine (e.g. amenorrhoea). Overall frequencies of the initial predominant presentation are hepatic (42 per cent), neurological (34 per cent), psychiatric (10 per cent), renal (1 per cent), or haematological/endocrinological secondary to hepatic dysfunction (12 per cent).

Diagnosis requires the presence of low serum caeruloplasmin levels and Kayser–Fleischer rings, or excess copper in liver biopsy; in practice the implications of the diagnosis are so great that patients are usually subjected to biopsy. Other cholestatic disorders (e.g. primary biliary cirrhosis) also cause excess hepatic copper deposition, but not to such a degree and usually in the face of increased caeruloplasmin.

Treatment is lifelong administration of penicillamine; hypersensitivity can usually be controlled by prednisolone. Withdrawal of penicillamine may be fatal. Patients with fulminant hepatic failure or progressive liver disease despite treatment may be considered for transplantation.

Answer 5

1   (b)

Explanation

Benign paraproteinaemia can be defined as the presence of a monoclonal protein without evidence of malignant disease. Up to 1 per cent of the population may have benign monoclonal proteins, the incidence increasing with age. Most are of the IgG class, but IgM and IgA paraproteins also occur. Diagnostically, the difficulty is in differentiating paraproteinaemia in an asymptomatic individual from early myeloma.

Between 10 and 20 per cent of benign paraproteinaemias develop into myeloma, but this may not be apparent for several years. Thus regular follow-up is recommended. Assessment of immune paresis and immunoglobulin production is the best method of follow-up.

Finally, some benign monoclonal proteins are the result of strong antigenic stimulus, such as persistent parasitic infection.

The following features help distinguish benign from malignant paraproteinaemias:

- The paraprotein concentration is less than 20 g/dL.
- There is no immune paresis, i.e. other immunoglobulin classes are not suppressed.
- There are no free light chains (Bence Jones protein) in the urine.
- The bone marrow contains less than 15 per cent plasma cells.
- There are no radiological bone lesions.
- There is no increase in paraproteinaemia with time.

Answer 6

1 (e)

The gadolinium-enhanced T1-weighted MR scan shows three meningiomata; in conjunction with the acoustic neuroma and the hereditary nature of the disease the diagnosis is neurofibromatosis type II (central nervous system manifestations; skin lesions and Lesch nodules occur rarely).

Answer 7

1 (a)
2 (d)

Essence

A young man with acute onset breathlessness and a systolic click.

Differential diagnosis

Answering this question depends on knowing that a systolic click can be heard following a pneumothorax. However, even without this piece of wisdom, you should be able to guess the answer. The patient is young and fit and has become breathless over the course of a day. There are very few causes of sudden dyspnoea in this age group, and although you might consider a pulmonary embolus, infection or asthma, you are given no

additional information to support these diagnoses, which more or less excludes infection and asthma. Pulmonary embolism remains possible, but is much less likely in this age group. Thus you are left to consider a condition which often affects young, healthy males with no prior warning and without other symptoms and signs. Put like that you should be able to arrive at pneumothorax. The only remaining problem is that you are not provided with any of the classical clinical features of pneumothorax. In fact, he is not very dyspnoeic and has a small pneumothorax. It would very possibly have been missed had it not been for the systolic click. Given the relatively minor nature of the dyspnoea, it is possible to argue that this may be one of the mild symptoms associated with mitral valve prolapse which also causes added systolic sounds.

Why pick pneumothorax rather than mitral valve prolapse? Why is it better to play down the lack of classical signs of pneumothorax rather than playing down the importance of the dyspnoea? This is one of the artefacts of the examination situation. The implications of sending the patient home with an undiagnosed pneumothorax are potentially more serious than failing to arrange an outpatient echocardiogram. In the real world this patient would have a chest x-ray whatever – but you only have one bite at the cherry in the exam.

Answer 8

1 (a), (e)

The differential diagnosis is that of a single expanded vertebra. Paget's is most common, then benign bone tumours such as haemangiomas, and occasionally hydatid disease. Sclerotic metastases (typically prostate or breast) do not expand the vertebra; osteoporosis gives usually multiple osteoporotic vertebrae, increasing in density if there is fracture and collapse; in ankylosing spondylitis vertebrae develop apparent squaring due to erosion of the 'corners' and so are not expanded.

Answer 9

1   (c)
2   (b)

Explanation

The family pedigree shows the characteristic features of autosomal dominant inheritance in which a monogenic disorder is passed on to offspring by one parent and the disease manifests itself clinically in the heterozygous state. Approximately ½ of offspring are affected, irrespective of whether they are male or female. Each generation is affected.

The probability of an affected offspring from the consanguineous marriage shown in the pedigree is still ½. In this disease, consanguinity is irrelevant, because we already know that one parent does not carry the abnormal gene and the other is heterozygous. The question is designed to fool you.

Answer 10

1   (c)

Cardiac sarcoidosis is relatively rarely a clinical problem, but heart block is the most common clinical manifestation when it occurs. An alternative diagnosis of cardiac failure causing pulmonary oedema is not really tenable because of the normal size of the heart shadow and the pattern of the pulmonary opacification. HOCM, for which pacemakers are used to cause delay in left ventricular contraction, does not explain the lung lesions. There are no features to suggest SLE (a cause of congenital heart block), nor of fibrosis to suggest amiodarone use and subsequent withdrawal.

Answer 11

1   (b)

Explanation

These diseases share a potential to cause widespread cystic change in the lung, with a predisposition to pneumothoraces. In histiocytosis X, infiltration by histiocytes and other cells produces a pattern of pulmonary function mimicking pulmonary fibrosis, but as cystic changes develop the pattern described above develops. Apart from the rarity of the other pulmonary diseases named, the polyuria suggests possible diabetes insipidus due to posterior pituitary histiocytic granulomata, which is why histiocytosis X is the best answer. Histiocytosis X occurs in three forms: eosinophilic granuloma, Hand–Schuller–Christian disease and Letterer–Siwe disease. The last presents in childhood. Lymphangio(leio)myomatosis is extremly uncommon in males. Causes of emphysema in a young patient (i.e. α-antitrypsin deficiency) are effectively rules out by the appearance of the chest x-ray.

Answer 12

1   (b)

While pallor is non-specific for any type of anaemia, the koilonychia seen here (along with stomatitis, papillary atrophy of the tongue, glossitis, thin and brittle lacklustre nails) is more specific for iron deficiency. Mild splenomegaly may be found, and the blood film shows varying degrees of microcytosis and hypochromasia with anisocytosis and poikilocytosis. Hookworm infection is the commonest cause in the tropics.

Answer 13

1   (e)

Explanation

There is a debate about whether or not this condition is associated with an increased risk of cerebrovascular and coronary artery disease. For the time being there is no indication for treatment of an otherwise asymptomatic individual. Venesection is appropriate when there is increase red cell mass and anticoagulation when there is a clear risk of thrombosis. Angiotensin-converting enzyme therapy is useful if there are inappropriately high levels of erythropoietin. Polycythaemia is discussed further in Exam A, Answer 99.

Answer 14

1 (d)

Typically, the facial skin is affected with crusting and bullous lesions. Impetigo is usually due to *Staphylococcus* but it is sometimes due to *Streptococcus* or even a mixture of both. It comprises multiple, discrete whitish-creamish lesions. The lesions may rupture, leaving a raw erythematous area with crusting.

Answer 15

1 (c), (f)

Explanation

This question concerns the differential diagnosis of 'pulmonary-renal syndromes', i.e. disorders which affect both kidneys and lungs. This is discussed in Exam B, Answer 60.

The history is typical for antiglomerular basement membrane disease, and this is the best-known acute disease to affect both lungs and kidneys.

Answer 16

1 (a)
2 (b)

The diagnosis is Friedreich's ataxia (FA), hypertrophic cardiomyopathy accounting for the abnormal ECG and pes cavus the problem with shoes. It is also associated with scoliosis, pyramidal tract involvement, distal wasting of lower limbs, large fibre sensory neuropathy and optic atrophy (although few patients have visual impairment). It is one of the causes of downgoing plantars and absent ankle jerks (a combination of peripheral neuropathy with a central lesion; the other causes are subacute combined degeneration of the spinal cord, motor neurone disease, conus lesion and tabes dorsalis). The gene for FA is on chromosome 9 and codes for a protein 'frataxin'. The predominant mutation is a trinucleotide (GAA) repeat in intron 1 of this gene. FA is the only triplet-repeat disease (others include Huntingdon's chorea, dystrophia myotonica, spinocerebellar ataxias) to be recessively inherited. Hence there is no family history.

Answer 17

1 (d)

Explanation

Respiratory (or pulmonary or lung) function tests are a favourite examination question. Usually, the relative change in FEV, and FVC (often expressed as FEV_1/FVC) will allow you to determine whether you are dealing with a predominantly restrictive or obstructive defect. In an obstructive defect, FEV, falls more than FVC and the ratio FEV_1/FVC decreases. In a restrictive defect, both fall and the ratio may be normal or increased.

In a patient with a restrictive defect, the next important question is whether the defect arises from pulmonary fibrosis (or oedema, which produces the same picture), or from abnormalities of the rib cage (used here to include the pleura, chest wall and respiratory muscles). To answer this, it is important to have an understanding of TL_{CO} and K_{CO}, as determined by carbon monoxide gas transfer.

A patient inhales a mixture of air, helium and carbon monoxide, holds his breath for 10 seconds and exhales. Helium is inert, so its dilution in a sample of exhaled air allows the volume of distribution of the gas mixture to be calculated.

Carbon monoxide diffuses rapidly across alveolar walls, so its dilution in the exhaled mixture depends on the volume of blood in contact with the alveolar volume, which in turn is a function of the nature of the alveolar walls, capillary volume and the pattern of ventilation and perfusion in the lungs. The carbon monoxide gas transfer for the whole or total lung (TLCO) is expressed as the uptake of the gas per unit partial pressure gradient of carbon monoxide (mmol/min/kPa). When this is corrected for the volume of distribution, the transfer coefficient, KCO (mmol/min/kPa/L), is obtained.

Pointers to pulmonary fibrosis are a reduced TLCO, reduced transfer factor (KCO) or low Pa_{O_2}, with normal or low Pa_{CO_2}. These changes are a manifestation of the thickening of alveolar walls and obliteration of alveolar capillaries by pulmonary fibrosis.

In extensive pleural disease, relatively small alveolar volumes are created by a rigid, constrictive pleural cage. However, alveolar walls are normal, allowing unimpaired gas transfer at the level of the single alveolus. As a result, single-breath carbon monoxide transfer (i.e. for the whole lung) is reduced, but when this is divided by the reduced value for alveolar volume to obtain the KCO, a raised value is obtained.

Causes of a raised KCO
- Pulmonary haemorrhage
- Polycythaemia
- Left-to-right shunts
- Bronchial asthma
- Pneumonectomy
- Neuromuscular weakness
- Skeletal deformity

In this question, FVC is reduced much more than FEV_1, suggesting a restrictive defect. The restriction may arise from pulmonary fibrosis or from extrapulmonary disease such as pleural thickening. The raised KCO suggests extrapulmonary disease with unimpaired gas transfer. The hint of asbestos-related disease may lead you to suggest mesothelioma as an underlying diagnosis, but although this tumour may present with this clinical picture due to pleural thickening, a pleural effusion is common. Mesothelioma is a possibility but is less precise in the absence of more characteristic evidence. Other diseases of the chest wall might also be in the differential, but the possibility of asbestos exposure in the occupational history is too strong for the examiners to ignore!

Answer 18

1 (b)

Classical pictures of the scleroderma hand demonstrate sclerodactyly with loss of finger pulp and ulceration. This view emphasizes the inflammatory component of the disease with periungual inflammation and oedema and loss of the distal interphalangeal skin folds.

Raynaud's phenomenon associated with other connective tissue disorders may give this appearance, but the gastrointestinal immotility and severity of digital involvement suggest scleroderma.

Answer 19

1 (d)

Explanation

In the normal heart, oxygen saturations in the right chambers and vessels should be uniformly lower than those on the left side. Abnormal saturations imply the presence of an abnormal communication between the two sides of the heart. When asked to interpret abnormal saturations, you should comment on two things – the level of communication and the direction of the shunt.

If a right-sided chamber or vessel has a saturation higher than expected, this implies blood has reached it through a shunt from the left. Similarly, a left-sided chamber or vessel with a lower saturation than expected implies a shunt from the right.

The anatomical level of the shunt can be determined by looking at the saturations in anatomical order. All right-sided measurements (SVC, IVC, RA, RV, and PA) should be more or less the same as each other, as should all left-sided measurements (LA, LV, and aorta). The first chamber to deviate from this rule is the site of the 'step-up' or 'step-down'.

In this question a step-up clearly occurs at the level of the right ventricle. This implies a left-to-right shunt at the level of the ventricles (a VSD) because well-oxygenated blood from the left ventricle has mixed with venous blood in the right ventricle. The step-up occurs as blood cannot flow from right ventricle to right atrium across the tricuspid valve. A step-down at the level of the left ventricle would also imply a VSD, but with a right-to-left shunt.

Answer 20

1   (e)

Usually a single well-defined lesion, red, scaly and often slightly pigmented, it looks not unlike a single patch of psoriasis. A third of patients have multiple lesions. In non-exposed areas, think of underlying arsenic poisoning.

> **Hint**
> If you think you are being shown a single patch of psoriasis, ask: could it be Bowen's disease?

Answer 21

1   (d)

Your duty is to the patient and therefore to not breach confidentiality, except with the consent of the patient. This consent must usually be express, although it is implied when we inform the multi-disciplinary team about a patient and his condition. Confidentiality may only otherwise be broken when required by statue law (e.g. notification of infectious disease) or by the common law principle of a wider public duty. In this situation the wider public interest is that a serious crime has been committed and the alleged perpetrator is still at large. However, without the cooperation of the victim there may no justification for breach of confidentiality. In this case you are aware that there is a clear potential other victim (the younger sister) and you can justify a breach of duty to the agency most able to help (social services), who will have a specialist child protection team.

Answer 22

1   (c)

The femur is abnormally shaped with coarsened trabeculae and a thickened medial cortex. The radiological distinction between active and inactive disease is irrelevant for Membership purposes. Sarcomatous change occurs in 10 per cent of patients with widespread Paget's disease, commonly osteosarcoma of femur, humerus or pelvis. The calcified projection around a metaphysis is a characteristic appearance.

Answer 23

1   (c), (e)

A 76-year-old man with a past history of arthritis and in need of a carer, has confusion ?cause. A common problem in A and E and all of the investigations are usually done, which may reflect doctor training rather than clinical need. Old people become confused for a variety of reasons, but the most common are also the most reversible:

- Infection – usually of the chest or the urine
- Infarction – of the heart or the head
- Metabolic disturbance
- Drug toxicity

Urine Dipstix is considered part of the examination and is not an investigation, although clearly this would be a necessary step.

The ECG shows normal sinus rhythm (and hence makes MI less likely).

The BM is normal (and hence hypo- or hyperglycaemia is unlikely).

The FBC is normal and therefore does not need rechecking as a first step.

He needs:

- U + E (to rule out metabolic disturbance affecting renal function)
- chest x-ray (to rule out pneumonia and pulmonary oedema).

Blood cultures take too long when compared to other available tests. With these results back, the next step would not be CT or drug levels, but to ring the GP and find out the PMH and drug history (the carer helped the patient to dress and thus it is still daytime).

Answer 24

1 (d)

The red cells show microcytosis and hypochromasia characteristic of an iron deficiency anaemia. In addition, there is an abundance of platelets with several giant platelets. This suggests that the underlying cause of the peptic ulcer is essential thrombocythaemia.

Causes of a microcytic anaemia are discussed in the answer to Exam C, Question 82.

Answer 25

1 (b)
2 (b)

Essence

Chronic early morning non-productive cough and exertional dyspnoea. Hyperinflated chest and low PEFR.

Differential diagnosis

The choice lies between reversible and irreversible airflow limitation, i.e. asthma and chronic obstructive airways disease. While there can be some fixed obstruction in asthma and reversibility in chronic airways disease, it is reasonable to allow the presence of significant reversibility to differentiate the two.

It is clear from the examination that he has a hyperinflated chest. The symptoms are entirely in keeping with either diagnosis. Indeed, part of the point of this question is to test whether or not you know that asthma can present predominantly with cough. The therapeutic interventions reported no longer help, but that does not make the differential diagnosis any easier. The dose of steroids is too low and the length of the course too short to be able to draw a conclusion of irreversibility. On the basis of the fact that the cough is dry, there is unlikely to be much disease of the bronchi and bronchioles, again limiting the type of chronic airflow limitation. However, in his thirties he had a disease that responded to bronchodilators – he had asthma. Particularly given the current inadequacy of treatment, there is no reason to postulate a second disease now. In addition, he is a non-smoker and is presenting at rather a young age for this to be chronic irreversible airflow limitation.

Investigation and therapy

If he had emphysema, gas exchange would be impaired, but not in asthma. Hence confirm the diagnosis with DLco. The single most effective therapeutic measure would be a prolonged course of high-dose steroids.

Answer 26

1 (c)

Knowledge of the sequence of events in rheumatoid allows early radiological diagnosis:

- Synovial inflammation shows as soft tissue swelling.

- Hyperaemia and disuse leads to periarticular osteoporosis.
- Destruction of cartilage causes loss of joint space.
- Destruction of bone at the margins of synovial pannus results in erosions.
- Finally, subluxation and deformity give way to fibrosis and ankylosis.

Answer 27

1 (a)

Hypoglycaemia is the commonest cause of fitting in diabetics and glucose may spontaneously normalize is these patients. Hence, there is no need to invoke any less common cause to explain this scenario.

Answer 28

1 (b)

The blood film shows more than 50 per cent oval cells (elliptocytes), which should lead to the diagnosis of hereditary elliptocytosis. The presence of pencil cells and other poikilocytes in the film is typical of this condition. Note that elliptocytes can also be seen in thalassaemias and iron-deficient anaemias. Conditions with 'hereditary' or 'familial' in the title are inherited in a dominant fashion – the presence of an inherited condition prior to modern genetic studies would only be noted if it was dominant. Also conditions with 'von' in the title (Germanic) are also inherited dominantly, such as von Recklinghausen, von Willebrand, von Herrenschwand, and von Hippel Lindau. Von Gierke is an exception in that it is a sporadic and not inherited condition.

Answer 29

1 (b)
2 (a)
3 (b)

Essence

Do you know how to manage a cardiac arrest? Previously candidates had the potential to be asked to conduct a mannequin resuscitation during their clinical exam. This has been abandoned at PACES in favour of SpR applicants needing a separate qualification in resuscitation, from the resuscitation council. Their website provides the latest algorithms used in resuscitation in the UK – for your and the written examiners' perusal: www.resus.org.uk.

Compressions should be carried out 15:2 even with two rescuers present as it leads to less disruption to the required number of cardiac compressions.

Following cardioversion, the monitor may initially show asystole, called electrical stunning. Later, despite there being electrical activity, the myocardium may not yet contract with sufficient force to give a detectable pulse, called myocardial stunning. Hence CPR should be continued for a total of 1 minute following defibrillation, and then the pulse rechecked.

If the pulse returns and at a later stage there is another indication for defibrillation, the energy selection returns to the beginning of the algorithm, as if a new cardiac arrest has occurred.

Answer 30

1 (c), (i), (m)

Explanation

As fluid loss is severe in hyperosmolar non-ketotic diabetic coma, this must be replaced, usually with hypotonic saline if the sodium is very high (above 155 mmol/L). Potassium supplements should be given (10 mmol/h is usually adequate). Administering more than 40 mmol/h is usually regarded as potentially dangerous. Blood glucose should be normalized with insulin, as for the management of ketoacidosis. These patients are not usually acidotic, however. As the risk of thrombosis is significantly increased, anticoagulation should be considered. Finally, an underlying or precipitating cause, such as pancreatitis or infection, should be sought.

Answer 31

1   (e)

Myasthenia gravis occurs in about 30 per cent of patients with thymic tumours. Strictly speaking, two views are required to localize a mass to a mediastinal compartment, but the answer here is in the history.

Mediastinal masses on chest x-ray
- Lymph nodes (lymphoma, metastases, granulomas, etc.)
- Thymic tumours and cysts
- Neural tumours
- Mediastinal goitres
- Teratomas
- Pericardial or pleuropericardial cysts
- Foregut duplication or cysts
- Meningocoeles
- Mediastinal abscesses
- Hiatus hernias
- Aortic aneurysms

Answer 32

1   (b)

Explanation

This is an example of an old favourite which is nevertheless worth repeating – seemingly abnormal values which are in fact due to the physiological changes of pregnancy. In a woman of child-bearing age, always keep pregnancy in mind if the diagnosis seems obscure.

Physiological changes in pregnancy
Cardiovascular
- Blood volume
- Cardiac output increases
- Peripheral resistance falls

Endocrine
- Increased thyroxine-binding globulin
- Increased levels of T3 and T4 (but free T3 and T4 remain in the normal range). Increased peripheral resistance to insulin
- Increased tendency to glycosuria

Haematological
- Red cell mass increases
- Haemoglobin concentration, packed cell volume and red cell count fall (Hb may fall further if iron deficiency also occurs)
- MCV rises slightly
- Platelet count may increase, but may also fall due to haemodilution. Serum ferritin falls
- Blood viscosity falls
- Concentrations of factors VII, VIII and X and fibrinogen increase

Renal
- Renal blood flow and glomerular filtration increase
- Clearance of urea, urate, creatinine increases (and plasma levels fall)

Respiratory
- Tidal volume increases
- $Pa\text{CO}_2$ and plasma bicarbonate fall

Immunological
- Serum immunoglobulin concentrations fall

Answer 33

1   (e)

The narrowing of the lumen with irregularity and shouldering of the mucosal outline suggests a malignant stricture. Benign strictures, including those found in scleroderma (where the stricture is secondary to reflux) usually have a smooth mucosal outline and no 'shouldering'. In achalasia, the rat-tail tapering distal to the dilatation and below the diaphragm may mimic a stricture.

Answer 34

1 (c)

Explanation

The differential diagnosis is that of a raised CSF protein and a lymphocytosis. This is much wider than that of a raised CSF protein alone. The examiners are therefore keen on this type of question, and will expect you to use all the clues they provide to make a definitive diagnosis. In this case, the clues suggest Lyme disease as the likely diagnosis.

Causes of raised CSF protein and CSF lymphocytosis

Infectious
- Lyme disease – diagnostic clues include rash, cranial nerve palsy, low CSF glucose
- Tuberculous meningitis – usually occurs in immigrants or immunosuppressed (AIDS); patients often have hydrocephalus with ataxia, drowsiness, high CSF pressure, and low glucose
- Fungal meningitis – usually immunosuppressed patients with low CSF glucose
- Syphilis – may be asymptomatic, presenting only with positive serum syphilis serology
- Viral meningitis – no focal neurological signs, normal CSF glucose and often normal protein
- Viral encephalitis – presents with abnormal behaviour often with convulsions; normal CSF glucose but raised protein

Non-infectious
- Sarcoidosis – usually some other clue such as a skin rash (glucose only slightly reduced)
- Multiple sclerosis – usually a classical clinical presentation (e.g. optic neuritis). CSF shows a slight lymphocytosis (less than 50 cells/mm³), normal glucose and only moderately elevated protein
- Leptomeningeal
- Secondary neoplasms

Others such as systemic lupus erythematosus and Behçet's disease are very unusual.

Answer 35

1 (b)

The picture shows a markedly erythematous, ulcerated mucosa covered by the exudative yellow-white membrane-like material found in pseudomembranous colitis, caused by toxins A and B of *Clostridium difficile*. It usually occurs a few days after the institution of antibiotic therapy. Clindamycin, ampicillin, tetracycline, lincomycin, and the cephalosporins have been causally linked. With no clues from the history, it is difficult to distinguish this from amoebic dysentery which produces similarly coloured mucosal ulceration. Both are initially treated with oral metronidazole.

The colonoscopic features of inflammatory bowel disease are usually somewhat different. Crohn's disease initially produces shallow intramucosal ulcers, but when they become as advanced as those in this picture, they are usually of bizarre shape with the surrounding mucosa forming pseudopolyps and a cobblestone picture. In ulcerative colitis, the picture is of a granular mucosa with polyps and mucosal bridges between the ulcers.

The presence of the membrane is not essential to make a diagnosis of pseudomembranous colitis, which can be confirmed by identifying the toxin in the stool. Culture of the organism is not useful since 5 per cent of the population carry *C. difficile*. Rectal biopsy usually demonstrates fairly characteristic changes.

Answer 36

1 (b), (d)
2 (a), (e)

Sputum for TB and fungi; aspergillosis precipitins are positive in mycetomas and negative in allergic aspergillosis, while skin tests are positive in allergic aspergillosis and negative in aspergillomas.

Answer 37

1   (c)
2   (b)

Explanation

In atrial flutter, the atrial rate is usually close to 300/min. Typically, 2:1 atrioventricular (AV) block results in a ventricular rate of 150. Thus whenever a patient has a ventricular rate of around 150, atrial flutter should be considered. With a high degree of AV block, atrial flutter is easy to diagnose. The rapid atrial activity produces regular F waves. Often these appear as the characteristic 'saw tooth' baseline appearance. With 2:1 block, diagnosis can be more difficult, as alternate F waves can be superimposed on T waves. Temporarily increasing the degree of AV block should aid diagnosis; this could also be attempted pharmacologically, but as carotid sinus massage is simple, it is the best initial manoeuvre and attracts most marks. The figure below shows the ECG appearance after carotid sinus massage.

Note that 'atrial flutter with 2:1 block' attracts more marks than 'atrial flutter' alone.

> **Interpreting ECGs**
> The ECG is one of the most important investigations to master for the exam section, since examples are often included in papers. As it is one of the most common investigations performed in clinical practice, the examiners can reasonably expect candidates to interpret difficult examples. For this reason, a detailed approach to the ECG is given in Appendix B. This will allow you to pick up most abnormalities.

Answer 38

1   (a)

Cervical lymphadenopathy, rash and sore throat can be due to several infectious agents: EBV, CMV, *Toxoplasma gondii*, *Streptococcus pyogenes* and rubella. They are also a feature of Kawasaki's disease in children. The age favours EBV, but this is a question about the most likely differential diagnosis.

Answer 39

1 (e)

Explanation

The key to this question lies in the disproportionately raised creatinine compared with the urea level. An additional clue is the greatly raised phosphate and potassium. Renal failure resulting in a urea of only 22 mmol/L would not be severe enough to cause hyperkalaemia. Raised creatinine, phosphate and potassium levels are usually the result of muscle breakdown. The presence in a diabetic of severe hypercholesterolaemia would lead a GP to prescribe a statin drug to lower the cholesterol with the side effect of rhabdomyolysis.

Diagnosis can be made by measurement of plasma creatine phosphokinase (CPK), which is usually markedly elevated.

Causes of raised creatine phosphokinase (CPK)
- Muscle trauma
- Rhabdomyolysis (bruises/contusion)
- Intramuscular injections
- Post DC shock
- Myocardial infarction [note cardiac isoenzymes (CK-MB) can be distinguished from skeletal muscle isoenzymes]
- Physical exertion
- Muscular dystrophy
- Muscle inflammation
- Polymyositis
- Dermatomyositis

Answer 40

1 (e)

The signs here are of a right complete and left incomplete ptosis with a normal pupil. The arched eyebrows, caused by an overactive frontalis muscle, demonstrate that the patient is trying to open her eyes. A third nerve palsy does cause a complete ptosis and there is no clue as to any ophthalmoplegia of the underlying eyeball. However, the position of the left eyeball makes a complete third nerve palsy unlikely, and the normal pupil excludes a Horner's syndrome. We are left with generalized muscle diseases, of which the most likely is myasthenia. The facial muscles are the earliest to be involved. Always think of myasthenia when presented with 'funny' ophthalmoplegias.

Answer 41

1 (c)
2 (b), (f)
3 (c), (i)

Essence

The questions provide the essential features of this illness and possible red herrings:

- previous late abortion
- worse in pregnancy
- arthropathy (never a firm diagnosis of rheumatoid, no deformities noted)
- dyspnoea (fibrosis/thromboembolic)
- renal disease
- ?endocarditis

Rheumatoid arthritis typically improves during pregnancy, while lupus worsens, and rheumatic disease and miscarriages should suggest lupus. Renal disease is unusual in rheumatoid except for amyloid (now rare) or drug effects. The GP was obviously concerned about pre-eclampsia but you are concerned about the lack of oedema, the murmur, evidence of peripheral vasculitis, and cytopenia.

For question 2, your investigations must aim to sort out your differential diagnoses. It is extremely rare for the ANA and anti-DNA antibody to be negative in active systemic lupus. Transthoracic echocardiography is insufficiently sensitive to exclude vegetations (which may anyway be present and sterile in lupus), and blood

Disease-modifying anti-rheumatic drugs

	Pregnancy	Breast feeding
Sulphasalazine	Safe	Safe
Antimalarials	Safe	Best avoided
Gold	Probably safe	Best avoided
Penicillamine	Probably safe	Best avoided
Azathioprine	Safe	Best avoided
Cyclosporin	Safe	Best avoided
Prednisolone	Safe	Safe <15 mg

cultures must be done to exclude SBE. The ESR is elevated by pregnancy, proteinuria, anaemia, large molecular weight proteins (e.g. fibrinogen and gammaglobulins, generally raised in SLE), as well as in inflammation, so will not differentiate. The CRP will be more discriminatory as it only rises in active inflammation such as infection or vasculitis but not in SLE without infection or active tissue damage. Anticardiolipin antibody in significant titre is a risk factor for miscarriage but in the absence of lupus is unlikely to explain the arthropathy and cytopenia.

Pregnancy and rheumatic disease are a particular problem as rheumatoid and SLE are diseases of women of child-bearing age, many drugs are at least theoretically risky, and pregnancy may affect disease and disease may affect pregnancy outcome. There are a few general rules. In rheumatoid, drugs are often not required during pregnancy, but NSAIDs are best avoided in the last trimester, as they have been associated with bleeding, pre-eclampsia and neonatal respiratory distress, although in practice NSAID suppression of premature labour is not associated with problems. NSAIDs achieve only low concentrations in breast milk and are probably safe, although short half-life agents are recommended.

Answer 42

1 (a)

The aortic 'knuckle' and descending aorta are seen on the right.

Answer 43

1 (c)

Explanation
The ECG shows the typical abnormalities associated with hyperkalaemia: peaked, tall T waves, widened QRS complexes and diminution of P-wave amplitude.

A discussion on non-cardiac ECG abnormalities can be found in the answer to Exam B, question 37.

Answer 44

1 (a)

Essence
An early middle-aged woman presents with jaundice. A moderate smoker and a heavy drinker, she has evidence of renal failure and intrinsic hepatic damage.

Differential diagnosis
This question hinges on the differential diagnosis of her hepatitis. By far the strongest clue favours an alcoholic aetiology. There are no positive features to suggest an infective or toxic cause. There are no positive features to suggest paracetamol

overdose, but it is always important to consider this cause of acute hepatic failure, so this answer would attract some marks. There has been no febrile phase and her urinalysis is normal, thereby ruling out leptospirosis. The onset of jaundice is too soon after her arrival in Ibiza to be linked to a viral hepatitis contracted there. It is more likely that she increased her alcohol intake on holiday. Given her lifestyle it would be appropriate to mistrust a negative drug history.

Hepatorenal syndrome is essentially a prerenal form of renal failure which mimics hypotension as a result of the accumulation of vasoactive substances. In order to maximize renal perfusion, the central venous pressure needs to be as high as possible. However, given the tendency to lose fluid from the intravascular compartment, it cannot be too high. For this reason these patients must be managed with a central venous line. Since hepatic failure is essentially a state of secondary hyperaldosteronism, the patient will be retaining sodium – indeed, measurement of urinary sodium, which will be very low in this case, is clinically helpful. In addition, this is the natural response to prerenal uraemia. Thus the patient should not receive exogenous sodium.

Answer 45

1 (a)

The section shows a classical giant cell granuloma. Granulomatous lesions involving the face are restricted to sarcoidosis, tuberculosis, syphilis, Wegener's granulomatosis and foreign bodies. Only those of TB will be caseating.

Nose lesions
– Lupus pernio (sarcoidosis)
– Lupus vulgaris (tuberculosis)
– Lupus erythematosus (SLE)
– Lepromatous leprosy (ENL or LL)
– Leishmaniasis (cutaneous or PKDL)
– Acne rosacea
– Rhinophyma

– Nasal diphtheria (perinasal crusting)
– Collapsed nasal cartilage

Wegener's granulomatosis
Syphilis
Lepromatous leprosy
Relapsing polychondritis

Answer 46

1 (c)

No patient well enough to remain an outpatient could have these blood results. There must be shum mistake shurely doctor! There is evidence of cell lysis from the high potassium and phosphate (normally intracellular). However, the low glucose implies continued metabolism (which is prevented by collecting it in a fluoride tube). These observations make it unlikely that this is merely a haemolysed sample. In fact, this specimen was analysed only after being left unattended for a whole weekend.

Answer 47

1 (b)

The high white cell count suggests a leukaemia. The blood film shows an excess of small, mature lymphocytes. The likely diagnosis is therefore CLL.

Answer 48

1 (c)

Explanation

The patient has a high plasma bicarbonate, low plasma potassium and low plasma chloride. The raised bicarbonate means the acid–base disturbance is either a metabolic alkalosis or a compensated respiratory acidosis. The low potassium favours metabolic alkalosis, which is caused by a primary rise in plasma bicarbonate.

In this case the likely diagnosis is pyloric stenosis. The hypochloraemia reflects gastric loss of chloride, which may result in a plasma chloride up to 80 mmol/L lower than plasma sodium (compared to the usual 40 mmol/L). Hypokalaemia results from the absence of hydrogen ions to compete for potassium secretion in the distal tubules of the kidney. Severe hypochloraemic alkalosis is now rare because pyloric stenosis is usually detected earlier.

Causes of a metabolic alkalosis
- Ingestion or infusion of alkali
- Sodium bicarbonate ingestion
- Forced alkaline diuresis (e.g. for salicylate overdose)
- Excess ingestion of alkali during therapy for acidosis
- Milk-alkali syndrome
- Pyloric stenosis
- Persistent self-induced vomiting
- Potassium depletion (except tubular acidosis)
- Chloride depletion
- Hyperaldosteronism
- Fulminant liver failure

Answer 49

1   (e)

A defect of smooth muscle lining lymph vessels, causing lymph to 'leak' into the pleural space and alveoli, the latter provoking fibrosis and the parenchymal fine honeycomb radiological changes, which are subtle on this film. Rare in males, and may respond to progesterones.

Answer 50

1   (b)
2   (a)

A symmetrical polyarthritis/arthralgia with elevated ESR and some evidence of a multisystem disease; proteinuria, postural hypotension and orthopnoea, dyspnoea, easy bruising. The lack of tenderness informs you that this is not an inflammatory arthritis, and that the elevated ESR may relate to abnormal plasma proteins, possibly secondary to proteinuria. It is difficult to think of an alternative chronic illness which would encompass all the clinical findings. AL amyloidosis (formerly primary) is a complication of the presence of a circulating monoclonal immunoglobulin ('L' refers to 'light chain'), most commonly as a monoclonal gammopathy of uncertain significance (MGUS), but also in myeloma. The clinical manifestations are very varied, affecting almost any extracranial tissue through extracellular deposition of amyloid fibrils, and disrupting normal function. Renal, cardiomyopathic and neuropathic (either compressive, polyneuropathy or autonomic) presentations are most common. Prognosis is poor but there may be some improvement with chemotherapy aimed at suppressing the production of the circulating paraprotein.

Answer 51

1   (c)

The diagnosis is made by virtue of the lack of scarring, the well-demarcated patches, and the 'exclamation mark' stumps of hair around the edges of the patches.

Answer 52

1   (a)

Essence

A young man presents with fever, weight loss and non-bloody diarrhoea. He has a diffuse, tender mass in the right iliac fossa.

Differential diagnosis

Superficially, this patient presents with a picture not unlike a subacute appendicitis with an appendix mass. (Remember the surgical diagnoses!) But appendicitis is usually associated with constipation. The combination of an acute illness with diarrhoea, abdominal pain, fever, weight loss, anaemia, a mass in the right iliac fossa, and hypoalbuminaemia suggests Crohn's disease. Even in patients with Crohn's colitis, rectal bleeding occurs in only 50 per cent; it is even less common in patients with ileal disease. Lymphomas and infections such as tuberculosis, actinomycosis, and *Yersinia enterocolitis* can mimic Crohn's but it is rare for ulcerative colitis to present with a mass in the iliac fossa. His low back pain is too non-specific to help.

In practice, you are likely to have drawn a blank on all other investigations before having the result of this culture (it takes 6 weeks). At this point you are likely to be proceeding to an exploratory laparotomy. However, when asked at this stage in the history about investigations, it would be inappropriate to suggest a laparotomy (unless you were looking for a malignancy) but entirely reasonable to suggest that you should be preparing to culture for tuberculosis at this early stage.

Answer 53

1   (c)

This rare condition used to arise most commonly in the context of congenital syphilis, but is now seen following viral infections such as mumps, measles, cytomegalovirus, Epstein–Barr and chickenpox, and after *Mycoplasma pneumoniae* infections and in lymphomas, and is associated with the presence of polyclonal complement-fixing IgM autoantibodies known as cold agglutinins. The condition can also develop spontaneously with recurrent attacks over many years. Acute intravascular haemolysis occurs on exposure to cold, resulting in abdominal pain, Raynaud's phenomenon, peripheral cyanosis, haemoglobinuria,

haemoglobinaemia and occasionally transient leukopenia. The recurrent form occurs mainly in adult males and the acute form in children. This is quite distinct from paroxysmal nocturnal haemoglobinuria, a clonal disorder characterized by intravascular haemolysis, venous thrombosis and marrow failure.

Answer 54

1   (b)
2   (a), (d)
3   (c), (e)

Essence

A young alcohol and IV drug abuser, with recent syphilis and recent travel to Morocco, presents with an acute febrile illness with features localizing to the chest, and jaundice.

Differential diagnosis

The clinical picture is of a respiratory tract infection in a high-risk individual with features characteristic of *Pneumocystis carinii* pneumonia (PCP): paucity of chest signs in relation to severity of illness, tachypnoea, cyanosis, hypoxia, and unresponsiveness to conventional antibiotic treatment for pneumonia. PCP is the most common infectious complication of HIV infection (for which this patient is also at risk) in Europe and the USA. There is no better explanation of the clinical features that would arise from either the history of syphilis or exotic travel. They should therefore be regarded as 'red herrings'. None of the other causes of pneumonia in the IV drug abuser fits the clinical picture so well. There is a possibility of *Mycoplasma* pneumonia in a patient who presents with a history of pneumonia that has not responded to amoxicillin. However, the history and the chest x-ray are far more in keeping with PCP. Amoxicillin can cause a hepatitis but the picture is of a transient transaminitis and not the picture seen here.

Although the diagnosis is a clinical one, confirmation by demonstration of the organism, is important. (*Pneumocystis carinii* is now classified as a fungus.) Sputum staining has a very low yield (although induced sputum is much better), but bronchial washings and biopsy allow silver or immunofluorescent antibody staining which has a much higher chance of identifying the organism. Diagnosis can also be achieved through the polymerase chain reaction (PCR). This clinical picture is of sufficient severity to need parenteral treatment. In such cases steroids are commenced immediately.

Pneumonia in the IV drug abuser
Lobar pneumonias
– Classical: *Pneumococcus*
– Other: *Klebsiella, Staphylococcus, Mycobacterium tuberculosis*

Atypical pneumonia: *Mycoplasma, Legionella, Chlamydia, Coxiella*
Fungal: *Candida, Aspergillus, Histoplasma, Cryptococcus*

Answer 55

1   (d)

Questions on the CSF are common and are easy to answer. It is important to have a list of causes of the common abnormalities. There are relatively few causes of a raised CSF protein with a normal cell count.

Causes of a raised CSF protein with a normal cell count
• Guillain–Barré syndrome
• Spinal block
• Lead encephalopathy
• Subacute sclerosing panencephalitis

In this question there is a raised CSF pressure. The student doing finals has been exposed to a toxin throughout his 3 years at university. Lead encephalopathy fits both the history and the data.

Answer 56

1   (b)

Essence

A young man is found unconscious having been well 4 hours earlier. He is shocked, hyperpyrexial and has fixed pupils.

Differential diagnosis

There are very few reasons for a young man suddenly becoming this ill. This is not a picture of diabetes. (You do not even need the blood glucose to tell you that.) The only infectious diseases which would make someone this ill are septicaemia, meningitis or encephalitis. The temperature is too high for a normal bacterial infection and he is unlikely to be shocked if he has a viral infection. A patient with profound immunosuppression could become this ill very quickly, but it would be extremely unusual for this to be the initial presentation of a myeloproliferative or lymphoproliferative disease or AIDS. The orofacial dyskinesia is known as 'bruxism'.

The most likely acute insult in this case is substance abuse and the picture is typical of the severe effects of 3,4-methylenedioxymethamphetamine (MDMA) or 'ecstasy' – or just 'E'. No other substance is likely to cause this syndrome. In fact this patient had taken three tablets and died a few hours after admission.

Causes of hyperpyrexia
• Infection
• Heatstroke
• Cerebrovascular accident
• Neuroleptic malignant syndrome
• Malignant hyperthermia
• Monoamine oxidase inhibitor overdose
• Substance abuse
• 'Ecstasy'
• Amphetamine
• Methamphetamine
• Cocaine

No other diagnosis fits as well. Malignant hyperthermia follows anaesthetic agents. Neuroleptic malignant syndrome is associated with muscle stiffness and there is no history of psychiatric illness. Cocaine would cause small pupils.

Answer 57

1 (b)

This is background diabetic retinopathy showing hard exudates and dot haemorrhage/microaneurysms; the significant changes are well lateral to the macula.
See answer to Exam C, Question 81.

Answer 58

1 (a)

Explanation
Potassium is a crucial investigation in the initial assessment of secondary hypertension.

Conn's syndrome
Questions about Conn's syndrome usually carry some hint towards the diagnosis other than hypokalaemia, e.g. nocturia or the typical biochemical picture of a hypokalaemic alkalosis and serum sodium of more than 140 mmol/L. The basis of most tests for Conn's syndrome is to demonstrate:

* hypokalaemic alkalosis
* increased plasma aldosterone in circumstances where aldosterone secretion would normally be suppressed
* low plasma renin activity.

Suppression of aldosterone secretion can be attempted by lying the patient down, infusing saline, administering a high salt diet or giving fludrocortisone. Aldosterone can be measured in plasma or urine. Plasma renin activity will fail to rise during volume depletion (e.g. standing up) if it is suppressed by autonomous aldosterone secretion. Many antihypertensive drugs may interfere with these tests. If antihypertensive medication cannot be stopped, nifedipine is probably the least disruptive agent.

Secondary hyperaldosteronism
The common stimulus in the various forms of secondary hyperaldosteronism appears to be reduced renal perfusion, due to renal artery stenosis or intravascular depletion. This results in the clinical syndrome of hypertension, oedema, low serum potassium and raised renin. The usual cause of renal artery stenosis in an elderly population is atheroma at the origin of the artery from the abdominal aorta. Occasionally the artery will be involved in an abdominal aortic aneurysm.

In this question the examiners are trying to get you to answer Conn's syndrome. However, there are pointers towards renal artery stenosis:

* there is oedema and the serum sodium is less than 140 mmol/L; both suggest secondary hyperaldosteronism;
* there is evidence of generalized atheroma. The mild renal failure does not help differentiate since hypertension of any cause may result in renal impairment.

Causes of hypokalaemia and hypertension
Diuretics
Primary hyperaldosteronism (Conn's syndrome)
    Adrenal adenoma
    Adrenal hyperplasia
    Adrenal carcinoma

Secondary hyperaldosteronism
    Renal artery stenosis
    Cirrhosis
    Nephrotic syndrome
    Renin-secreting juxtaglomerular tumour

Mineralocorticoid effect of excess glucocorticoids
    Cushing's disease and syndrome
    Steroid therapy

Answer 59

1   (d)

The publication by the Royal College some years ago of a book about organophosphate poisoning led to much speculation about such a question.

The question shows a number of points. Phrases such as 'unremarkable observations' lull you into a false sense of security. There is nothing normal about a blood pressure of 95/60 and in the context of this question a pulse of 60 should alert you to the possibility of cholinergic excess.

The lung function tests may have caught your eye early and suggested a restrictive disease and led you down the wrong list. Remember that in order for the test to be interpretable the patient must comply properly – in this case the patient is too weak to give a proper breath and hence the obscure results.

This man has organophosphate poisoning from exposure to pesticide, although recent concern has been raised by a more potent organophosphate, Sarin, a chemical warfare agent. The poisons inhibit cholinesterases, causing build-up of Ach at cholinergic nerve endings. Patients present with muscarinic effects (nausea, vomiting, abdominal colic, diarrhoea and hypersalivation) and then nicotinic effects (flaccid paralysis of limb, respiratory and extraocular muscles). Treatment is aimed at removal of the source (removing clothing, washing the body, gastric lavage and activated charcoal if poison swallowed) and blocking the Ach receptors with atropine and reactivating cholinesterase with pralidoxime.

A small proportion may go on to develop intermediate syndrome of cranial nerve problems and peripheral neuropathy together with respiratory problems.

Answer 60

1   (b)

The picture shows rose spots (distinct discrete pinkish macules or maculopapules) that are typical of typhoid fever and may appear towards the end of the first week and up to the twentieth day. They occur in 50 per cent of adults with typhoid and less frequently in children. The rash is distributed over the abdomen, chest and back. Adequate volume blood culture is the standard diagnostic test and has higher sensitivity than the other options, the sensitivity and specificity of the Widal serological tests varying widely. Bone marrow culture is still more sensitive than blood culture because of the larger numbers of micro-organisms in marrow. The College might be fussy about stool cultures in constipated patients!

Answer 61

1   (b), (e)

Essence

Following surgery, a young woman has a severe recurrent intra-abdominal arterial bleed and develops renal failure. She has a fever and thrombocytopenia, and fails to respond to antibiotics.

Management

Questions about management will usually be testing principles. This woman has had instrumentation to and bleeding within the abdomen and has intravenous cannulae. The problem now is one of unexplained fever and thrombocytopenia. The differential diagnosis of the fever lies between a resolving haematoma and a collection of pus. Even if she does have a resolving haematoma, it may very well be infected. A drug fever is less likely given the haematological abnormalities. Certainly she has been too ill for too long to work on that basis. You must assume that she has an infection. Infected lines may be impossible to sterilize so should be changed. If that fails, it may be necessary to stop her antibiotics in order to repeat cultures when there is a higher chance of their growing an organism. It is reasonable to consider organisms that may not be responsive to the chemotherapy used – particularly fungi, although the other measures would be carried out first. Finally, attempts to localize collections of pus should start with ultrasound and move on to CT scanning. If all else fails she will need an exploratory laparotomy.

Answer 62

1 (c)

The classic face of the patient with Graves' disease should be instantly recognizable. The condition, which has an autoimmune basis, most often affects women in the third or fourth decades. Although the eye signs are predominant, do not forget to look at the neck if it is visible – is there a goitre or a thyroidectomy scar? Other photographic features which may occur in Graves' disease include pretibial myxoedema, vitiligo (occasionally hyperpigmentation), alopecia, onycholysis, palmar erythema and spider naevi.

Note that it is not possible from this photograph to say whether the patient is hyperthyroid, euthyroid or hypothyroid. There may be other clues that might suggest thyroid status, such as 'this is a 43-year-old woman with a tachycardia' in the question, but in general be careful about over-interpretation. Although in PACES one only diagnoses exophthalmos or proptosis after examining the eyes from over the forehead (without which the most one can say is that the patient has lid retraction), in the written paper it is acceptable to make such a likely assumption.

Answer 63

1 (a)

This soft tissue mass of leukaemic cells, a chloroma, has greenish discoloration around a bruise-like lesion. This is the only pathognomonic lesion of any of the leukaemias, named for its green colour (which is due to myeloperoxidase in the cells of acute granulocytic leukaemia).

Answer 64

1 (d)

Explanation
Clinical features of SLE include the following manifestations in the approximate frequency shown in parentheses: musculoskeletal (95 per cent), cutaneous (80 per cent), fever (77 per cent), splenomegaly (70 per cent), CNS (60 per cent), renal (50 per cent), pulmonary (50 per cent), cardiovascular (40 per cent) and normocytic normochromic anaemia (25 per cent).

Nearly 80 per cent of patients with SLE have antinuclear antibodies. Anti-double-stranded DNA antibodies are more specific in diagnosis. Forty per cent of patients with SLE have rheumatoid factor and about 10 per cent give a false-positive VDRL test. Complement levels are usually decreased in active SLE.

Answer 65

1 (b)

Although this young man does not have florid prominent neurofibromatoses, he has many *café-au-lait* spots. The presence of six or more in an adult, greater than 1.5 cm in diameter, is diagnostic of neurofibromatosis until proven otherwise. The other causes of multiple *café-au-lait* spots are too rare to be encountered in the examination.

Answer 66

1 (c)

Explanation
On the basis of the fact that IgM does not cross the placental barrier, any IgM detectable in the baby must be in response to an active infection. IgM synthesis does not normally begin until 6 months of age but in neonatal infections synthesis

begins earlier. Hence the diagnosis is confirmed by requesting IgM fluorescent treponemal antibody (FTA) test. This is much more sensitive than either culture or smear.

Answer 67

1 (c)
2 (e)

The intravenous pyelogram shows calyceal clubbing and calcification in the right kidney. The combination of unilateral scarring and calcification is typical of tuberculosis. Sterile pyuria suggests tuberculosis, incomplete antibiotic treatment of a urinary tract infection, or analgesic nephropathy

Answer 68

1 (e)
2 (c)

The 'negative' image tells you this is MR angiography; moving material (blood) leaves a signal void and so acts as a contrast medium. The carotid siphons are readily identifiable as are the two anterior cerebral arteries close to each other in the bottom of the picture. The two vertebral arteries join to form the basilar almost at the centre of the picture. The middle cerebral arteries branch laterally from the carotids and on one side there is a dilatation which, on this view, is difficult to distinguish from the internal carotid itself; it is not arising from the PCA. The patient had suffered a subarachnoid haemorrhage but you can only see the aneurysm.

Answer 69

1 (b)

Questions about adolescent medicine will be asked. Young patients with Crohn's disease do not present with the more usual abdominal pain and per rectal bleeding. In this case there are several hints that this girl has non-organic disease – she complains of ankle pain but can still go dancing, she has become unwell at the time of exams and may be unhappy at the prospect of leaving school. However, she also has a normocytic anaemia and raised platelets. Given this, the rash becomes a possibility for erythema nodosum and the ankle pain the arthritis that can be associated with Crohn's.

Answer 70

1 (a)

The bone marrow shows an increased number of plasma cells (>10 per cent), many with abnormal forms, in part reflecting their immaturity. If accompanied by typical clinical features (osteolytic lesions, anaemia, renal insufficiency and recurrent bacterial infections) these bone marrow abnormalities have high diagnostic value, especially if there is evidence of monoclonal immunoglobulin production (in the serum or light chains in the urine). Light chains only appear in the serum if there is severe renal impairment. The peripheral blood film often shows marked rouleaux formation, and contains occasional plasma cells in about 15 per cent of cases.

Answer 71

1 (d)

Explanation

Not all appearances of acute MI are due to coronary thrombosis. In this case the patient had a subarachnoid haemorrhage, and hence it is important for a full history to be taken before giving treatment. It is considered that release of endothelin-1 in the area of vessel damage causes vasospasm elsewhere.

Answer 72

1 (c)

Essence

A middle-aged man presents with intermittent dilation of both pupils without other neurological signs and a bizarre gait.

Differential diagnosis

The flavour of this case, with one single objective feature, strongly suggests a non-organic aetiology. This single feature is accompanied by nothing else that would help place it in a recognizable clinical scenario. It is almost inconceivable that a central cause of bilateral mydriasis would have no other features. Given the associated feature of the bizarre gait, suggesting an unusual personality, the most likely diagnosis is that he was doing this to himself. In the event, we identified homatropine in his tears and he admitted to self-administration.

Answer 73

1 (b)

Explanation

Clinical and laboratory features suggest malabsorption, and an itchy rash on the buttocks is therefore dermatitis herpetiformis (DH) in associ-

Apart from nutritional deficiencies, complications of coeliac disease include:
* Development of malignancy
   increased risk of all GI malignancies
   T-cell lymphoma of small bowel

* Myopathy
* Neuropathy
* Splenic atrophy

ation with coeliac disease (CD) until proven otherwise. The investigations are consistent with malabsorption and the rash suggestive of DH. DH responds to a gluten free diet or treatment with dapsone. Both DH and CD have a strong association with HLA-B8 and HLA-DR3.

Serological confirmation of a diagnosis of CD [i.e. answer (b)] would be the single most useful test. Skin biopsy shows characteristic IgA deposition at the dermoepidermal junction, but does not confirm CD.

A general guide to the investigation of malabsorption is given in the answer to Exam B, Question 52.

Answer 74

1 (c)

Essence

A young woman with an acute febrile illness associated with widespread mucocutaneous lesions.

Differential diagnosis

With all the classical features of the Stevens–Johnson syndrome – a systemic illness with mucocutaneous lesions in the mouth, conjunctiva and genitals – this is a clinical diagnosis. The combination of skin and mucosal lesions is relatively uncommon and none of the other causes usually presents in this florid fashion. The combination of oral and conjunctival ulcers is also uncommon, suggesting Behçet's syndrome; however, there are no other features to support this diagnosis. The term Stevens–Johnson syndrome tends often to be used to denote a severe form of erythema multiforme. In fact, it was originally described as being the syndrome of erythema multiforme, systemic illness and ulceration of at least two mucosal surfaces.

This case conforms to this definition, so Stevens–Johnson syndrome is a better answer than erythema multiforme.

> **Commonest causes of Stevens–Johnson syndrome**
> <u>T</u>etracycline
> <u>A</u>spirin
> <u>R</u>
> <u>G</u>libenclamide
> <u>E</u>pileptic: barbiturates
> <u>T</u>rimoxazole and other sulphonamides
>
> <u>L</u>ymphoma
> <u>E</u>levated calcium
> <u>S</u>LE
> <u>I</u>nfections: herpes
> <u>O</u>rf
> <u>N</u>ycoplasma
> <u>S</u>treptococcus

> **Causes of bullous lesions of the skin**
> • Drug sensitivity, e.g. barbiturates
> • Dermatitis herpetiformis
> • Pemphigus vulgaris
> • Pemphigoid
> • Erythema multiforme
> • Insect or snake bite

Answer 75

1   (e)

African trypanosomiasis can be caused by two morphologically indistinguishable trypanosome species: *Trypanosoma brucei rhodesiense* (East and Central Africa) or *Trypanosoma brucei gambiense* (West Africa). These are transmitted by the bite of a tsetse fly (*Glossina* spp.).

African sleeping sickness is also called by the name 'Nagana'. South American trypanosomiasis (Chagas' disease) is caused by *Trypanosoma cruzi* and is transmitted by bugs belonging to the Reduviidae family, infective faeces being rubbed into skin or conjunctiva. Since both forms can be present in the blood, contaminated blood can very rarely be a source of infection. (In the presence of complete ignorance, this would have been a good

guess, with nothing to be lost.) African trypanosomiasis is distinguishable from South American by the geographical origin of the patient and by the morphological appearance of the parasite: *T. cruzi* is slightly larger, has a prominent kinetoplast at the end and is C-shaped.

Answer 76

1   (a)

Explanation
This patient clearly has a systemic disease, and you are being called on to recognize a syndrome. The biggest clue is the positive antineutrophil cytoplasmic antibody (ANCA), which suggests an autoimmune disease, particularly a vasculitis. The non-vasculitic causes of a positive ANCA generally give a perinuclear staining pattern, pANCA (as here), but anti-myeloperoxidase antibodies are not present. A more detailed discussion of ANCA is to be found in Exam C, Question 74.

The purpuric skin lesion represents a cutaneous vasculitis. The history of nasal involvement, eosinophilia and the lack of any renal impairment or an active urinary sediment suggests either Churg–Strauss syndrome or classical polyarteritis nodosa (PAN); the history of asthma makes the former much more likely.

Answer 77

1   (d)

This small bowel enema shows the bowel wall is thickened (witnessed by the increase distance between bowel loops), there is thickening of the valvulae conniventes (due to lymphoid hyperplasia causing obstructive lymphoedema of bowel wall), destruction of the normal mucosal pattern, which could be called rose-thorn (in profile) ulcers. There are no skip lesions, but this could not be ulcerative colitis in view of the sparing of the large bowel with small bowel involvement.

Answer 78

1 (b)

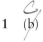

Cutaneous larva migrans is characterized by this serpiginous, raised, erythematous pruritic skin lesion. None of the other lesions mentioned look like this.

Answer 79

1 (a), (g)

Investigations

Anti-mitochondrial IgM antibodies are found in up to 94 per cent of patients and titres of >1:80 make the diagnosis more likely. Hence this makes the first preferred investigation an easy choice. The second one is more difficult to choose. Liver biopsy is ultimately necessary to confirm a diagnosis of primary biliary cirrhosis. Bile duct damage is shown by swelling and proliferation of epithelial cells and the ducts are surrounded by an infiltrate of lymphocytes, plasma and epithelioid cells. Granulomata, when seen, imply a good prognosis. There is a marked increase in copper-binding protein on biopsy.

However, in real clinical practice, you would not perform a liver biopsy without having first undertaken imaging of the liver to ensure there are no dilated ducts. However, none of the imaging investigations (ultrasound, CT or ERCP) will make the diagnosis of PBC. They will exclude other causes of obstructive jaundice. Only biopsy will allow the definitive confirmation of PBC. The words used here in the stem are important.

Answer 80

1 (a)

The slide shows dextrocardia in an otherwise normal chest x-ray. It is tempting to organize a CT chest in order to check that there is no evi-dence of bronchiectasis, but as the CXR is normal it is better to do nothing at all rather than expose the patient to unnecessary radiation.

The ability to identify a normal CXR is a requirement of the exam – just because you are shown a CXR does not confirm that there is pathology. However, be sure that what looks like a normal CXR really is normal. Commonly missed lesions include:

- **S**itus inversus
- **E**mphysema
- **P**ancoast
- **T**errible Ts (Teratoma, Thymoma, T-cell lymphoma, Thyroid)
- **E**levated hemiD / **E**mpyema
- **M**astectomy
- **B**order of heart
- **E**sophagus
- **R**ibs

- **C**lavicles
- **L**ooser zone
- **U**nilateral signs
- **B**oney mets

Answer 81

1 (b)

Explanation

We included this question because it demonstrates that you may be able to work out more than you think you know.

This child is sick. The possibilities are that he has a treponemal infection (most likely congenital syphilis) or that this is a 'false-positive VDRL' associated with another symptomatic condition that he has acquired. Considering the causes of a positive VDRL, none except syphilis is likely to be associated with this clinical syndrome. This means that he is most likely to have congenital syphilis.

Other neonatal infections to consider are tox-oplasmosis, rubella, herpes simplex, CMV and HIV.

> **Causes of positive VDRL**
> - Infections
>   Syphilis
>   Yaws
>   Leptospirosis
>   Hepatitis A
>   EBV
>   *Mycoplasma*
>   Bacterial endocarditis
>
> - Tropical disease
>   Leprosy
>   Malaria
>   Trypanosomiases
>   Filariasis
>
> - Autoimmune diseases
>   SLE
>   Sjögren's disease
>   Hashimoto's thyroiditis
>   Haemolytic anaemia
>
> - Old age

Answer 82

1 (c), (j)

A young man with arthralgia but no true arthritis, possible respiratory disease, evidence of poor dental hygiene at a young age, a history of a painful ?purpuric rash, and a polyclonal rise in gammaglobulins with resultant high ESR but normal CRP. The findings are highly suggestive of primary Sjögren's syndrome. The rash may have been due to primary vasculitis or associated with cryoglobulins.

You are asked to **organize** tests, which may be an additional free clue as it suggests a little more than filling out a form: samples for cryoglobulins have to be collected into a pre-warmed tube. The other test would be for extractable nuclear antigens (ENA).

ENA (subset of ANA)

nRNP	MCTD/SLE
Sm	diagnostic but insensitive for lupus
Ro/La	Sjögren's, SLE, neonatal lupus

Cryoglobulins
A globulin that precipitates at <37°C.

Cryoglobulinaemia presents with purpura, Raynaud's, sensorimotor peripheral neuropathy, membranoproliferative glomerulonephritis.

Type	Cryoglobulin	Underlying disorder
I	Ig paraprotein, usually IgM	Lymphoproliferative disease
II	Various Igs with a RhF paraprotein (Ig directed against Fc portion of IgG)	HCV; macroglobulinaemia, Sjögren's (lymphoma)
III	Mixed polyclonal Igs	Many infections and autoimmune disorders

Answer 83

1 (c)

The difficulty in this question is simply spotting the abnormality. When an immediate diagnosis is not apparent, develop a systematic routine for examining the projected material, whether it be a chest x-ray, a pair of hands or a face. What is important is not that you follow a particular routine, but that you devise one in the first place – and learn to stick to it. We offer one such routine for examining chest x-rays. Another method was given above in answer 80.

Places to look on the chest x-ray for subtle abnormalities

- Behind the heart (?prosthetic valves, increased densities air shadows)
- Hilar regions (?left higher than right as is normal, ?symmetrical density)
- Costophrenic angles
- Look along both diaphragms and up the sides of the lungs (?calcification, pleural plaques)
- Mediastinum
- Particularly scrutinize the region of clavicles and suprasternal notch (?tracheal compression, ?retrosternal goitre, erosions of the medial ends of the clavicles)
- Lung apices
- Bones of the thoracic cage (?fracture, rib notching, ribs missing, cervical ribs)
- Breast shadows
- Check both arms are present!
- Any abnormality below diaphragm

Answer 84

1 (a)

Explanation

Candidates often complain that Membership examinations (particularly Part 1) have little to do with the kind of medicine they deal with on a day-to-day basis. Questions can crop up which are completely outside the experience of most candidates. We would be surprised if you were asked a question on population genetics. Nevertheless, we have included this question to illustrate that sometimes it is possible to answer questions from first principles, provided you have a clear mind. Unfortunately, clear minds are at a premium during the examination, so it pays to have a plan of action designed for this type of question. Remember, if the question is difficult, leave it until you have answered the other questions. You are then under less pressure and can think straighter.

To answer this question, first work out the frequencies of the two alleles L^M and L^N.

The frequency of L^M, which we can call p, is $1400/2000 = 0.7$. The frequency of L^N, which we can call q, is $600/2000 = 0.3$. Note that $p + q$ must equal 1.

During random mating, it can be assumed that the contribution of each allele to the next generation will reflect their frequency in the initial population, i.e. the ratio of L^M gametes to L^N gametes will be 0.7:0.3. This ratio will be the same irrespective of whether the gamete is an egg or sperm. The next generation will thus be produced by the following mating combinations:

The frequency of $L^M L^M$ genotypes will thus be $p^2 = 0.49$.
The frequency of $L^M L^N$ genotypes will thus be $2pq = 0.42$.
The frequency of $L^N L^N$ genotypes will thus be $q^2 = 0.09$.

Note that the allele frequencies in the new population are once again $p = 0.7$ and $q = 0.3$. Thus if this second-generation population was to undergo random mating to produce a third generation, the genotype frequencies would be identical to the second generation! This is called Hardy–Weinberg equilibrium (HWE).

Blood group	Genotype	No. of individuals	No. of L^M alleles	No. of L^N alleles
M	$L^M L^M$	450	900	0
N	$L^M L^N$	500	500	500
N	$L^N L^N$	50	0	100
Total		1000	1400	600

HWE is defined by a set of genotype frequencies p^2 of AA to $2pq$ of Aa to q^2 of aa, where A and a represent two alleles of a locus and p and q are the frequencies of A and a. If the ratio of AA:Aa:aa is p^2:$2pq$:q^2 then the population is in HWE. When this is the case, genotype and allele frequencies do not change from one generation to the next. In this question the genotype ratios of the initial population were 450:500:5 (L^ML^M:L^ML^N:L^NL^N) whereas the ratio p^2:$2pq$:q^2 was 0.49:0.42:0.9, so the population was not in HWE. But after one generation of random mating the genotype frequencies (L^ML^M:L^ML^N:L^NL^N) did equal 0.49:0.42:0.9, so the next generation was in HWE.

This illustrates a principle of population genetics. If a population is not in Hardy–Weinberg equilibrium, then it takes only one generation of random mating to establish Hardy–Weinberg equilibrium.

Thus candidates who manage to remember this principle could quickly answer the question by working out the allele frequencies in the initial population (p and q) and realizing that the genotype frequencies in the next population would be p^2, $2pq$ and q^2 – a process which should take under a minute. However, less fortunate candidates could still derive the answer by working it out in the manner shown above!

Answer 85

1 (d)

Kayser–Fleischer ring of Wilson's disease – a rare, truly pathognomonic physical sign.

Answer 86

1 (c)

Explanation

Cushing's syndrome is defined by hypersecretion of cortisol. This can be demonstrated by a reliable 24-hour urine collection which contains more than 200 nmol of free cortisol or an elevated plasma cortisol level at 9 a.m. after administration of 1 mg dexamethasone 9 hours earlier. Having established cortisol hypersecretion, it is necessary to establish its cause.

Other types of Cushing's syndrome, such as hypothalamic-driven or the recently described adrenal hypersensitivity to gastrointestinal peptide, are rare.

Causes of Cushing's syndrome
- Cushing's disease
  Excess corticotrophin (ACTH) from pituitary adenoma

- Ectopic source of ACTH
  Small cell carcinoma of the bronchus
  Small, undetectable carcinoid tumour
  Adenoma or carcinoma of the adrenal gland

- Corticosteroid or ACTH administration
- Alcohol excess

Diagnosis is classically sought on the basis of suppression by exogenous steroids.

Corticotrophin-driven Cushing's from a pituitary source will not be suppressed by low-dose dexamethasone (0.5 mg 6-hourly for 2 days) but will be suppressed by high doses (2 mg 6-hourly for 2 days). Ectopic corticotrophin-driven Cushing's and adrenal Cushing's will usually not suppress. However, these tests may be unreliable as 20 per cent of pituitary-driven hypersecretion may not suppress, while benign ectopic sources may suppress.

Further refinement is possible by monitoring the corticotrophin response to intravenous ovine corticotrophin-releasing hormone (CRH), providing the laboratory has a reliable corticotrophin assay. Cushing's disease is usually associated with an exaggerated rise in corticotrophin, while ectopic tumours do not respond. The most reliable method of detecting a pituitary source is to sample the inferior petrosal sinuses for corticotrophin and compare the ratio of the central to the peripheral level. Sensitivity is further increased by simultaneous infusion of the ovine releasing hormone.

The best way to image the pituitary fossa is by magnetic resonance imaging. Scanning the abdomen is useful if adrenal disease is suspected, and a chest x-ray may suggest an ectopic source.

The most likely diagnosis in this case is Cushing's disease, the usual cause of hypercortisolism in young women. The potassium is quite low for a patient with Cushing's disease, but the suppression of cortisol secretion with high-dose dexamethasone is very suggestive of a pituitary source.

Definitive treatment for Cushing's disease is surgical. Medical therapy to control adrenal hypersecretion (metyrapone, ketoconazole or mifepristone) is used prior to surgery. Transient cranial diabetes insipidus is almost invariable for about 1 week postoperatively. No other complications are common.

Questions on Cushing's syndrome test your understanding of the pituitary adrenal axis. The questions are unlikely to be complicated provided the scheme outlined above is understood.

Answer 87

1   (b)

There is a single low attenuation area in the right lobe of the liver. Hepatic amoebic abscesses are usually single masses in the right lobe containing anchovy sauce-like material. The clinical picture is usually of swinging fever, abdominal pain and leucocytosis. Diagnosis is suggested by ultrasound, CT appearances and positive serology. Surgical drainage may be required in some cases not responsive to metronidazole or impending rupture. Diloxanide furoate is given together with metronidazole to clear the colonic cysts.

Most other causes of solitary hepatic lesions (including hydatid cysts) are unlikely to have such uniform attenuation pattern on CT. The fever suggests an infective cause, but the foreign travel favours amoebiasis over a pyogenic abscess.

Causes of space-occupying liver lesions
- Abscesses
  Amoebic pyogenic
  Infected cysts/tumours

- Cysts
  Hydatid
  Congenital

- Tumours
  Primary
  Malignant (hepatoma)
  Secondaries

Answer 88

1   (c)

Essence

A young woman with chronic bruising and nose bleeds and who is a heavy drinker has mild thrombocytopenia and no disorders of clotting.

Differential diagnosis

Pathological bleeding is due to abnormal vessels, platelets or clotting factors. There is nothing to suggest a problem with her vasculature and tests show her clotting system is normal. She has thrombocytopenia, but it is too mild at the time of testing to cause spontaneous bleeding. However, that does not exclude fluctuating thrombocytopenia, and indeed the type of bleeding is characteristic of that due to platelet deficiency. The platelet defect may be absolute, due to reduced numbers, or functional, due, for example, to aspirin or sulphinpyrazone therapy, hypergammaglobulinaemia, uraemia, or liver disease. The platelets produced in myeloproliferative disease may be functionally abnormal.

The most important diagnosis to exclude must be a proliferative disorder, but the absence of any other abnormality clinically or in the blood picture makes a leukaemia or lymphoma very unlikely. Thus an isolated platelet deficiency is probably the cause and given the history is very unlikely to be a congenital problem. Beyond that there are few clues, which makes this a difficult question. A normal prothrombin time makes significant liver disease less likely.

Answer 89

1 (c)

Primary skin diseases do not usually have associated lymphadenopathy, so the question tells you to look for a systemic disease. Of the causes for lymphadenopathy the only one likely to cause this type of lesion is syphilis in its secondary stage.

Causes of lymphadenopathy
- Inflammatory
  Pyogenic
  Non-pyogenic infection
  Autoimmune disease

- Granulomatous
  Sarcoidosis
  Tuberculosis
  Syphilis
  Toxoplasmosis
  Systemic fungal infection (e.g. histoplasmosis)

- Malignant
  Lymphoma
  Leukaemia
  Carcinoma
  Melanoma
  Sarcoma

- Drugs
  Phenytoin

- Endocrine
  Addison's disease
  Thyrotoxicosis

- Congenital
  Lymphangioma
  Cystic hygroma

Answer 90

1 (b)
2 (a)

IgA nephropathy is the commonest primary glomerulonephritis and most commonly presents in young-to-middle-aged men with intermittent macroscopic haematuria. An associated tonsillitis is common, but far from invariable. Post-streptococcal glomerulonephritis is probably much less common and does not usually present with macroscopic haematuria. Nor is this a common presentation for Wegener's granulomatosis, when, in any case, the upper respiratory tract involvement is more commonly sinusitis. While a diagnosis of leukaemia is superficially seductive, tonsillitis is very common and, only rarely reflects the immunosuppression of leucopenia. Finally, although a benign bladder tumour may be one of the commonest causes of macroscopic haematuria, it is uncommon in young men and does not explain the tonsillitis.

The investigations follow from the most likely diagnosis. Nephrotic range proteinuria is uncommon in IgA nephropathy and presentation at end stage is rare, as is acute renal failure. Stems a and b both include normal urinalysis. This would be commoner in IgA nephropathy than either nephrotic-range proteinuria or oligouria. (However, it should be said that minor urinary abnormalities, such as microscopic haematuria or sub-nephrotic proteinuria would be commoner still. But these are not offered in this question!) Choosing between a normal and elevated serum creatinine is less easy. Either is possible, although it would be much commoner, after a single episode of macroscopic haematuria, for the disease to be relatively early in its natural history and thus have no evidence of an impaired GFR.

Answer 91

1 (c)

The commonest cause of bilateral ptosis is myasthenia gravis, for which the best diagnostic test would be (c). Acetylcholine receptor antibody assays take a long time to get a result, and have low sensitivity (40 per cent negative). Bilateral ptosis occurs in some muscle dystrophies, e.g. dystrophia myotonica, mitochondrial myopathies (chronic progressive external ophthalmoplegia), and may be seen in the elderly due to disinsertion of the levator palpebrae muscle. The Argyll–Robertson pupil of meningovascular syphilis is associated with ptosis due to third cranial nerve involvement in the basilar area. However, bilateral third nerve palsies are rare, usually with less severe ptosis. Note the contracted frontalis in an attempt to compensate for the ptosis.

Answer 92

1 (d)

Explanation

The respiratory function tests show the characteristic features of the obstructive defect of asthma: an obstructive defect with a raised K_{CO}. In addition, they show reversibility – defined as an improvement of 15 per cent or greater in FEV, after bronchodilators.

The second question can be rephrased as this: could it be anything other than asthma? The occupational history is compatible with a diagnosis of farmer's lung, a form of extrinsic allergic alveolitis (EAA). However, even acute EAA with wheezing is usually associated with a restrictive defect on respiratory function testing. In addition, the reversibility of the airways obstruction argues against EAA where reversibility of any obstruction present may be attenuated because of the predominance of inflammation over bronchospasm. The overall respiratory picture is more in keeping with atopic asthma which may indeed present only with a dry cough. The history of hay fever confirms atopy.

Answer 93

1 (d)

There is fine calcification joining two vertebrae which represents ossification of the annulus fibrosus. This is a syndesmophyte, characteristic of spondylitis, and if extensive gives rise to a bamboo spine (as illustrated in Exam A, Question 95). The main differential is alkaptonuria. It should be compared to diffuse idiopathic skeletal hyperostosis in which there is coarse calcification of the anterior longitudinal ligament, often with a gap between that arising from each vertebra and often with calcification in the disc. It is probably unfair to expect a Membership candidate to differentiate this from seronegative arthritides (Reiter's, psoriatic) in which the ossification is coarser, and paravertebral with a gap between the calcification and the disc/vertebra. Tuberculosis may be associated with paraspinal calcification but the main changes are of vertebral and disc destruction and collapse.

Answer 94

1 (d)

Explanation

The R waves and depressed ST segments in the anterior leads represent the changes of acute infarction in the posterior wall viewed, as it were, from behind, and hence reversed. The physiological Q waves sometimes seen in V1 in a normal ECG are lost. Dominant R waves in V1 might suggest right ventricular hypertrophy, but there is no right axis deviation, and the T waves in the left ventricular leads are upright.

> **Causes of a dominant R wave in V1**
> - Posterior myocardial infarction
> - Right bundle branch block
> - Wolff–Parkinson–White type A
> - Right ventricular hypertrophy
> - Mirror image dextrocardia

Answer 95

1 (e)

Answer 96

1 (b)

In order for an advance directive to be valid it must be signed by an adult patient who has mental capacity to understand the consequences of their directive, and the contents of the directive must predict the clinical circumstances that have now arisen. This advance directive is not valid as you do not know the mental state of the patient when it was signed. The tempting answer would be to contact the consultant but this would waste valuable time which should be spent by you treating the patient. Treatment can always be withdrawn at a later stage if it turns out to have been the wrong thing to do.

Answer 97

1 (c)

Explanation
The water deprivation test is straightforward in principle. It is essentially a hormone stimulation test performed when there is a suspicion of a functional deficit of antidiuretic hormone (vasopressin; ADH), just as the Synacthen test is used in Addison's disease. The test is performed in two parts. In the first part, water deprivation is used as the stimulus to assess the patient's ability to produce ADH; in the second part, ADH is given (in the form of DDAVP) to assess the patient's ability to respond appropriately. In both parts the presence of effective ADH is determined by an ability to concentrate urine and thus increase urinary osmolality.

In theory, the interpretation of the test is also straightforward:

If there is normal urine concentration in both parts of the test, the diagnosis is primary polydipsia. The absence of a concentrating response to water deprivation (the first part) is diagnostic of diabetes insipidus (DI). If the second part is normal, you can conclude that the patient will respond to ADH, but is just not producing it himself: this is cranial diabetes insipidus. If the second part is also abnormal (i.e. he still fails to concentrate urine), you can conclude that his kidneys are unable to respond to ADH: this is nephrogenic diabetes insipidus.

In practice, however, there are complicating factors:

- There may be inadequate stimulus to ADH release; therefore, the test includes measurement of plasma osmolality. This must rise to at least 290 mOsm/kg for the stimulus to ADH to be adequate. For this reason it is important to continue with the first part of the test, i.e. the water deprivation for as long as possible. Since this can be dangerous, it is essential to weigh the patient hourly and discontinue the test if the weight falls by more than 3 per cent.
- There may not be an adequate concentration gradient in the renal parenchyma because of prolonged polyuria. This would make urinary osmolality a poor index of ADH function. If adequate urinary concentration does occur at any stage in the test, then this cannot be a problem. If the urine does not concentrate at

Urinary concentration in response to water deprivation	Urinary concentration in response to exogenous ADH	Diagnosis
+	+	Psychogenic polydipsia
−	+	Cranial diabetes insipidus
−	−	Nephrogenic diabetes insipidus

any point, then one cannot exclude an inadequate concentration gradient and the test may be difficult to interpret. In other words, the diagnosis of nephrogenic diabetes insipidus is difficult to make with certainty.

- In cranial diabetes insipidus there may only be a partial deficit of ADH release. In this case there may be some concentration in the first part of the test. There is usually an obvious step-up in concentrating ability with the administration of DDAVP, which does not occur in patients without diabetes insipidus. However, in mild cranial diabetes insipidus, this may be difficult to interpret with confidence in a specific case.

In these situations one may be left with equivocal results. Clearly any test must be interpreted in its clinical context, but if doubt remains, a hypertonic saline challenge test may be used to increase the serum osmolality and correlate it with measured ADH levels. In the Examination, unless you are specifically asked a question about the reliability of your conclusions, assume that a failure to concentrate urine in response to water deprivation and DDAVP is diagnostic of nephrogenic DI.

In this particular question the patient could be polyuric because of steroid-induced diabetes mellitus. Hence the initial investigation should be a blood glucose. Alternatively, he could have cranial diabetes insipidus or hypothalamic polydipsia due to cerebral lymphoma; or he could have nephrogenic diabetes insipidus because his manic-depressive illness is being treated with lithium. Everything depends upon the water deprivation test which offers the correct diagnosis of cranial diabetes insipidus, caused in this case by a retro-orbital mass of lymphomatous tissue which had spread posteriorly.

Answer 98

1   (a)

There is a partial duplex of the right kidney. This is the most common anomaly of the urinary tract

and is found in about 4 per cent of individuals. It is usually unilateral and more common on the left side than the right. Options (c) to (e) were complications of diseases that are commonly shown as 'incidental' findings on membership IVUs. These include bamboo spine (ankylosing spondylitis), sacroiliitis (IBD) and aortic aneurysms.

Answer 99

1   (a)

Explanation

The patient has a raised haemoglobin and red cell count. These are both expressed as a concentration. The red cell mass is normal; therefore the plasma volume must be decreased. This means the diagnosis must be pseudopolycythaemia.

There are other clues that exclude other diagnoses. Given the clinical setting and normal blood gases, it is reasonable (in the examination) to exclude all the secondary causes of polycythaemia. Similarly, with normal white cell and platelet counts and no features of myeloproliferative disease, there is no suggestion of polycythaemia rubra vera. (A lone raised RBC may be an early preneoplastic condition, in which case it is called benign (or idiopathic) erythrocytosis.) Pseudopolycythaemia is a poorly defined condition in which the red cell mass tends to the upper limit of normal, the plasma volume tends to the lower limit of normal and hence haemoglobin and red cell counts are elevated. Individuals with this condition tend to be middle-aged obese men with mild hypertension. There is a debate about whether or not this condition is associated with an increased risk of cerebrovascular and coronary artery disease. For the time being there is no indication for treatment of an otherwise asymptomatic individual.

Causes of polycythaemia
True polycythaemia
    Primary
        Polycythaemia rubra vera
        Benign (idiopathic) erythrocytosis
    Secondary
        Chronic hypoxia
            Altitude
            Lung disease
            Cyanotic congenital heart disease
            Haemoglobinopathies
            Decreased production of 2,3-DPG
        Inappropriately high erythropoietin
        secretion
            Renal pathology
                Tumour
                Cyst
                Hydronephrosis
                Post-renal transplant
            Other tumours
                Hepatoma
                Cerebellar haemangioblastoma
                Uterine fibroma
            Genetic abnormality of erythropoietin
            control
        Endocrine (mechanism unknown)
            Cushing's disease
            Phaeochromocytoma
Pseudopolycythaemia (synonyms: stress
polycythaemia, relative polycythaemia,
Gaisbock's syndrome)

Answer 100

1   (d)

Essence

An elderly man becomes breathless after receiving a non-steroidal anti-inflammatory drug (NSAID).

Discussion

You are given so little information that this question can be reduced to the side effects of ibuprofen. NSAIDs and Cox-II-specific anti-inflammatory drugs, not only aspirin, can precipitate bronchospasm by their inhibition of the metabolism of arachidonic acid by cyclo-oxygenase. Production of bronchodilator prostacyclins is inhibited and bronchospasm ensues. Asthma is a reversible and intermittent condition, so that respiratory function tests may be normal. NSAIDs also cause fluid retention alone or, as a result of renal failure. The latter may be due to acute interstitial nephritis or acute tubular necrosis. NSAIDs also cause a picture of minimal change nephropathy with interstitial nephritis which may present with nephrotic syndrome.

NSAIDs are always well known causes of GI haemorrhage. This may be insidious and present with dyspnoea secondary to anaemia.

Examination B

Questions

Question 1

A 6-year-old boy was referred with swelling of his left knee. He had played football in his school playground 48 hours before and had not noticed any problems until the morning of referral. He had had no other problems. There was no family or personal history of significance.

On examination, an otherwise well-looking boy had a red swollen knee which was warm and moderately painful to move. He was not systemically unwell and had a pyrexia of 37.3°C.

Results of investigations were as follows:

Hb	11.8 g/dL
WBC	6.9×10^9/L
Platelets	405×10^9/L
Bleeding time	normal
Prothrombin time	13 s *(normal range 11–15)*
Activated partial thromboplastin time	60 s *(control 25–34)*
Factor VIII level	123 per cent

1 What is the diagnosis?
   (a) Von Willebrand's disease
   (b) Factor VIII deficiency
   (c) Factor V (Leiden) mutation
   (d) Factor IX deficiency
   (e) Protein C deficiency

Question 2

A 20-year-old Caucasian woman was referred with persistent severe acne and hirsutism. Her menses were infrequent, irregular and heavy. She was on no medication and used barrier methods of contraception. Her mother also had irregular menses.

On examination, she was obese, had moderately severe acne, greasy skin, and excessive amounts of body hair in a male pattern distribution. The distribution of her obesity was uniform. Her visual fields were normal. There were no other abnormalities on examination or urinalysis.

Results of investigations were as follows:

Plasma luteinizing hormone	20 IU/L *(normal range 3–8)*
Plasma follicle stimulating hormone	6 IU/L *(normal range 2–8)*
Plasma prolactin	423 IU/L *(normal range <600)*
Plasma thyroxine	98 nmol/L *(normal range 70–140)*
Plasma testosterone	11 nmol/L *(normal range 1–3)*
Dehydroepiandrosterone sulphate (DHAS)	6 μmol/L *(normal range 3–7)*
Urinary 17-oxosteroids	39 μmol/L *(normal range 14–59)*

1   What is the diagnosis?
   (a) Congenital adrenal hyperplasia
   (b) Anabolic steroids
   (c) Pituitary adenoma
   (d) Polycystic ovary syndrome
   (e) Cushing's syndrome

2   How would you confirm this?
   (a) MRI pituitary
   (b) 24-hour urinary cortisol
   (c) Pelvic ultrasound scan
   (d) CT abdomen and pelvis
   (e) LH suppression test

Question 3

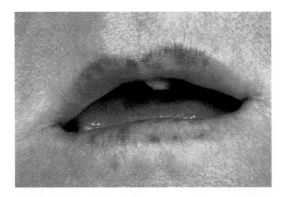

1   What is the diagnosis in this patient with a positive faecal occult blood test?

   (a) Hereditary haemorrhagic telangiectasia
   (b) Systemic sclerosis
   (c) Chronic liver disease
   (d) Carcinoma of the colon
   (e) Peutz–Jegher's syndrome

Question 4

A 44-year-old clerk presents with anorexia and painless jaundice. On examination there is hepatosplenomegaly and a single axillary lymph node is palpated. He is sent home with a diagnosis of infectious hepatitis and seen in the outpatient department 2 weeks later. At this time he has a fever with ascites and ankle oedema.
Investigations show:

Hb	12.8 g/dL
WBC	14.6×10^9/L
Neutrophils	85 per cent
Lymphocytes	7 per cent
Monocytes	5 per cent
Eosinophils	1 per cent
Serum albumin	23 g/L
Plasma bilirubin	125 µmol/L
Plasma alkaline phosphatase	380 IU/L *(normal range 30–100)*
Plasma alanine aminotransferase	38 IU/L *(normal range 5–35)*
Faecal fat	60 g/24 h *(normal range 11–18)*

1   What is the likely diagnosis?
   (a) Alpha-chain disease
   (b) Whipple's disease
   (c) Intestinal tuberculosis
   (d) Intestinal lymphoma
   (e) Crohn's disease

Question 5

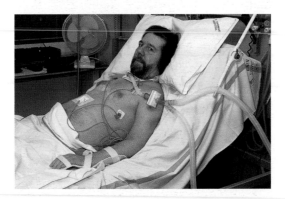

1   Other than a mild gastroenteritis, this man was well until 3 days ago. What investigation would be most likely to support your diagnosis?

(a) Blood culture
(b) Treponemal serology
(c) Stool culture
(d) Chest x-ray
(e) Tensilon test

Question 6

A 23-year-old man is admitted with a severe exacerbation of his asthma. He is treated with 5 mg nebulized salbutamol, 500 μg nebulized ipratropium and 15 litres of oxygen via a re-breathing mask.

	Pretreatment	Post-treatment
Po_2	6.6	7.6
Pco_2	3.5	3.7
pH	7.35	7.30
PEFR	100	150

1 The next stage in his management according to the British Thoracic Society guidelines is:
   (a) Intravenous salbutamol
   (b) Intravenous magnesium
   (c) Intravenous aminophylline
   (d) Intravenous suxamethonium and ventilation
   (e) Intravenous hydrocortisone

Question 7

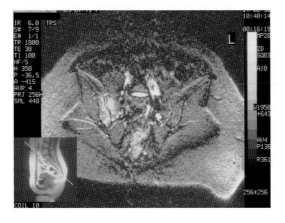

This woman complains of back pain.

1   What does the T2-weighted MR scan of her pelvis show?
   (a) Endometrial tumour
   (b) Unilateral sacroiliitis
   (c) Effusion in the right hip
   (d) Paget's disease of the pelvis
   (e) Multiple metastases

Question 8

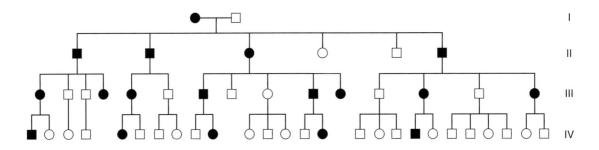

1   Which modes of inheritance are compatible with this pedigree?
   (a) X-linked recessive
   (b) X-linked dominant
   (c) X-linked dominant with incomplete penetrance
   (d) Autosomal recessive
   (e) Autosomal dominant
   (f) Autosomal dominant with incomplete penetrance
   (g) Polygenic inheritance
   (h) Mitochondrial inheritance
   (i) Random inheritance

2   What is the probability of a son of individual III^8 inheriting the disease?
   (a) 1:1
   (b) 1:2
   (c) 1:3
   (d) 1:4
   (e) 1:8

Question 9

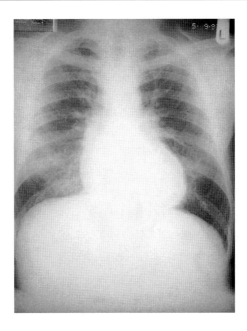

1   What is the diagnosis?
    (a) Left ventricular aneurysm
    (b) Misplaced ventricular pacing wire
    (c) Right lower zone pneumonia
    (d) Tuberculous pericarditis
    (e) Left lower zone bulla

Question 10

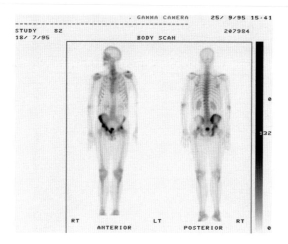

1   What is the diagnosis?
     (a) Paget's disease
     (b) Prostatic carcinoma
     (c) Osteosarcoma of the pelvis
     (d) Osteomalacia
     (e) Renal osteodystrophy

Question 11

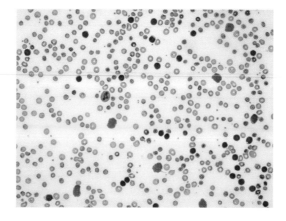

A 65-year-old tramp who frequently visits the A and E department is proving more difficult to eject than normal. He is noted to have widespread lymphadenopathy.
     Haematological examination:

Hb	9.8 g/dL
WBC	$123 \times 10^9/L$
Platelets	$195 \times 10^9/L$
MCV	109 fL

1   What tests would you arrange to confirm the cause of his macrocytosis?
   (a) B_{12} level
   (b) Red cell folate level
   (c) Blood alcohol
   (d) Thyroid-stimulating hormone
   (e) Blood film

Question 12

A 10-year-old Greek boy presents with lethargy and reduced exercise tolerance. His mother says that he often complains of stomach pains.
   Investigations show:

Hb	9.8 g/dL
WBC	$7.8 \times 10^9/L$
MCV	65 fL
Platelets	$430 \times 10^9/L$

1   Give two likely diagnoses.
   (a) Thalassaemia trait
   (b) α-Thalassaemia trait
   (c) β-Thalassaemia trait
   (d) Hookworm infection
   (e) *Ascaris* infection
   (f) Familial Mediterranean fever
   (g) Crohn's disease
   (h) Coeliac disease
   (i) Sickle cell trait
   (j) Sickle cell disease

Question 13

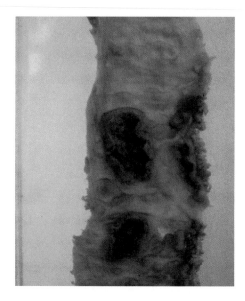

This post-mortem specimen shows a section of ileum from a patient who died after an acute febrile illness.

1   What was the post-mortem diagnosis?
   (a) Typhoid
   (b) Schistosomiasis
   (c) Carcinoid
   (d) Tuberculosis
   (e) Crohn's disease

Question 14

A 56-year-old man presents with a 6-month history of back pain and recent nausea and vomiting. He is now anuric. Investigations show:

Plasma sodium	146 mmol/L
Plasma potassium	5.7 mmol/L
Plasma urea	56 mmol/L
Plasma creatinine	1020 µmol/L
Plasma calcium	2.95 mmol/L
Plasma phosphate	1.1 mmol/L
Serum total protein	96 g/dL
Serum albumin	32 g/dL
Hb	9.4 g/dL

1   What is the likely underlying diagnosis?
    (a) Carcinoma of the prostate
    (b) Metastatic cancer, unknown primary
    (c) Multiple myeloma
    (d) Parathyroid adenoma
    (e) Medullary carcinoma of the thyroid

2   What two investigations will be helpful in reaching a diagnosis?
    (a) Concurrent serum parathormone and calcium levels
    (b) Serum prostate specific antigen
    (c) Serum protein electrophoresis
    (d) Serum angiotensin converting enzyme level
    (e) Bone marrow aspirate/trephine
    (f) Ultrasound of thyroid
    (g) Bence Jones protein
    (h) Ultrasound of abdomen
    (i) Chest x-ray
    (j) Sestamibi scan

Question 15

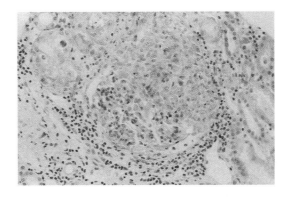

1   The likely underlying diagnosis is:
    (a) Diffuse glomerulosclerosis
    (b) Diffuse membranoproliferative glomerulonephritis
    (c) Minimal change glomerulonephritis
    (d) Focal segmental proliferative glomerulonephritis
    (e) Crescentic glomerulonephritis

Question 16

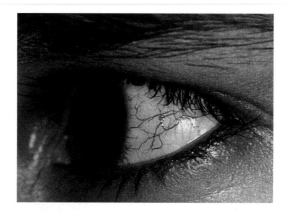

This patient is ataxic.

1 What is the mode of inheritance?
(a) Autosomal recessive
(b) Autosomal dominant
(c) X-linked dominant
(d) X-linked recessive
(e) Triplet repeat disorder

Question 17

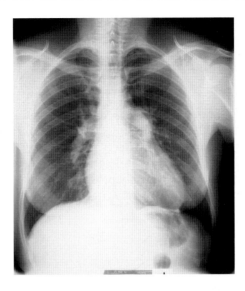

A 39-year-old woman with mild Raynaud's disease complains of breathlessness on minimal exertion. The houseman finds no abnormality on examination and arranges a chest x-ray and pulmonary function tests, and shows them to you.

FVC	2.29 (2.71)
FEV_1	1.88 (2.31)
FEV_1/FVC	74 (85)
PEFR	550 (6.96)
TLC	4.91 (4.3)
DL/VA	1.00 (1.2)
DL_{CO}	6.75 (3.83)

1   What is the diagnosis?
   (a) Primary pulmonary hypertension
   (b) Mitral stenosis
   (c) Pulmonary emboli
   (d) Extrinsic allergic alveolitis
   (e) Sarcoidosis

2   What two further investigations would you organize?
   (a) Echocardiography
   (b) Pulmonary angiography
   (c) Cardiac catheterization
   (d) CT spiral angiography
   (e) VQ scan
   (f) High resolution CT scan
   (g) Serum ACE

(h) Serum precipitins
(i) Coagulation screen including D-dimer
(j) Calcium and ESR

Question 18

A GP rings you on a Monday morning for some advice. He has with him in his surgery a 69-year-old male patient with osteoarthritis. The patient had OA diagnosed several years ago and had a left knee replacement 6 months ago that was complicated by a postoperative MI. He is awaiting a right knee replacement and has experienced further pain in this knee. His usual prescription of paracetamol did not provide relief so the patient bought himself some ibuprofen from the local petrol station. He wants the GP to give him ibuprofen on prescription.

1   Would you recommend:
    (a) Ibuprofen 200 mg t.d.s.
    (b) Ibuprofen 400 mg t.d.s.
    (c) Celecoxib 100 mg b.d.
    (d) Ibuprofen 400 mg t.d.s. and lansoprazole 30 mg o.d.
    (e) Celecoxib 100 mg b.d. and lansoprazole 30 mg o.d.

Question 19

A heart murmur is investigated by cardiac catheterization.

Site	Pressure (mmHg)	Oxygen saturation (per cent)
Superior vena cava		60
Inferior vena cava		66
Right atrium (mean pressure)	5	88
Right ventricle	60/5	90
Pulmonary artery	15/4	89
Pulmonary wedge (mean pressure)	6	

1   Which of the following best describes the abnormalities?
    (a) Ventricular septal defect with left-to-right shunt plus pulmonary stenosis
    (b) Atrial septal defect with right-to-left shunt plus pulmonary stenosis
    (c) Atrial septal defect with left-to-right shunt plus tricuspid stenosis
    (d) Atrial septal defect with left-to-right shunt plus mitral stenosis
    (e) Atrial septal defect with left-to-right shunt plus pulmonary stenosis

2   Which of the following may be associated with this situation?
   (a) Down's syndrome
   (b) Noonan's syndrome
   (c) Turner's syndrome
   (d) Kawasaki's syndrome
   (e) Libman–Sachs' syndrome

Question 20

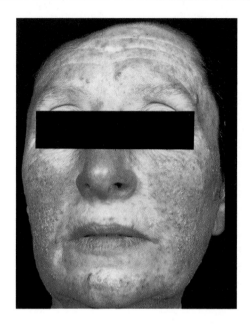

1   What is the diagnosis?
   (a) Dermatitis
   (b) Acne
   (c) Systemic lupus erythematosus
   (d) Rhinophyma
   (e) Rosacea

Question 21

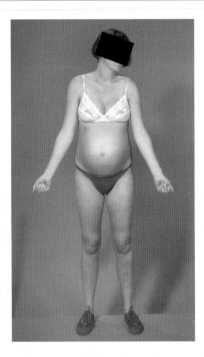

This woman presented with abdominal pain. Three days earlier she had a tender rash on her shins. On examination she was noted to be anaemic.

1   The first diagnostic test would be:
   (a) CT abdomen
   (b) Plasma hormone level
   (c) Colonoscopy
   (d) Blood cultures
   (e) Serum glucose

Question 22

The day after returning from a 6-week holiday to the Philippines, Nepal and India, a 28-year-old doctor developed diarrhoea, abdominal pain and anorexia. He prescribed kaolin and morphine for himself. Ten days later the diarrhoea had become worse, producing bloodless, pale, foul-smelling stools. He also had borborygmi, flatulence, anorexia and lethargy and had lost 5 kg in weight. He had taken the recommended course of antimalarial chemoprophylaxis and prior to departure had received typhoid, hepatitis B, yellow fever and rabies vaccination as well as human normal immunoglobulin. Whilst in India he had been treated for *Shigella* dysentery with co-trimoxazole.

On examination he looked chronically ill, thin, pale, and fluid depleted. His temperature was 36.8°C. He had pitting of the nails and small patches of psoriasis on the forearm and back. His abdomen had stretch marks and was not distended or tender. The liver and spleen were not palpable. The bowel sounds were increased in frequency and duration. The stools were pale, soft and yellow. Sigmoidoscopy and urinalysis were normal.

Investigations performed revealed the following results:

Hb	12.7 g/dL
WBC	6.2 × 101/L
Plasma sodium	140 mmol/L
Plasma potassium	4.1 mmol/L
Plasma urea	5.5 mmol/L
Serum albumin	26 g/L
Serum total protein	81 g/L
Plasma aspartate aminotransferase	20 IU/L *(normal range 4–20)*
Plasma alanine aminotransferase	42 IU/L *(normal range 2–17)*
Serum bilirubin	6 μmol/L
Serum immunoglobulins:	
IgG	14.0 g/L *(normal range 7.2–19.0)*
IgM	1.3 g/L *(normal range 0. 5–2. 0)*
IgA	6.5 g/L *(normal range 0.8–5. 0)*
Blood film	negative for malaria and filaria
Stool culture	no significant bacterial pathogens isolated
72-hour faecal fat	140 g/L *(normal range 11–18)*

1   Which two of the following are the most likely diagnoses?
(a) *Clostridium difficile*
(b) Adult coeliac disease
(c) Giardiasis
(d) Amoebiasis
(e) Schistosomiasis
(f) Typhoid
(g) Inflammatory bowel disease
(h) Irritable bowel syndrome
(i) Ischaemic colitis
(j) Tropical sprue

2   Which single investigation would be most useful?
(a) Stool microscopy and culture
(b) Abdominal ultrasound
(c) Endomysial antibodies
(d) Duodenal aspirate and biopsy
(e) CT abdomen

Question 23

A 30-year-old woman with schizophrenia was admitted 3 days after a routine outpatient appointment. Unusually, she has been increasingly withdrawn over the past 48 hours and has been brought to A and E because her family is worried that she is now running a temperature. There is no further history available.

On examination, she has a temperature of 39.3°C, with a mild impaired level of consciousness and generalized muscle rigidity. There are no other physical signs.

1   What is the best treatment?
    (a) Intravenous ceftazidime
    (b) PR paracetamol
    (c) Intravenous dantrolene
    (d) Oral dantrolene
    (e) Intravenous suxamethonium

Question 24

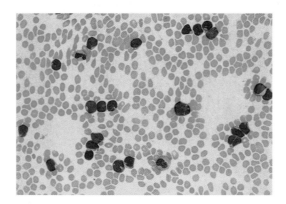

This is the peripheral blood film of a 4-year-old boy who has presented with mucous membrane bleeding.

1   What is the diagnosis?
    (a) Acute lymphoblastic leukaemia
    (b) Autoimmune thrombocytopenia
    (c) Acute myeloid leukaemia
    (d) Haemolytic uraemic syndrome
    (e) Sickle cell disease

Question 25

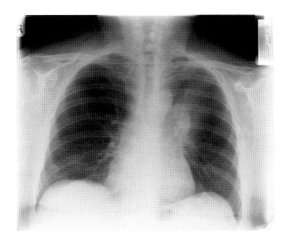

1   A 53-year-old man presents with cough and leg pain. What does the chest x-ray show and what is the likely diagnosis?
   (a) Collapse of the right lower lobe due to bronchogenic carcinoma
   (b) Right middle lobe collapse due to bronchogenic carcinoma
   (c) Secondary tumour of the lung from osteosarcoma of the femur
   (d) Aortic coarctation with claudication
   (e) Collapse of left upper lobe due to bronchogenic carcinoma

Question 26

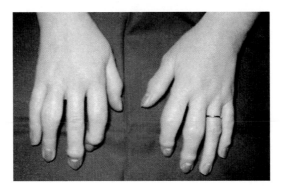

1   List two abnormal signs:
   (a) Joint subluxation
   (b) Ulnar deviation
   (c) Heberden's node
   (d) Z-shaped thumb
   (e) Gouty tophus

(f) Bouchard's node
(g) Soft tissue swelling
(h) Swan neck deformity
(i) Gottron's papules
(j) Nail pitting

Question 27

A woman has been admitted with breast cancer. She has bone and brain metastases that have failed to respond to chemotherapy. The analgesics that she had been prescribed have failed to control her pain. These were paracetamol 1 g q.d.s., codeine phosphate 60 mg q.d.s., tramadol 50 mg t.d.s., Voltarol 50 mg t.d.s.

She would like you to start diamorphine 'to put me out of my misery'.

1 You would prescribe:
   (a) 20 mg diamorphine over 24 hours with the intention of ending the patient's life
   (b) 20 mg diamorphine over 24 hours with the intention of ameliorating pain
   (c) 20 mg diamorphine over 24 hours with the intention of ameliorating pain and ending the life of the patient
   (d) 20 mg MST over 24 hours with the intention of ameliorating pain
   (e) 20 mg MST over 24 hours with the intention of ending the patient's life

Question 28

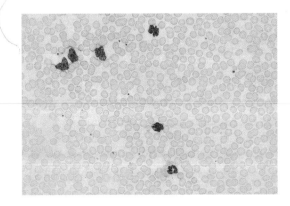

1 What is the diagnosis in this 30-year-old with lymphadenopathy?
   (a) Iron deficiency anaemia
   (b) Viral infection
   (c) Leukaemia
   (d) Cold agglutinin disease
   (e) Lymphoma

Question 29

A 54-year-old female has been treated with insulin for diabetes for the past 10 years. She has been referred for investigation of recently diagnosed hypertension. She is currently taking 40 units of insulin in the morning and 30 in the evening and is also taking 8 mg perindopril.

Examination shows her to be obese with a blood pressure of 180/100 mmHg, measured using a large cuff.

Results of investigations were as follows:

Plasma sodium	136 mmol/L
Plasma potassium	4.1 mmol/L
Plasma creatinine	130 µmol/L
Plasma glucose	11.0 mmol/L
Serum HDL	0.7 mmol/L *(normal range >0.91)*
Urinalysis	protein ++

1   What management change would you suggest to her GP?
    (a) Change perindopril to an angiotensin II blocker
    (b) Addition of a thiazide diuretic
    (c) Addition of a calcium channel blocker
    (d) Addition of a beta-blocker
    (e) Weight loss

Question 30

A man with known multiple endocrine neoplasia type II has diarrhoea.

1   Which of the following is unlikely to be the cause of the diarrhoea in this man?
    (a) Medullary carcinoma of the thyroid
    (b) Phaeochromocytoma
    (c) Vasoactive intestinal peptide secretion
    (d) Hyperparathyroidism
    (e) Myenteric neuromas

Question 31

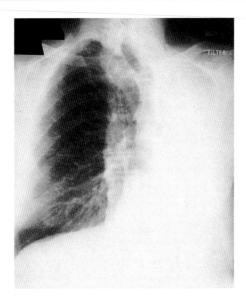

This is the CXR of a patient who had lung carcinoma 15 years previously. He is now short of breath.

1   What is the diagnosis?
    (a) Left pleural effusion
    (b) Left pneumonectomy
    (c) Left-sided consolidation
    (d) Left phrenic nerve palsy
    (e) Left complete collapse

Question 32

A 73-year-old man refuses an intravenous cannula through which you wish to administer antibiotics for a chest infection. His daughter insists you insert the cannula, as he is just being difficult. You determine that he is confused and disoriented in time and place.

1   The correct course of action is:
    (a) To accede to the patient's stated wish and withhold treatment
    (b) To accede to the daughter's wish and force treatment on him because she is the only competent relative
    (c) To apply to the court for an order to permit treatment
    (d) To administer drugs you believe to be in his best interests irrespective of his incompetent opinion or that of his daughter
    (e) To conclude that his quality of life is so poor from your contemporaneous assessment of his mental state and thus withhold medication as an act of kindness

Question 33

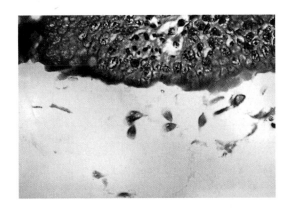

This patient has diarrhoea.

1   How would you treat this patient?
    (a) Vancomycin
    (b) Metronidazole
    (c) Gluten-free diet
    (d) Mesalazine
    (e) Doxycycline

Question 34

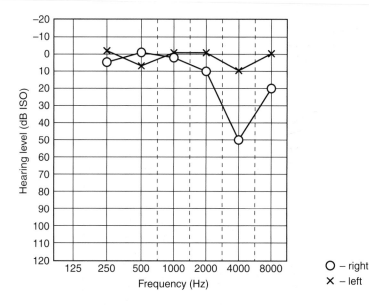

This is an audiogram of a left-handed gamekeeper who complained of hearing loss. There is no air–bone gap.

1   What is the likely aetiology?
    (a) Cerebellopontine angle tumour
    (b) Ear wax
    (c) Ménière's disease
    (d) Noise-induced hearing loss
    (e) Age-related hearing loss

Question 35

A 68-year-old woman with rheumatoid arthritis who has been on a stable dose of methotrexate for 5 years has had two recent episodes of pneumonia. Her only other medication is folic acid and a recently introduced non-steroidal anti-inflammatory drug. Investigations show:

Hb	10.1 g/dL
MCV	89 fL
WBC	1.7×10^9/L
Neutrophils	0.6×10^9/L
Platelets	53×10^9/L
ESR	25 mm in first hour
CRP	10 mg/L
Plasma aspartate aminotransferase	100 IU/dL
Plasma alkaline phosphatase	200 IU/L

1   What is the most likely diagnosis?
     (a) Felty's syndrome
     (b) Septic myelosuppression
     (c) Methotrexate bone marrow suppression
     (d) Idiosyncratic reaction to non-steroidal drug
     (e) Intercurrent viral infection

Question 36

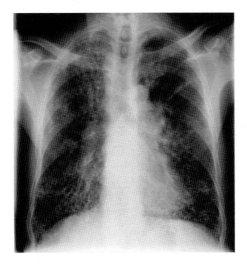

This man is increasingly breathless and clubbed.

1   What complication has arisen?
     (a) Malignant transformation
     (b) Mitral stenosis
     (c) Aspergilloma
     (d) Pulmonary hypertension
     (e) Tuberculosis

Question 37

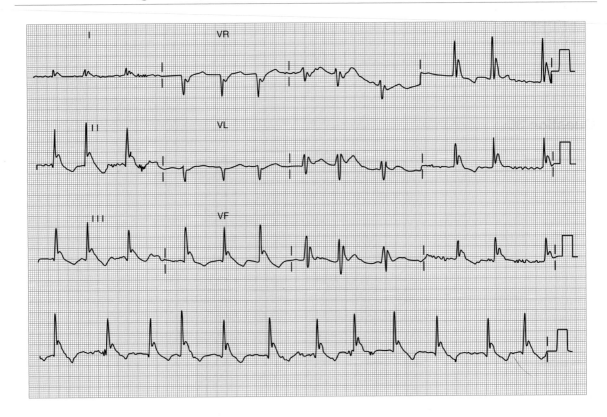

This is the ECG of a 38-year-old unconscious male.

1   Give three abnormalities.
   (a) J waves
   (b) Delta waves
   (c) Alpha waves
   (d) U waves
   (e) Prolonged PR interval
   (f) Prolonged QT interval
   (g) Atrial fibrillation
   (h) Atrial flutter
   (i) Paroxysmal atrial tachycardia
   (j) Misplacement of chest leads
   (k) Reversal of arm leads
   (l) Anterior T-wave inversion
   (m) Reversal of leg leads
   (n) Lateral ST elevation
   (o) Muscle tremor artefact

2   What is the diagnosis?
   (a) Hypothermia
   (b) Hypercalcaemia
   (c) Hypocalcaemia
   (d) Parkinsonism
   (e) Hypokalaemia

Question 38

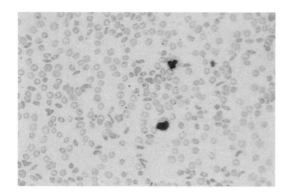

This is the peripheral blood film of a 12-year-old girl with anaemia.

1   What is the diagnosis?
   (a) Infectious mononucleosis
   (b) Malaria
   (c) Hereditary elliptocytosis
   (d) Hereditary spherocytosis
   (e) Sickle cell disease

Question 39

The following table summarizes the immunological data on three patients awaiting renal transplantation and one donor.

1   Based on this information, which of these patients would be appropriate recipients for this kidney?
   (a) Patient 1
   (b) Patient 2
   (c) Patient 3
   (d) Patients 1 or 2
   (e) Patients 2 or 3

	Patient 1 (GG)	Patient 2 (RA)	Patient 3 (FG)	Donor
Age	19	44	39	32
Sex	F	M	F	M
Cause of renal failure	Anti-GBM disease	Diabetic nephropathy	Polycystic kidney disease	–
Blood group	B+	B+	A+	B+
HLA type	A2, 30	A1	A2, 29	A1, 2
	B8, 40	B8, 17	B12, 22	B12, 35
	Cw7	Cw6, 7	Cw3	Cw4
	DR3, 6	DR3, 4	DR7, 13	DR3, 11
	DRw52	DRw52	DRw52	DRw52
	DQ1, 2	DQ2, 8	DQ5, 7	DQ2, 7
Cross-match with donor cells	+	–	Not tested	
Previous failed transplant				
Blood group		B		
HLA type		A1, 2		
		B8, 44		
		DR3, 4		

Question 40

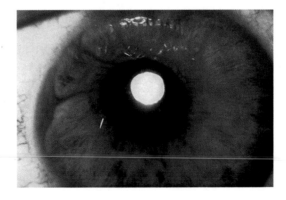

1 What is the underlying disease?
   (a) Diabetes mellitus
   (b) Wilson's disease
   (c) Previous uveitis
   (d) Rheumatoid arthritis
   (e) Reiter's disease

Question 41

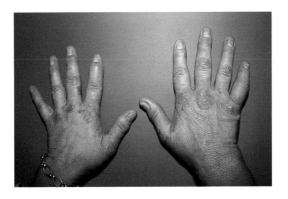

1   What is the diagnosis?
    (a) Tinea
    (b) Psoriatic arthritis
    (c) Osteoarthritis with eczema
    (d) Rheumatoid arthritis with eczema
    (e) Parvovirus arthritis

Question 42

A 28-year-old American marine presents with fever, red eyes, backache and swelling and pain in his right knee and left ankle following a trip to Thailand. His mother had psoriasis and an aunt diabetes mellitus. On examination he is febrile, and there is warmth, swelling and tenderness of the right knee and left ankle. There are mouth ulcers, nail pitting and a rash on his soles, and conjunctivitis.

1   Which of the following is your first investigation?
    (a) Joint aspiration
    (b) Rheumatoid factor
    (c) Serum urate
    (d) Measurement of inflammatory markers
    (e) Urethral smear

2   What is the diagnosis?
    (a) Gonococcal arthritis
    (b) Psoriatic arthritis
    (c) Non-gonococcal septic arthritis
    (d) Reiter's syndrome
    (e) Osteomyelitis

Question 43

Following the death of his 39-year-old brother from a myocardial infarction, a 42-year-old man requests analysis of his serum lipids.
Investigations show:

Plasma cholesterol	5.8 mmol/L *(normal range 4.7–6.2)*
Plasma HDL cholesterol	2.9 mmol/L *(normal range 0.96–2.0)*
Plasma LDL cholesterol	4.1 mmol/L *(normal range 2.4–5.0)*
Plasma triglycerides	8.1 mmol/L *(normal range 0.74–2.1)*

1   What is the likely diagnosis?
 (a) Primary hypertriglyceridaemia
 (b) Familial hypercholesterolaemia
 (c) Familial hypertriglyceridaemia
 (d) Familial combined hyperlipidaemia
 (e) Secondary hypertriglyceridaemia

Question 44

A 49-year-old woman presented to her GP with a 2-day history of severe epigastric pain and vomiting. She had been drinking with friends to celebrate her birthday. The pain responded to a proprietary antacid. She visited her GP again with recurrent heartburn and epigastric pain. When seen in the gastroenterology outpatient clinic she gave a 3-week history of weight loss and diarrhoea. Her maternal aunt had a history of peptic ulcer. There were no abnormalities on physical examination.

An outpatient endoscopy showed two deep duodenal ulcers, one extending beyond the first part of the duodenum, but no *Helicobacter pylori* was detected. Sigmoidoscopy was normal. She was prescribed omeprazole but at her next clinic appointment 8 weeks later she complained of persisting diarrhoea and epigastric pain.

1   Which two further diagnostic tests would you perform?
 (a) Abdominal ultrasound
 (b) Selective angiography of the pancreas
 (c) CT scan of the abdomen
 (d) Upper GI endoscopy
 (e) Fasting plasma gastrin levels
 (f) Barium meal and follow-through
 (g) Urinary omeprazole metabolites
 (h) Colonoscopy
 (i) Trial of IV omeprazole
 (j) Secretin gastrin stimulation test

2   What is the diagnosis?
     (a) Failure to comply with medication
     (b) Zollinger–Ellison syndrome
     (c) Gastrinoma
     (d) Carcinoma of the pancreas
     (e) Alcoholic gastritis

Question 45

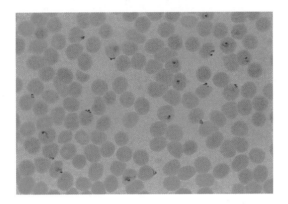

1   What is the diagnosis?
     (a) Sideroblastic anaemia
     (b) Splenectomy
     (c) *Plasmodium ovale* malaria
     (d) *Plasmodium falciparum* malaria
     (e) Heinz bodies

Question 46

A 15-year-old girl presents with breathlessness. Blood gas analysis shows:

pH	7.49
P_{CO_2}	6.4 kPa
P_{O_2}	4.8 kPa
Plasma bicarbonate	15 mmol/L

1   What is your next investigation?
     (a) Serum salicylate level
     (b) Ethylene glycol level
     (c) Blood glucose
     (d) Chest x-ray
     (e) Repeat blood gas analysis

Question 47

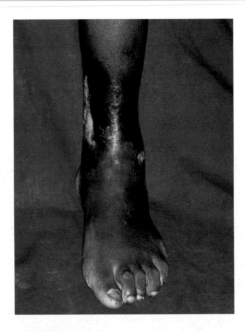

1   What is the likely cause of this lesion?
    (a) Venous ulceration
    (b) Sickle cell disease
    (c) Diabetes mellitus
    (d) Leishmaniasis
    (e) Cellulitis

Question 48

A 58-year-old Asian male alcoholic, who had been resident in the UK for the past 18 years, presented with a 3-month history of myalgia, low back pain and difficulty in walking.
    Investigations showed:

Fasting plasma glucose	3.8 mmol/L
Plasma calcium	2.10 mmol/L
Plasma phosphate	0.48 mmol/L
Serum albumin	34 g/L
Plasma aspartate aminotransferase	44 IU/L *(normal range 5–35)*
Plasma alkaline phosphatase	220 IU/L *(normal range 30–100)*
Hb	10.8 g/dL
WBC	7.2 × 10⁹/L
MCV	102 fL
ESR	12 mm in first hour

1   What is the likely cause for his gait symptoms?
    (a) Renal tubular acidosis
    (b) Osteomalacia
    (c) Dermatomyositis
    (d) Subacute-combined degeneration of the cord
    (e) Hypoparathyroidism

Question 49

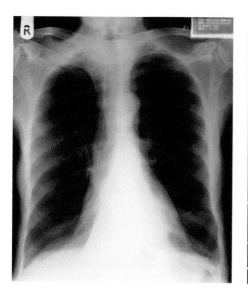 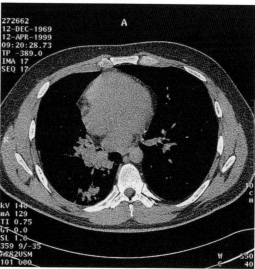

A 47-year-old referred with asthma. Examination shows a monophobic wheeze. Chest x-ray and CT scan are shown.

1   What is the radiological diagnosis?
    (a) Right upper lobe collapse with para-aortic lymphadenopathy
    (b) Right lower lobe collapse with bronchial tumour
    (c) Inferior mediastinal mass
    (d) Left middle lobe mass
    (e) Left lower lobe collapse

Question 50

A 45-year-old woman has had seropositive arthritis for the past 10 years. After 5 years of treatment with gold she developed a rash and was subsequently managed with an alternative disease-modifying drug, an anti-inflammatory and small dose of prednisolone. She is referred for urgent review because of a 'flare'. Her history is of worsening mobility, increasing stiffness and being unable to use her arms for more than a few minutes without dropping things. A relative promises to bring in her drugs later. She looks unwell, with stigmata of rheumatoid, including nodules. Both knees and elbows are hot and painful, with patchy sensory loss distally in the upper limbs. Power was difficult to assess because of deformities but reflexes were intact.

1 Give three likely possible causes of her recent deterioration:
   (a) Rheumatoid flare
   (b) Loss of effect of disease-modifying drug
   (c) Alcoholic neuropathy
   (d) Septic arthritis
   (e) Systemic vasculitis
   (f) Non-compliance
   (g) Adrenal crisis after discontinuing steroid
   (h) Cervical myelopathy
   (i) Avascular necrosis
   (j) Steroid-induced diabetes

   Initial investigations:

Hb	9.6 g/dL
WCC	1.9×10^9/L
Platelets	150×10^9/L
ESR	105 mm/h
Urinalysis	protein ++
U+E	normal
LFTs	albumin 25 g/L

2 Which possible diagnosis best explains all the abnormal tests?
   (a) Rheumatoid vasculitis
   (b) AA amyloidosis
   (c) Septic arthritis
   (d) Penicillamine adverse reaction
   (e) Methotrexate adverse reaction

Question 51

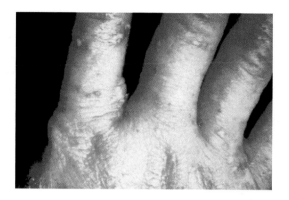

1   What is the agent?
   (a) *Sarcoptes scabiei*
   (b) Human papillomavirus
   (c) Varicella-zoster virus
   (d) Herpes simplex virus
   (e) Human herpesvirus 8

Question 52

A 30-year-old Turkish Cypriot waiter presents with fever, diarrhoea, abdominal pain, weight loss and arthritis. He has had several similar episodes in the past. On examination, he is thin with clinical evidence of a small left pleural effusion and marked ankle oedema. Investigations show:

Hb	13.2 g/dL
MCV	101.3 fL
Serum albumin	25 g/L
CRP	55 mg/L
Urinary xylose excretion after 25 g oral load	3.2 mmol/5 h *(normal range 8.0–16/24 h)*
Urinalysis	protein +++

1   What is the diagnosis?
   (a) Familial Mediterranean fever
   (b) AL amyloidosis
   (c) Tropical sprue
   (d) Whipple's disease
   (e) Rheumatoid arthritis

2   Which is the most helpful next investigation?
    (a) Rectal biopsy
    (b) Renal biopsy
    (c) Faecal fat collection
    (d) 24-hour urinary protein
    (e) Serum B_{12} level

3   What treatment would you consider?
    (a) Prednisolone
    (b) Cyclophosphamide
    (c) Cyclosporin A
    (d) Colchicine
    (e) Low-fat diet

4   What contributes to the development of the pleural effusion?
    (a) Pleural infiltrates
    (b) High output cardiac failure
    (c) Fluid retention due to renal impairment
    (d) Low serum albumin
    (e) Pleurisy

Question 53

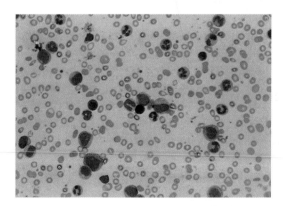

This is the blood film of a 50-year-old woman with anaemia and splenomegaly.

1   What is the diagnosis?
    (a) Acute lymphoblastic leukaemia
    (b) Malaria
    (c) Leukaemoid reaction
    (d) Chronic myeloid leukaemia
    (e) Multiple myeloma

Question 54

A 40-year-old Argentinean waiter presented to his GP complaining of a 6-month history of progressive exertional dyspnoea and swelling of his ankles. Direct questioning revealed mild dysphagia and regurgitation as well as intermittent constipation. He was a moderate smoker but did not drink. He was on no medication other than the diuretic. He had previously had falciparum malaria. He had come to the UK at the age of 24 years and had returned to Argentina only twice since then.

On examination he was thin but apyrexial. His pulse was 98/min at rest. His blood pressure was 100/50 mmHg. His JVP was raised to the angle of his jaw. He had dependent oedema to the sacrum. His cardiac impulse was diffuse and displaced to the mid-axillary line. Heart sounds were normal. Respiratory and neurological examinations were normal. In the abdomen, he had non-pulsatile hepatomegaly. Urinalysis was normal.

His chest radiograph showed gross cardiomegaly. The lungs appeared normal. Echocardiography showed globally hypokinetic left and right ventricles. There were no valvular abnormalities. ECG showed an intraventricular conduction defect with numerous ventricular ectopics. Twenty-four hour continuous ECG monitoring revealed four brief episodes of ventricular tachycardia. Barium swallow showed a dilated and poorly contracting oesophagus.

1   What is the diagnosis?
    (a) Chagas' disease
    (b) Dilated (congestive) cardiomyopathy
    (c) Systemic sclerosis
    (d) Tuberculous constrictive pericarditis
    (e) Loeffler's endomyocardial fibrosis

Question 55

A 19-year-old trainee Buddhist monk complains of progressive numbness in his feet over the past 6 months. Neurophysiological studies show the following:

Sural sensory action potential	6 μV *(normal >15)*
Median nerve sensory action potential	4 μV *(normal >20)*
Common peroneal nerve motor conduction velocity	47 m/s *(normal >45)*

1   What abnormality does this suggest?
    (a) Multiple mononeuropathy
    (b) Chronic demyelinating peripheral neuropathy
    (c) Traumatic nerve palsy
    (d) Chronic axonal peripheral neuropathy
    (e) Non-specific peripheral neuropathy

2   What are possible aetiologies?
   (a) Diabetes mellitus
   (b) Hereditary sensorimotor neuropathy type I
   (c) Hereditary sensorimotor neuropathy type II
   (d) Alcohol
   (e) Pressure from Lotus position
   (f) Vitamin B$_{12}$ deficiency
   (g) Drugs
   (h) Renal failure
   (i) Guillain–Barré syndrome
   (j) Idiopathic

Question 56

A 28-year-old industrial worker presents to A and E with a 2-day history of abdominal pain, nausea and vomiting. His past medical history is unremarkable apart from intermittent high alcohol consumption. Investigations show:

Plasma sodium	138 mmol/L
Plasma potassium	5.1 mmol/L
Plasma urea	18.3 mmol/L
Plasma creatinine	392 μmol/L
Plasma calcium	2.3 mmol/L
Plasma phosphate	1.9 mmol/L
Plasma bilirubin	53 μmol/L
Plasma aspartate aminotransferase	32 543 IU/L *(normal range 5–35)*
Plasma alkaline phosphatase	178 IU/L *(normal range 30–100)*
Serum albumin	44 g/L
Hb	14.7 g/dL
WBC	8.3 × 10^9/L
Platelets	210 × 10^9/L

1   What is the most likely diagnosis?
   (a) Chronic active hepatitis
   (b) Acute alcoholic hepatitis
   (c) Chronic hepatitis C infection
   (d) Salicylate poisoning
   (e) Carbon tetrachloride poisoning

Question 57

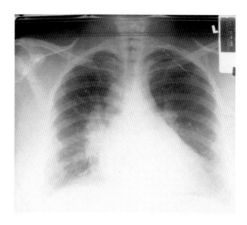

A 30-year-old West Indian male bus driver presented with a 40-month history of tiredness and polyarthralgia. One year previously he had had arthritis affecting the knee and ankle associated with a rash over the right shin. This had responded well to treatment with non-steroidal anti-inflammatory drugs. During the past 2 months he had used over-the-counter eye drops for itchy eyes. During the past week his right wrist joint had become swollen and painful and he had noticed breathlessness on climbing stairs. He gave a history of polyuria and polydipsia for the past 2 months. His last trip overseas was 3 years ago. He drank socially at weekends and smoked 15 cigarettes a day. There was no family history of sickle cell disease.

On examination, he was afebrile. There was conjunctival injection but examination of the fundus was normal. There was a red lesion with a crusty rim on the margins of the right nostril and small papular lesions on the chest. The right wrist joint was swollen and tender. There was hepatomegaly (4 cm below the costal margin) and inspiratory crackles in the left midzone of the chest. Urinalysis was normal.

The results of investigations performed were as follows:

Hb	11.8 g/dL
WBC	7.6×10^9/L
Neutrophils	56 per cent
Lymphocytes	40 per cent
Platelets	182×10^9/L
ESR	38 mm in first hour
Plasma glucose	5.1 mmol/L
Joint fluid	Gram stain negative
Chest x-ray	as shown
Sputum	negative for culture
	negative stain for acid-alcohol-fast bacilli

1   What are the two causes of his polyuria?
    (a) Diabetes mellitus
    (b) Craniogenic diabetes insipidus
    (c) Nephrogenic diabetes insipidus
    (d) Hyponatraemia

(e) SIADH
(f) Hypercalcaemia
(g) Psychogenic polydipsia
(h) Illicit drug use
(i) Proximal renal tubular acidosis
(j) Distal renal tubular acidosis

2 What two investigations would be most useful to guide initial therapy?
(a) Antinuclear antibody/factor
(b) Urea and electrolytes
(c) Serum calcium
(d) 24-hour urine calcium collection
(e) Biopsy of skin lesions
(f) Serum angiotensin-converting enzyme levels
(g) Gallium scan
(h) Bronchoscopy with transbronchial biopsy and bronchoalveolar lavage
(i) Bone marrow biopsy
(j) CT thorax

Question 58

A 28-year-old woman has been on carbimazole for 1 year. She has recently noticed that her menses have become less frequent and shorter. She is attempting to divorce her husband, and appears anxious, with sweaty palms.

Thyroid function tests show the following:

Thyroxine	75 nmol/L *(normal 50–150)*
TSH	0.2 mU/L *(normal 0.5–5)*

1 What is the definitive treatment?
(a) Propranolol
(b) Increase carbimazole dose
(c) Radioiodine
(d) Referral for counselling
(e) Propylthiouracil

Question 59

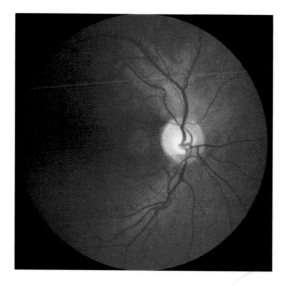

This man has had an episode of left arm weakness in the past.

1 What is the diagnosis?
  (a) Angioid streaks
  (b) Friedreich's ataxia
  (c) Optic atrophy in a Negroid fundus
  (d) Optic neuritis in a Negroid fundus
  (e) Retinal artery occlusion

Question 60

Two months prior to admission, a 66-year-old woman presented to her GP with a 1-month history of malaise. In the preceding week she had experienced an ache in her nose and under the right eye. In the 10 days before admission she had become increasingly tired and nauseated. On the day before admission she had become breathless and coughed up a small amount of blood. She was a non-smoker.

On examination she was afebrile, her pulse was 100/min and regular, her blood pressure 145/90 mmHg. Her jugular venous pressure was not raised and she had no oedema. Heart sounds were normal with no added sounds or murmurs. There were bilateral coarse crackles in both lungs. The urine contained blood (+++) on urinalysis.

Results of investigations were as follows:

Plasma sodium	140 mmol/L
Plasma potassium	6.6 mmol/L
Plasma urea	45 mmol/L
Plasma creatinine	1134 μmol/L
Chest x-ray	bilateral diffuse alveolar shadowing; normal heart size

Questions: Exam B

1   What is the diagnosis?
     (a) Subacute bacterial endocarditis
     (b) Systemic lupus erythematosus
     (c) Wegener's granulomatosis
     (d) Churg–Strauss syndrome
     (e) Sarcoidosis

Question 61

A 24-year-old woman presented to her GP with influenza-like symptoms. She was prescribed amoxicillin. Two weeks later she was suffering from headaches and had vomited several times.
     CSF obtained at lumbar puncture showed:

Protein	1.1 g/L
Cells	80/mm^3 (50 per cent lymphocytes)
Glucose	6 mmol/L
No organisms seen on Gram stain and no growth on culture	
Plasma glucose	20 mmol/L

1   Of the possible diagnoses, which two are the likely clinical diagnoses?
     (a) Partially treated bacterial meningitis
     (b) Demyelination
     (c) Diabetes mellitus
     (d) Tuberculous meningitis
     (e) Cerebral abscess
     (f) Viral meningitis
     (g) Spinal block due to tumour
     (h) Guillain–Barré syndrome
     (i) Cushing's disease
     (j) Cerebral vasculitis

Question 62

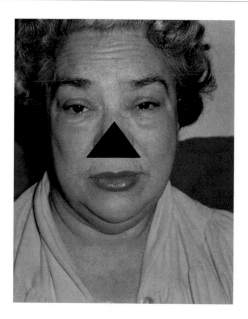

1 What is the diagnosis?
   (a) Polycystic ovary syndrome
   (b) Hypothyroidism
   (c) Acromegaly
   (d) Acute nephritis
   (e) Myasthenia gravis

Question 63

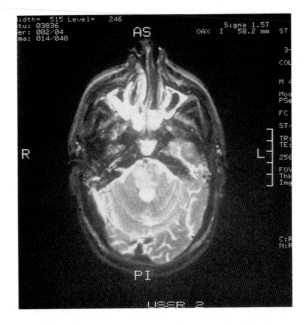

1   What diagnostic abnormality does this MRI scan show in a previously well man who suddenly became obtunded?
(a) Deviated nasal septum
(b) Haemorrhage within a hydrocephalic aqueduct of Sylvius
(c) Central pontine myelinosis
(d) Temporal lobe haematoma
(e) Pontine haemorrhage

Question 64

A 32-year-old renal transplant recipient attends a routine 3-month appointment at the transplant clinic. Since his last appointment, he has been well apart from several episodes of gout which have been managed by his GP.
    Investigations show:

Plasma sodium	134 mmol/L
Plasma potassium	4.7 mmol/L
Plasma urea	14 mmol/L
Plasma creatinine	154 µmol/L
Plasma bicarbonate	23 mmol/L
Plasma urate	0.43 mmol/L
Hb	12 g/dL
WBC	0.9×10^9/L

1   What is the treatment for his low WBC count?
   (a) Change immunosuppressive agent
   (b) Lower immunosuppressive dose
   (c) Investigate for malignancy
   (d) Stop other medication
   (e) Commence broad-spectrum antibiotics

Question 65

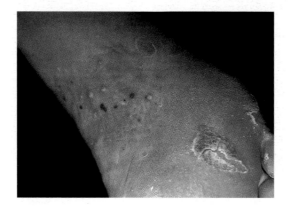

1   What is the diagnosis?
   (a) Pustular psoriasis
   (b) Tinea pedis
   (c) Diabetic sensory neuropathy
   (d) Granuloma annulare
   (e) Verruca

Question 66

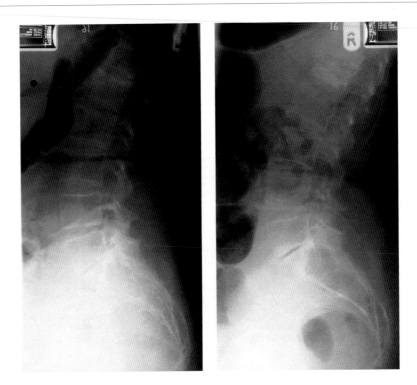

This woman had suffered steadily worsening back pain for some months; these two films are 5 months apart. She has an elevated ESR and other routine investigations are normal.

1   What is the likely diagnosis?
   (a) Repeated osteoporotic vertebral fracture
   (b) Tuberculosis
   (c) Ankylosing spondylitis
   (d) *Salmonella typhi* osteomyelitis
   (e) *Staphylococcus aureus* paraspinal abscess

Question 67

A 19-year-old woman is referred for investigation of headaches. These had started 2 months previously and were worse in the mornings. She had previously been well, having visited her GP previously only for treatment of severe acne. She had been referred to the local dermatologist. At that time the doctor had also given her contraceptive advice.

Examination showed her to be obese with an unsteady gait and some blurring of the optic disc margins. Her acne was very well controlled.

1   What is the likely drug that the dermatologist prescribed?
(a) Nitrofurantoin
(b) Prednisolone
(c) Isotretinoin
(d) Trimethoprim
(e) Tetracycline

Question 68

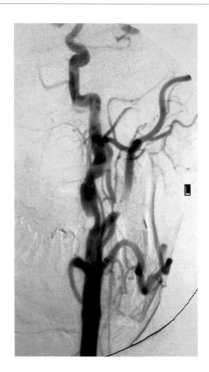

This man presented with a brief but complete episode of visual loss in one eye.

1   What does the investigation show?
(a) Dissection of the internal carotid artery
(b) Aortic stenosis
(c) Takayasu's disease
(d) Internal jugular thrombosis
(e) Complete occlusion of the internal carotid artery

Question 69

A previously healthy 58-year-old security guard working at a building site was admitted having collapsed at home. Five days previously he had become ill with malaise, anorexia, nausea, a dry cough and dysuria. He was prescribed trimethoprim by his doctor. Two days before admission he developed diarrhoea and headache. He smoked 30 cigarettes a day. There was no history of recent travel or contact with someone with similar symptoms. The family owned a pet dog and a parrot.

On examination he was unkempt, febrile (38.4°C), mildly dehydrated, dyspnoeic and cyanosed with a blood pressure of 100/60 mmHg. He was disorientated and had mild neck stiffness but a negative Kernig's sign and there were no focal neurological signs or papilloedema. There was bronchial breathing in both midzones and inspiratory crackles at the right base. The urine contained a trace of blood and protein ++.

Intravenous amoxicillin, metronidazole and gentamicin were commenced by the admitting doctor. His condition worsened the next day.

The results of investigations performed were as follows:

Hb	13.1 g/dL
WBC	14×10^9/L
Neutrophils	86 per cent
Lymphocytes	10 per cent
ESR	56 mm in first hour
Plasma sodium	126 mmol/L
Plasma potassium	4.4 mmol/L
Plasma urea	9.6 mmol/L
Plasma glucose	5.4 mmol/L
Serum albumin	32 g/L
Plasma aspartate aminotransferase	100 IU/L *(normal range 4–20)*
Plasma bilirubin	14 µmol/L
Plasma alkaline phosphatase	130 IU/L *(normal range 30–100)*
Chest x-ray	patchy shadowing both midzones; reticular shadowing right base

1   What is the most likely diagnosis?
   (a) Psittacosis
   (b) *Mycoplasma* pneumonia
   (c) *Legionella* pneumonia
   (d) Ornithosis
   (e) Pigeon fancier's lung

2   Name two diagnostic investigations you would perform:
   (a) *Chlamydia* serology
   (b) *Mycoplasma* serology
   (c) Urine *Legionella* antigen
   (d) Sputum culture
   (e) Blood culture
   (f) CT chest
   (g) Bronchoscopy with bronchoalveolar lavage

(h) Blood gases
(i) Lumbar puncture
(j) Stool microscopy and culture

3   What additional drug treatments would you administer?
(a) Amphotericin
(b) Imipenem
(c) Cefuroxime
(d) Erythromycin
(e) Tetracycline

Question 70

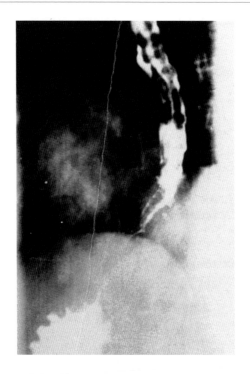

1   What is the abnormality on this barium swallow?
(a) Oesophageal *Candida*
(b) Oesophageal carcinoma
(c) Cytomegalovirus oesophagitis
(d) Oesophageal varices
(e) Oesophageal web

Question 71

A woman who is in the 30th week of her second pregnancy is admitted because of ankle swelling and hypertension.

Investigations show:

Plasma sodium	137 mmol/L
Plasma potassium	4.2 mmol/L
Plasma urea	11.7 mmol/L
Plasma creatinine	138 µmol/L
Hb	9.8 g/dL
WBC	10.5×10^9/L
Platelets	40×10^9/L
Urinalysis	protein +++
	blood ++
	glucose +++

Investigations at antenatal clinic 18 weeks earlier:

Hb	12.6 g/dL
WBC	10.7×10^9/L
Platelets	190×10^9/L
Blood glucose	4.5 mmol/L
VDRL	positive

1   What is the most helpful diagnostic procedure?
   (a) Anti-double-stranded DNA antibody titre
   (b) Serum urate level
   (c) Delivery
   (d) Assess response to antihypertensive
   (e) Serum complement levels

Question 72

A 77-year-old man with a long-standing bipolar affective disorder, managed on lithium, is found to be hypertensive by his GP, who commences drug therapy. Three weeks later the patient is confused and off his food.

Results of investigations show the following:

Plasma sodium	136 mmol/L
Plasma potassium	3.3 mmol/L
Plasma creatinine	95 μmol/L
Serum lithium	2.3 mmol/L *(therapeutic range: 0.3–1.3)*

1   What medication did the GP prescribe?
   (a) Ramipril
   (b) Atenolol
   (c) Amlodipine
   (d) Bendroflumethazide
   (e) Moxonidine

Question 73

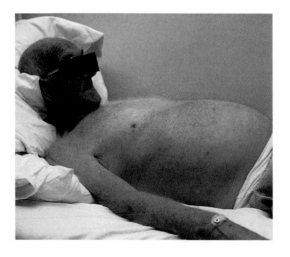

1   What illness has given rise to this man's distended abdomen?
   (a) Haemochromatosis
   (b) Alcoholic liver disease
   (c) Jaundice
   (d) Wilson's disease
   (e) Carcinoma of the stomach

Question 74

A 22-year-old man presented with severe central abdominal colicky pain. He had vomited three times and was constipated. Two days earlier he had developed stiffness in his left shoulder and was finding it difficult to lift items.

On examination, he was distressed and had a pyrexia of 38.0°C. His pulse was 145/min and his blood pressure was 190/105. His abdomen was tender but there was no rigidity. He had weakness (grade 4) of both shoulders, particularly affecting abduction. Power was not obviously affected more distally. Bulk and tone were normal, but both triceps reflexes were absent. Pinprick sensation was lost around the left shoulder. The lower limbs were normal, as were his cranial nerves, save for the finding of papilloedema.

Results of investigations were as follows:

Plasma sodium	124 mmol/L
Plasma potassium	4.5 mmol/L
Plasma urea	5.5 mmol/L
Hb	13.5 g/dL
WBC	8.8×10^9/L
Urinalysis	protein ++
	blood –
	glucose –

1   What is the diagnosis?
    (a) Guillain–Barré syndrome
    (b) Alcohol abuse
    (c) Lead poisoning
    (d) Acute intermittent porphyria
    (e) Carcinoma of the colon

2   What are two most likely explanations for his hyponatraemia?
    (a) Large bowel obstruction
    (b) Syndrome of inappropriate ADH secretion
    (c) Pancreatitis
    (d) Polydipsia
    (e) Excessive vomiting
    (f) Diabetes insipidus
    (g) Craniopharyngioma
    (h) Prolactinoma
    (i) Heavy metal deposition in pituitary
    (j) Diarrhoea

Hint
Do not be tempted to try to pull together a disparate collection of complications of a common disease and its therapy when a single rare disease would do as a unifying diagnosis. It does not work in clinical practice and it certainly does not work in the Membership.

Question 75

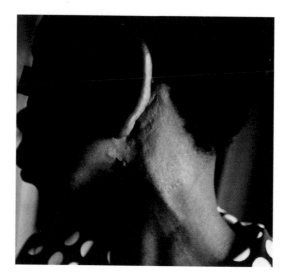

1   What is the likely causative organism?
   (a) *Mycobacterium leprae*
   (b) *Mycobacterium tuberculosis*
   (c) HIV
   (d) *Treponema pertenue*
   (e) *Treponema pallidum*

Question 76

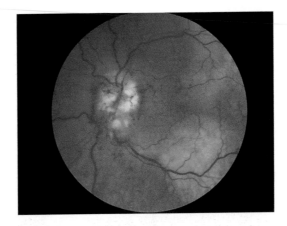

1   What two abnormalities are shown?
   (a) Background diabetic retinopathy
   (b) Grade I hypertensive retinopathy
   (c) Papilloedema
   (d) Diabetic maculopathy
   (e) Pigmented fundus
   (f) Choroidal naevus
   (g) Photocoagulation scars
   (h) Choroidal metastasis
   (i) Optic atrophy
   (j) Optic disc cupping

Question 77

A patient whose epilepsy had initially been difficult to control but who had had no change in her anticonvulsants presented with her first fit in 5 years.

1   What is the most likely cause?
   (a) Head trauma
   (b) Pregnancy
   (c) Introduction of another medication
   (d) Space-occupying lesion
   (e) It is likely no cause will be found

Question 78

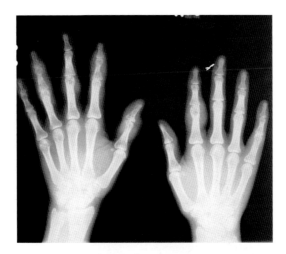

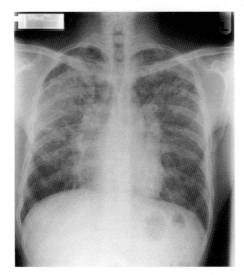

This man is a builder and keen cyclist. He feels he is having a little more difficulty cycling up the long hill leading to his place of work. He also has painful hands.

1 What is the diagnosis?
    (a) Ankylosing spondylitis
    (b) Rheumatoid arthritis
    (c) Systemic sclerosis
    (d) Sarcoidosis
    (e) Carcinoma of the bronchus with hypertrophic pulmonary osteoarthropathy

Question 79

A 33-year-old nurse had been an insulin-dependent diabetic since the age of 16. She had managed her diabetes attentively and had remained in good health. She developed a 'flu-like' illness while on a strenuous walking holiday in the Lake District. Several days later, she noticed that she had developed shortness of breath on exertion and returned home several days early. However, she became increasingly breathless and was admitted to hospital.

On examination, she was well at rest but became mildly dyspnoeic on minimal exertion. She was apyrexial. She had a few crepitations at her right base but her left hemithorax was clear. She had a pulse of 108/min at rest and a blood pressure of 115/65 mmHg. She had mild ankle oedema and her JVP was raised 4 cm with normal waveform. Urinalysis was normal.

Her chest x-ray showed some shadowing at the right base and a cardiac silhouette at the upper limit of normal. Her ECG showed minor T-wave inversion in all the chest leads. On admission, the results of initial investigations were as follows:

Plasma sodium	131 mmol/L
Plasma potassium	3.4 mmol/L
Plasma urea	12.6 mmol/L
Hb	14.4 g/dL
WBC	7.2×10^9/L
Platelets	335×10^9/L

1   What is the most likely diagnosis?
   (a) Ischaemic heart disease
   (b) Pulmonary embolism
   (c) Viral pericarditis
   (d) Viral myocarditis
   (e) Diabetic nephropathy

2   What two further investigations would be most useful to guide further management?
   (a) Cardiac troponin
   (b) Serum creatinine + 24-hour urine collection
   (c) Echocardiogram
   (d) Viral serology
   (e) VQ scan
   (f) D-dimer
   (g) Arterial blood gas
   (h) Serial ECGs
   (i) Coronary angiography
   (j) CT pulmonary angiogram

Question 80

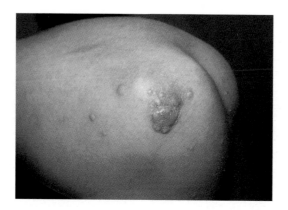

1   What are these lesions?
    (a) Dermatitis herpetiformis
    (b) Herpes simplex
    (c) Pemphigus
    (d) Xanthomata
    (e) Tophi

Question 81

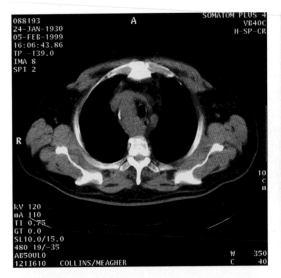
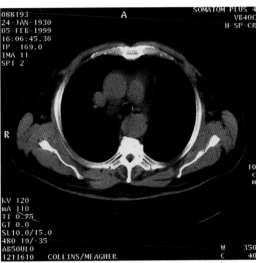
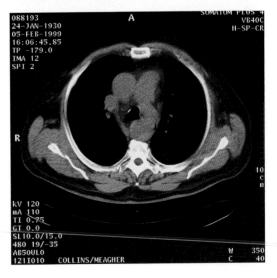
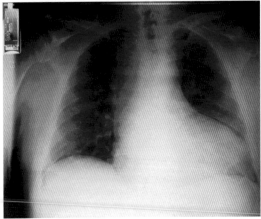

1   What is the congenital abnormality?
  (a) Right-sided aortic arch
  (b) Absent lingula
  (c) Coarctation of the aorta
  (d) Ventricular septal defect
  (e) Kartagener's syndrome

Question 82

A GP has taken two blood samples 10 minutes apart from the same nursing home resident. The results show:

	First sample	Second sample
Hb	13.7 g/dL	14.4 g/dL
WBC	7.4×10^9/L	8.0×10^9/L
Platelets	344×10^9/L	401×10^9/L
Plasma sodium	139 mmol/L	137 mmol/L
Plasma potassium	4.2 mmol/L	4.1 mmol/L
Plasma calcium	2.30 mmol/L	2.52 mmol/L
Serum albumin	42 g/L	47 g/L
Plasma glucose	4.3 mmol/L	4.5 mmol/L

1   What is the most likely explanation of the difference between the two sets of results?
    (a) Normal variability in test
    (b) The patient has gone from lying to standing between the two tests
    (c) The first sample is taken uncuffed, the second sample cuffed
    (d) First specimen taken from same arm as IV drip
    (e) The first sample is taken cuffed, the second sample uncuffed

Question 83

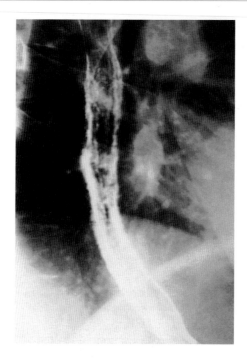

This barium meal was performed on a 44-year-old man.

1   What is the likely diagnosis?
   (a) Reflux oesophagitis
   (b) Oesophageal candidiasis
   (c) CMV oesophagitis
   (d) Benign stricture
   (e) Varices

Question 84

A 33-year-old man presented with a 3-year history of increasing deafness and tinnitus in his left ear. He thought it dated from an occasion when his infant daughter had screamed into it very loudly. He was otherwise fit and on no medication. He smoked 20 cigarettes a day.

On examination he appeared well. The auditory acuity was severely impaired on the left but the external ear and tympanic membrane look normal. On Rinne's test air conduction was greater than bone conduction. There was no nystagmus and balance was normal. His left corneal reflex was absent.

1   What is the most likely diagnosis?
(a) Acoustic neuroma
(b) Basilar artery aneurysm
(c) Meningioma
(d) Multiple sclerosis
(e) Astrocytoma glioma

Question 85

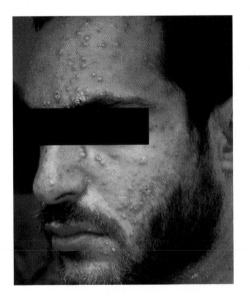

1   What is the diagnosis?
(a) Molluscum contagiosum
(b) Shingles
(c) Chickenpox
(d) Herpes simplex
(e) Acne vulgaris

Question 86

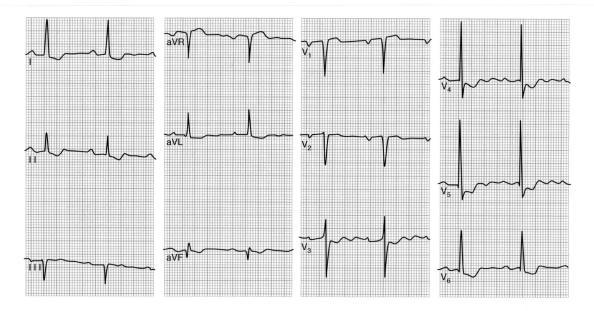

1 What is the electrocardiographic diagnosis?
  (a) First-degree heart block
  (b) Digoxin toxicity
  (c) Left atrial hypertrophy
  (d) Cardiac ischaemia
  (e) Hypokalaemia

Question 87

A 60-year-old woman is investigated for mild splenomegaly. Investigations show:

Hb	8.7 g/dL
MCV	100 fL
WBC	9.7×10^9/L
Platelets	187×10^9/L
Serum iron	44 µmol/L *(normal range 13–32)*
Serum ferritin	465 µg/L *(normal range 15–300)*
Blood film	normochromic and hypochromic erythrocytes

1 How would you confirm the likely diagnosis?
  (a) Haemoglobin electrophoresis
  (b) Bone marrow biopsy
  (c) Chromosomal analysis
  (d) Family history
  (e) Desferrioxamine suppression test

Question 88

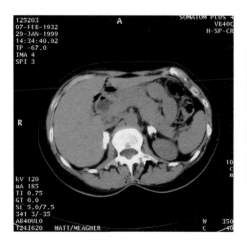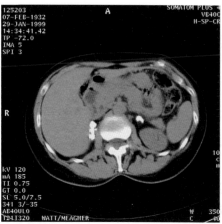

This woman is being investigated for general malaise and nausea.

1   Suggest the two likely diagnoses:
    (a) Addison's disease
    (b) Tuberculosis
    (c) Conn's adenoma
    (d) Hyperparathyroidism
    (e) Histoplasmosis
    (f) Metastatic disease
    (g) Congenital adrenal hyperplasia
    (h) Renal cell carcinoma
    (i) Renal artery stenosis
    (j) Old splenic haemorrhage

Question 89

A diabetic presents with intractable vomiting. Upper GI tract endoscopy is normal. Blood glucose control appears to be good from her meticulously presented records.

1   The most likely explanation is:
    (a) Hypoglycaemia
    (b) Ketoacidosis
    (c) Hyperosmolarity
    (d) Renal failure
    (e) Autonomic neuropathy

Question 90

A 29-year-old man presented with a 3-week history of non-bloody diarrhoea. He had no other GI symptoms. He had a similar episode 5 years previously. It had resolved spontaneously. He had had three episodes of bronchitis in the past 6 years although he was a non-smoker. He had not recently been abroad. On examination, he looked well and was afebrile. It was possible to feel the tip of his spleen. There were no other physical signs.

Results of investigations were as follows:

Hb	10.4 g/dL
MCV	103 fL
MCHC	33 g/dL
WBC	6.4 × 10⁹/L
Neutrophils	5.3 × 10⁹/L
Lymphocytes	0.7 × 10⁹/L
Eosinophils	0.4 × 10⁹/L
Platelets	87 × 10⁹/L
Plasma sodium	141 mmol/L
Plasma potassium	4.9 mmol/L
Plasma urea	5.0 mmol/L
Serum albumin	28 mmol/L
Serum total protein	56 mmol/L
Plasma aspartate aminotransferase	30 IU/L *(normal range 4–20)*
Plasma alkaline phosphatase	115 IU/L *(normal range 30–100)*
Serum immunoglobulins	
IgG	1.9 g/L *(normal range 7.2–19.0 g/dL)*
IgA	0.1 g/L *(normal range 0.8–5.0 g/dL)*
IgM	0.15 g/L *(normal range 0.5–2.0 g/dL)*
Upper gastrointestinal endoscopy	gastritis
Gastric biopsy	chronic inflammatory gastritis
Jejunal biopsy	villous atrophy
no *Giardia* seen or grown	
Small bowel enema	normal
Sigmoidoscopy	mild focal colitis
Rectal biopsy	cryptitis with eosinophilic infiltrate

1   What is the diagnosis?
   (a) Common variable immunodeficiency
   (b) Lymphoma
   (c) Coeliac disease
   (d) Whipple's disease
   (e) Primary hypogammaglobulinaemia

Question 91

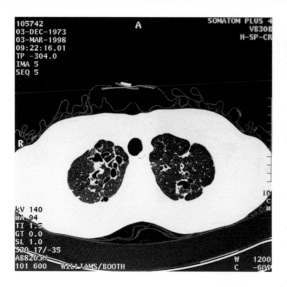 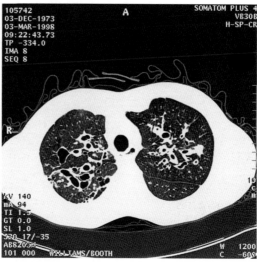

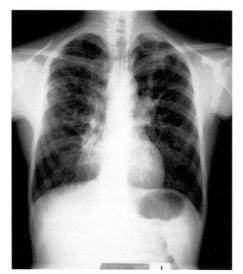

1   What is the radiological diagnosis?
  (a) Cystic fibrosis
  (b) Fibrosing alveolitis
  (c) Sarcoidosis
  (d) Histiocytosis X
  (e) Bronchiectasis

Question 92

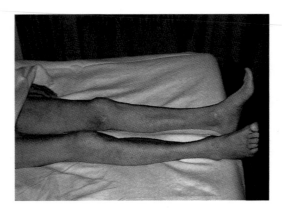

This patient is bed-bound.

1 What is the skin lesion?
   (a) Psoriasis
   (b) Pemphigus
   (c) Erythroderma
   (d) Folliculitis
   (e) Eczema

Question 93

A 7-year-old boy presents with growth retardation. Investigations were as follows:

Plasma sodium	142 mmol/L
Plasma potassium	4.2 mmol/L
Plasma urea	4.9 mmol/L
Plasma calcium	2.3 mmol/L
Plasma phosphate	0.3 mmol/L
Plasma alkaline phosphatase	175 IU/L *(normal range 30–100)*
Plasma glucose	4.3 mmol/L
Hb	12.9 g/dL
WBC	9.2×10^9/L
Platelets	333×10^9/L
ESR	9 mm in the first hour

After 1 year of treatment with vitamin D he has grown 3 cm. Alkaline phosphatase is now 150 IU/L.

1   What is the diagnosis?
     (a) Parental neglect
     (b) Vitamin D-dependent rickets
     (c) Vitamin D-resistant rickets
     (d) Osteomalacia
     (e) Ethnic variant

2   What would your next step be?
     (a) Referral to child protection team
     (b) 24-hour urine calcium collection
     (c) 24-hour urine phosphate collection
     (d) Bone scan
     (e) Serum vitamin D levels

Question 94

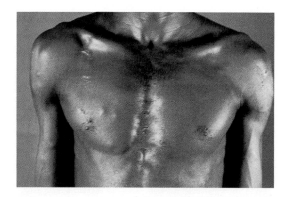

This patient has developed epilepsy and was noted to have an eosinophilia.

1   What is the diagnosis?
     (a) Cysticercosis
     (b) Toxoplasmosis
     (c) Schistosomiasis
     (d) Churg–Strauss vasculitis
     (e) Strongyloidiasis

Question 95

A healthy 33-year-old female patient asks your advice concerning cystic fibrosis. She had an 18-year-old brother who died of the disease. The patient and her two sisters, both of whom are also in their thirties, are unaffected. A younger brother died at the age of 5 years in a road traffic accident.

As she is planning to get married and start a family, she wishes to know the probability of her own children developing the disease. The patient is unrelated to her future husband.

1 Assuming the frequency of the cystic fibrosis gene in the general population is 1/25, what is that probability?
(a) 1/25
(b) 1/75
(c) 1/100
(d) 1/150
(e) 1/625

Question 96

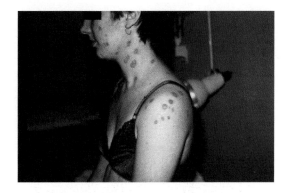

1 What is this skin lesion?
(a) Tinea corporis
(b) Erythema multiforme
(c) Plaque psoriasis
(d) Bowen's disease
(e) Erythema migrans

Question 97

Following a routine insurance medical, a 32-year-old man is referred for investigation of a raised bilirubin. Investigations show:

Hb	13.6 g/dL
Plasma sodium	140 mmol/L
Plasma potassium	4.2 mmol/L
Plasma urea	5.2 mmol/L
Plasma bilirubin	37 µmol/L
Plasma alkaline phosphatase	81 IU/L *(normal range 30–100)*
Plasma aspartate aminotransferase	30 IU/L *(normal range 5–35)*
Serum albumin	41 g/L
Urinalysis	no abnormality

1   What management would you advise?
(a) Blood film
(b) Ultrasound of liver and gallbladder
(c) Autoimmune screen
(d) Liver function tests for immediate relatives
(e) Reassurance

Question 98

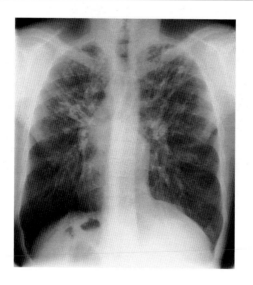

A 35-year-old of normal build presents with persistent cough. The chest x-ray is shown.

1   What is the diagnosis?
(a) Cystic fibrosis
(b) Aspergillosis
(c) Sarcoidosis
(d) Chronic extrinsic allergic alveolitis
(e) Alveolar cell carcinoma

Question 99

A 35-year-old man complains of gradual weakness and increasing dyspnoea on exertion.
Investigations show:

Plasma sodium	137 mmol/L
Plasma potassium	4.1 mmol/L
Plasma urea	5.7 mmol/L
Plasma creatinine	98 µmol/L
Plasma bilirubin	52 µmol/L
Plasma aspartate aminotransferase	21 IU/L *(normal range 5–35)*
Plasma alkaline phosphatase	75 IU/L *(normal range 30–100)*
Hb	9.1 g/dL
WBC	2.1×10^9/L
Neutrophils	0.7×10^9/L
Platelets	50×10^9/L
MCV	98 fL
Reticulocytes	10 per cent
Haptoglobins	1.2 mg/dL *(normal range 50–320)*
Hb electrophoresis	normal

1   How would you confirm the diagnosis?
(a) Ham's test
(b) CD59 count
(c) Bone marrow biopsy
(d) Complement levels
(e) CT chest

Question 100

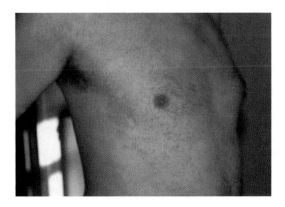

1   What is this scaly papular rash?
    (a) Pityriasis versicolor
    (b) Acne rosacea
    (c) Mycoses fungoides
    (d) Pityriasis rosea
    (e) Drug eruption

Answers

Answer 1

1   (d)

Essence

A 6-year-old boy presents with a painful, red, swollen knee. There is no evidence of systemic infection but he has a prolonged APTT with normal factor VIII levels

Differential diagnosis

The clinical history suggests a differential diagnosis of haemarthrosis or septic arthritis. However, the prolonged APTT make this a haemarthrosis. The normal bleeding time and platelet level make this a defect of the clotting cascade, and the APTT and prothrombin time put it in the intrinsic pathway. The most common defect, factor VIII deficiency or haemophilia A, is excluded; the answer is the next most likely, factor IX deficiency or haemophilia B. The lack of a family history is of no significance as one-third of patients carry new mutations.

Answer 2

1   (d)
2   (c)

Essence

A young obese woman with irregular menses presents with acne and hirsutism. There is a family history of this problem and she has raised LH and testosterone.

Differential diagnosis

If hirsutism is not associated with menstrual irregularities you are unlikely to find an underlying cause. This woman does have menstrual irregularity. However, there are specific reasons to exclude most of the differential diagnoses. Her corticosteroid production is normal (DHAS and 17-oxysteroids) which make adrenal causes unlikely. Similarly, there are no other clinical features of pituitary disease, making acromegaly unlikely, Cushing's is excluded by the clinical clue of the uniform distribution of the obesity, and the thyroxine level is normal. She is on no medication and there are no features of systemic disease.

The cause is likely to be ovarian. A malignant disease is very rare and unlikely, whereas polycystic ovary syndrome (Stein–Leventhal syndrome) is common – it is the cause of 80 per cent of all cases of oligomenorrhoea and 25 per cent cases of amenorrhoea. It is classically associated with greasy skin and acne as well as obesity and a family history is common. Levels of LH are raised, FSH normal or low, and testosterone/ DHAD at the upper limit of normal or raised. It can be confirmed with a pelvic ultrasound scan; a CT is unnecessary and has a high radiation dose.

Excess androgens cause the hirsutism and masculinization and excess oestrogens inhibit FSH and stimulate LH, leading to failure of ovulation.

Causes of hirsutism
Adrenal
–   Congenital adrenal hyperplasia
–   Cushing's syndrome
–   Adrenal carcinoma

Ovarian
–   Polycystic ovary syndrome
–   Ovarian tumour
        Arrhenoblastoma
        Hilar cell tumour
        Krukenberg tumour
        Luteoma of pregnancy

Pituitary
–   Acromegaly

Thyroid
- Juvenile hypothyroidism

Drugs
- Phenytoin
- Diazoxide
- Minoxidil
- Cyclosporin A
- Corticosteroids
- Anabolic steroids
- Testosterone
- Progesterones
- Psoralens

Porphyria
Anorexia nervosa (lanugo hair)
Menopause
Idiopathic
Constitutional
- Familial
- Racial (e.g. Indian)

Answer 3

1   (e)

Peutz–Jegher's syndrome is characterized by intestinal polyposis and freckles on the lips and oral mucosa and autosomal dominant inheritance. There may be massive gastrointestinal haemorrhage and malignant transformation of the polyps. This picture shows freckles rather than telangiectasia (a and b) or spider naevi (c).

Faces and gastrointestinal disease
Jaundice/spider naevi/parotids
- Liver disease

Pigmentation of lips and oral mucosa
- Peutz–Jegher's syndrome (polyps)
- Addison's disease (anorexia, nausea, vomiting, diarrhoea)

Telangiectasia
- Hereditary haemorrhagic telangiectasia (gut bleeding)

- Scleroderma (dysphagia)

White hair and lemon tinge
- Pernicious anaemia (hypochlorhydria)

Exophthalmos, stare, lid retraction
- Thyrotoxicosis (diarrhoea)

Coarse facial features, sparse hair, etc.
- Hypothyroid facies (constipation)

Heliotrope rash
- Dermatomyositis (dysphagia, carcinoma)

Answer 4

1   (d)

Explanation
The data strongly suggest biliary obstruction, but the marked hypoalbuminaemia suggests disease of the intestinal mucosa in addition. Because of the lymphadenopathy, lymphocytosis and hint of intermittent fever, the likely diagnosis is a lymphoma of the intestine with obstructive jaundice due to nodes at the porta hepatis. The only diagnostic test is tissue biopsy, although ultrasound will confirm biliary obstruction and the appearances of a barium meal and follow-through may be characteristic.

Alpha-chain disease is an immunoproliferative disorder of plasmacytoid cells of the small intestine, producing incomplete heavy chains of IgA. They may undergo malignant transformation to a lymphoma. A lymphoma would also be suggested by a history of dermatitis herpetiformis.

Whipple's disease is a rare infectious disease tending to occur in middle-aged Europeans with polyarthritis, malabsorption, lymphadenopathy, fever, skin pigmentation and neurological disease both peripheral and central. It is characterized by macrophages containing a bacillus in the lamina propria of the intestinal mucosa. They are *Tropheryma whippelii* and disappear slowly, along with resolution of the disease, on prolonged treatment with tetracyclines. The arthritis does not respond to NSAIDs. It is a rare Membership-type disease, but there is insufficient clinical evidence to support the diagnosis here.

It is important to consider the acquired immunodeficiency syndrome, where numerous pathogens may cause malabsorption although an aetiological agent in the gut may not be identified. The multisystem manifestations of the disease make it a consideration here, but some risk factor is likely to be specified.

A guide to malabsorption is given in the answer to Exam B, Question 52.

Answer 5

1   (c)

The slide shows a man who appears well except that he requires respiratory support via a tracheostomy. This suggests muscular disease. The history is short, and he does not look as though he has myasthenia, where the indication for tracheostomy is more usually to protect the airway rather than to support ventilation. Guillain–Barré is the likely diagnosis, with characteristically high CSF protein and normal cell count. A rapidly progressive pure motor syndrome with progression to ventilatory dependence in less than 3 days is commonly associated with preceding *Campylobacter jejuni* infection.

Answer 6

1   (e)

The answer is (e) even though this will not have a physiological effect for several hours. Be aware that questions about specifics of management are increasingly common, and hence the guidelines about common conditions should be well known by candidates. Clearly combinations of (a)–(c) will be urgently needed, but the question is asking about specifics of a guideline. The internet provides a very useful way of keeping up to date with guidelines, that may well have changed after pub-

lication of this textbook (see the Cochrane Collection, www.cochrane.org).

Answer 7

1   (b)

There is extra water (white on T2) on either side of the right sacroiliac joint.

On plain films sacroiliitis develops initially in the lower and middle thirds of the joint, and follows the same progression as inflammatory arthritis elsewhere (Exam A, Question 26); periarticular osteopenia and erosion leads to apparent widening of the joint space, and the subchondral sclerosis progresses to ankylosis of the joint.

The classical teaching is that unilateral sacroiliitis is infection until proven otherwise; this is still the correct answer but with the advent of MR scanning, inflammatory sacroiliitis is now recognized at an earlier asymmetrical stage.

Answer 8

1   (b), (e)
2   (b)

Explanation

The great majority of X-linked disorders are recessive, but a few are dominant. The following criteria apply to all X-linked disorders:

* Male-to-male transmission never occurs as a father cannot pass on his X chromosome to his son.
* All daughters of an affected male will receive the abnormal gene. If the disease is X-linked recessive they will be carriers; if the disease is X-linked dominant they will all be affected.
* Unaffected males never transmit the disease to sons or daughters.
* If X-linked recessive, half the sons of female carriers will be affected; similarly if X-linked dominant, half the sons of affected females will be affected.

- Half the daughters of carrier females will be carriers; in X-linked dominant disease, half the daughters of affected females will be affected.

This family tree may superficially resemble a pattern of autosomal dominant inheritance. However, closer inspection reveals that the disease is never transmitted from father to son, characteristic of X-linked inheritance. Furthermore, all the daughters of affected males are also affected, indicating X-linked dominant inheritance.

On the basis of a pedigree alone, it is difficult to distinguish between the two modes of inheritance. Although the presence of male-to-male inheritance in a pedigree excludes X-linked inheritance, the converse is not true. X-linked dominant disorders are rare enough for you to be wary of claiming this mode of inheritance even if no cases of male-to-male inheritance are seen in a large pedigree.

Answer 9

1   (d)

Either you see it or you don't!

Answer 10

1   (a)

The bone scan shows diffuse uptake in the right hemipelvis (as well as excretion of isotope into the bladder). Neither infection nor tumour is likely to produce such a diffuse picture. Prostate cancer might, but you would expect lesions elsewhere. Metabolic bone disease would also occur in other parts of the skeleton (especially axial skeleton and proximal long bones). Such bone scans should be interpreted with plain films to help exclude these possibilities.

Answer 11

1   (b)

In this case any vitamin deficiency is likely to be dietary, and folate is a more likely culprit than vitamin B_{12}.

Explanation

Chronic lymphocytic leukaemia is the most common leukaemia in the West, and its incidence increases with age. The important features for the Membership examination are that it is usually a B-cell leukaemia, where the prognosis depends on tumour bulk, as is reflected in the staging. Where disease load is small (e.g. few nodes involved, Hb >10 g/dL, platelets >100 × 10^9/L) the prognosis is no worse than that of matched controls. The important complications are autoimmune haemolytic anaemia (5 per cent of patients have positive direct antiglobulin tests) and infections, as the patients have depressed humoral and cell-mediated immunity.

It is worth remembering the causes of macrocytosis – they are relatively few, and the abnormality is likely to occur in Membership questions.

In this case the elevated MCV is most likely due to alcohol consumption (which causes macrocytosis through its effects on lipid metabolism and hence the erythrocyte membrane) and megaloblastic anaemia due to poor diet.

Causes of macrocytosis
- Megaloblastic anaemia
- Reticulocytosis
- Alcohol
- Liver disease
- Hypothyroidism
- Myelodysplasia

Less common causes in the Membership examination
- Multiple myeloma (due to associated B_{12}/folate deficiency and haemolysis)
- Acquired sideroblastic anaemia

- Aplastic anaemia
- Drugs, e.g. azathioprine, phenytoin, methotrexate

Answer 12

1 (a), (d)

Explanation

There is no excuse for getting this question wrong and a similar case is presented in Exam C, Question 82. By now you should recognize that this question should be approached via the differential diagnosis of a microcytic anaemia. Abdominal pain in a child from the Mediterranean with microcytic anaemia is sufficient evidence to suggest chronic blood loss from hookworm infestation and thus iron-deficient anaemia; it is estimated that hookworm is responsible for the loss of 700 litres of blood per day around the world. The second likely cause in this patient is thalassaemia trait. Note there are insufficient data here to distinguish between α- and β-thalassaemia.

As discussed elsewhere, plasma ferritin, total iron-binding capacity (TIBC), and marrow iron are measures of iron stores; in iron deficiency, ferritin and marrow iron fall while TIBC rises. In thalassaemia they are normal or may indicate increased iron stores. The blood film is the most basic and simplest of investigations; although it may not be possible to distinguish iron deficiency and thalassaemia trait, pencil cells and anisocytosis are more pronounced in the former and target cells in the latter.

The thalassaemias are a popular subject because the data test your understanding of basic pathophysiology. What follows is a greatly simplified summary of the essential information. Most adult haemoglobin is HbA, consisting of two β chains and two α chains. Fetal haemoglobin, HbF, has two α and two γ chains. A small proportion of adult haemoglobin is HbA_2, with α and β chains. Thalassaemia major is where there is a deletion or mutation of both β genes; the proportion of HbF rises to compensate and there is transfusion-dependent anaemia with haemolysis. These patients often develop transfusion-induced haemochromatosis. In β-thalassaemia trait, only one β gene is absent (i.e. the patient is heterozygous) and there is mild hypochromic anaemia, as here, with slight elevations of HbA_2 and HbF.

Two α-chain genes exist, α1 and α2, giving a total of four per individual, any number of which may be absent. Single gene deletions are usually clinically silent. Two gene deletions results in α-thalassaemia trait, with the same haematological picture as its β counterpart. Haemoglobin H disease results from triple gene deletion; there is variable anaemia with splenomegaly and a typical thalassaemia blood picture. Deletion of all four genes is incompatible with life as α chains are a component of all three major haemoglobin types.

Haemoglobin electrophoresis at an alkaline pH allows the proportions of HbA, HbA_2 and HbF to be determined and hence the likely diagnosis, e.g. HbA_2 is typically elevated in β-thalassaemia trait but not α trait. However, a definitive diagnosis requires a globin chain synthesis study.

Answer 13

1 (a)

Whilst the rule for ulcers is 'longitudinal ulcers for typhoid' and 'transverse ulcers for tuberculosis', this is not hard and fast. Small bowel ulcers can also occur in Crohn's disease. However, typhoid remains the best answer, because neither tuberculosis nor Crohn's qualify as the acute febrile illness of the history. *Yersinia* would have been a good alternative.

Answer 14

1 (c)
2 (c), (e)

Explanation

This question provides a good example of basing a differential diagnosis on a combination of key abnormalities. The constellation of abnormalities to consider here are: renal failure, hypercalcaemia and elevated serum protein. Base the diagnosis on the causes of hypercalcaemia.

The only cause that will produce a raised total protein of this degree and renal failure is myeloma. The history fits this diagnosis.

Renal failure usually presents with hypocalcaemia, not hypercalcaemia; tertiary hyperparathyroidism will cause a raised calcium, but only after long-standing renal failure (the patient here has probably developed renal failure over a course of months); sarcoidosis can occasionally cause renal failure and raised gammaglobulins.

Causes of hypercalcaemia
- Primary hyperparathyroidism
- Tertiary hyperparathyroidism
- Malignancy with ectopic hormone production
- Myeloma
- Sarcoidosis
- Thyrotoxicosis
- Milk-alkali syndrome
- Vitamin D overdosage
- Artefactual (venous stasis during collection)

Answer 15

1 (e)

The apparently empty spaces around the edges of the picture could either be for air or for urine. In fact, these are normal tubules – they would be very pathological pulmonary alveolar walls. Having established that this is kidney, it should become obvious that the pathological lesion in the centre of the field is a glomerulus. So what type of glomerulonephritis is this? There are three main cell types potentially involved: (a) the connective tissue cells of the supporting matrix – mesangial cells; (b) the endothelium of the glomerular capillaries; and (c) the epithelium of the Bowman's capsule – the blind-ending sac of the nephron. If either or both of the first two is involved, it is usually possible to make out the slim edge of the glomerulus made up of the epithelial cells. Here, the surrounding epithelial cells have enlarged, multiplied and encroached on the rest of the glomerulus. Since they surround the glomerulus circumferentially, epithelial lesions tend to grow in a crescentic fashion; hence crescentic glomerulonephritis. This is the best answer. Its usual clinical manifestation is as rapidly progressive glomerulonephritis, but the question asks for a histological diagnosis.

Answer 16

1 (a)

The picture shows telangiectasia in the eye. The question gives you the other half of the answer. Ataxia telangiectasia (AT) is an autosomal recessive disorder associated with selective IgA deficiency, cerebellar ataxia and oculocutaneous telangiectasia.

Telangiectasia of the conjunctiva may be prominent from a very early age which makes it a very useful feature for distinguishing AT from other causes of ataxia. Telangiectasia occur all over the body, not just in sun-exposed sites.

Answer 17

1 (a)
2 (a), (b)

Lung function is normal. The chest x-ray shows a large pulmonary outflow tract, especially on the left; the right may be slightly enlarged (upper limit of normal 15 mm). The small aortic knuckle might lead you to suspect a cardiac cause of pulmonary hypertension.

Primary pulmonary hypertension (PPH) is a disorder of unknown aetiology in which there is pulmonary hypertension without evidence of parenchymal lung disease, pulmonary emboli or primary cardiac disease. There is usually smooth muscle hypertrophy and intimal hyperplasia of small pulmonary arteries. The clinical picture is typically of a young woman with any combination of dyspnoea, precordial pain and exertional syncope. Examination may show tachypnoea and elevated neck veins but other signs such as a loud P2 are late and difficult to elicit. Investigations exclude interstitial lung disease (lung function), cardiac disease (e.g. mitral valve disease – echocardiography), and pulmonary emboli. The latter is difficult to exclude even with pulmonary angiography, although this will usually show some defects, while it will be normal in PPH.

Answer 18

1   (d)

At times you will need to interpret information and make assumptions. A man who has had an MI 6 months ago is likely to be on aspirin at least, if not also on clopidogrel. He wishes to be given a NSAID and there is a risk of GI bleed that is increased by the concomitant use of aspirin. Should he be given a Cox II inhibitor instead?

The National Institute for Clinical Excellence (NICE) was set up to appraise new and existing technologies that include drugs. NICE does not advise on drug safety – that process is carried out before a drug receives its licence. NICE analyses trial data to examine the true cost effectiveness of proposed interventions for the NHS. Such an analysis was published for the use of Cox II inhibitors. NICE did advise that patients needing long-term NSAIDs who were at high risk of GI bleeding should receive Cox II inhibitors – high-risk patients include those over the age of 65. However, NICE also advised that the concomitant use of Cox II inhibitors and PPI has no evidence so (e) becomes the wrong answer. NICE also identified that the VIGOR trial identified an increased cardiovascular event risk with one Cox II inhibitor, so that many would not prescribe any Cox II following an MI and so (c) is discounted. Without prescribing a PPI, there is a real danger of GI morbidity with the concomitant use of long-term ibuprofen and aspirin.

Answer 19

1   (e)
2   (a), (b)

Explanation

A guide to the interpretation of cardiac catheterization data is given in the answer to Exam A, Question 19.

A primum ASD may be associated with Down's, Noonan's or Klinefelter's syndromes.

Answer 20

1   (e)

This woman has diffuse facial erythema with papules and pustules. Her skin looks tense and shiny, and (although difficult to see) she has numerous telangiectasia. This is the characteristic appearance of rosacea. Thirty per cent of patients have associated keratoconjunctivitis.

Answer 21

1   (b)

The patient has erythema nodosum and may well be pregnant. These tender lesions, characteristically occurring on the shins, are a vasculitic response to a variety of insults, the most common of which are drugs (contraceptive pill, sulphonamides, penicillin), infections (streptococcal, mycobacterial, *Yersinia*, brucellosis and fungi), a variety of systemic disorders such as inflammatory bowel disease, sarcoidosis and Behçet's disease, and pregnancy.

Answer 22

1   (a), (c)
2   (d)

Essence

A young man returned from the Far East, where he had dysentery, and continues to have non-bloody diarrhoea and malabsorption.

Differential diagnosis

Persistent non-bloody diarrhoea following a course of co-trimoxazole is suggestive of a parasite infestation of the small bowel such as giardiasis, strongyloidosis or capillariasis. Giardiasis is the most common and has no systemic effects, although that may also be true of other infestations. Since the stools are not bloody, both amoebiasis and shigellosis are very unlikely. Colitis due to *Clostridium difficile* is also possible since it may follow treatment with any antibiotic. It is not possible to differentiate an infestation from tropical sprue on the basis of the given information. Adult coeliac disease is difficult to distinguish from tropical sprue in the early stages.

Investigations

Duodenal aspirate and biopsy has supplanted jejunal investigation in many centres, although both are still acceptable answers. This investigation has the highest chance of detecting the histological appearances of sprue or coeliac disease and is more reliable than stool microscopy or culture for the detection of parasites.

Answer 23

1   (c)

Essence

A young schizophrenic becomes obtunded and febrile with muscle stiffness over a period of days. She has recently been to her psychiatrist.

Differential diagnosis

It would be reasonable to consider a primary psychiatric explanation for the lack of communication. However, in the presence of fever and muscle stiffness it is important to exclude an organic cause, particularly since fever is a potent cause of an acute confusional state. Although infection would be the most likely cause of the fever, there are no localizing clinical features. It may be difficult to detect pneumonia or urinary tract infection clinically and encephalitis, although compatible with the fever and obtunded state, would be very unusual. There is also no reason to believe she has a deep-seated infection such as endocarditis. Fevers associated with malignant and autoimmune disease are rarely this high.

We are left with the rare causes of fever, and this question relies on your recognition of a syndrome: fever, confusion and muscle stiffness over a period of days following a precipitating drug – the neuroleptic malignant syndrome (NMS).

NMS is an idiosyncratic response to phenothiazines, thioxanthenes and butyrophenones, and carries a mortality rate of up to 30 per cent. The differential diagnosis includes encephalitis, catatonia and malignant hyperpyrexia. Malignant hyperthermia and NMS must be treated promptly with the use of intravenous agents, and avoiding the oral route owing to the concurrent risk of aspiration pneumonia.

Answer 24

1   (a)

In Membership, the combination of this history and a blood film is suggestive of acute leukaemia! This is confirmed by the film which shows an excess of undifferentiated blast cells. The difficulty usually lies in discriminating between acute myeloid and acute lymphocytic leukaemias. Here the cells are morphologically lymphocytes and the age is right for ALL.

Answer 25

1   (e)

The signs of collapse depend in part on the degree of collapse. The signs to look for are increased opacification on that side, left deviation of the trachea, vessel spreading and distortion of the pulmonary artery outline, and loss of some of the left heart border due to collapse of the lingula. In combination with the leg pain, a tumour is the likely cause.

Answer 26

1 (c), (f)

These eponymous nodes are, in fact, osteophytes.

Commonly illustrated hand lesions

Joints
• Arthritis mutilans (psoriasis)
• Rheumatoid arthritis
• Osteoarthritis (Heberden's and Bouchard's nodes)
• Gout
• Jaccoud's arthropathy (SLE)

Fingers
• Rash over knuckles
• Dermatomyositis
• Granuloma annulare
• Thick hands of acromegaly
• Marfan's fingers
• Claw hand
• Vasculitis/digital gangrene
• Calcinosis
• Sclerodactyly

Other
• Small muscle wasting (motor neurone disease/T1 lesion)
• Wasting of first dorsal interosseous (Pancoast's tumour)
• Vitiligo
• Psoriatic rash
• Palmar erythema
• Palmar xanthoma

Answer 27

1 (d)

The doctrine of double effect was first discussed in the criminal trial of Dr John Bodkin Adams who was accused of prescribing morphine in toxic doses to patients living on the south coast of England in the 1950s. This permits patients to be given doses of drugs to alleviate suffering, even if these doses happen to shorten the life of the patient. What is not permitted is to give drugs to end the life of a patient – this is murder, even if the patient so requests and even if the dose is the same as the palliative care dose. The key is not in the dose itself but in the intention of the prescription.

On account of the codeine and tramadol, this patient is not 'opiate shy' and therefore a high dose of 20 mg may be started – if the patient is still in pain, it is imperative that PRN doses of morphine are given. In this case the patient is able to swallow, as you are not given information to the contrary, so MST is the correct answer.

Answer 28

1 (b)

The blood film shows the abnormal ('atypical') lymphocytes (often called mononuclear cells) of a viral infection. Given the history and these cells, it is impossible to distinguish infectious mononucleosis and cytomegalovirus (or, less likely, toxoplasmosis) infection. Note that the cells are more pleomorphic than leukaemic cells, with which they might be confused. The cytoplasmic enhancement seen when the lymphocyte membrane lies adjacent to red blood cells also helps to make the distinction.

Answer 29

1 (c)

Essence

An obese diabetic on insulin develops hypertension. She has a mildly raised creatinine and proteinuria.

Differential diagnosis

Some knowledge of recent publications and the precise management of other conditions is expected. There has been considerable interest recently in the 'syndrome' of insulin resistance, hyperinsulinaemia, and associated hypertension, coronary artery disease and obesity. In syndrome X it is proposed that insulin acts as a growth factor for vascular endothelium, promoting atherosclerosis, and may cause hypertension through a renal sodium-sparing effect. There is a characteristic fall in HDL. Without this knowledge, this is an extremely difficult question, although you should appreciate that the onset of insulin-dependent diabetes is unusual at the age of 44.

An additional complication is the fact that the term 'syndrome X' has also been used in cardiology to denote ischaemic heart disease in the presence of normal coronary arteries.

The other piece of knowledge which you are being asked to demonstrate is that careful blood pressure control slows the progress of diabetic nephropathy, particularly if ACE inhibitors are used. If one ACE inhibitor is already being used at full dose, then the addition of another antihypertensive agent is appropriate. In such a situation a simple guide to hypertensive agents is to initially choose from A/B or from C/D. If a single agent does not control the BP then add in a second from the group not selected for first line therapy. For example, if a beta-blocker was initially commenced then a second-line agent should be selected from group C/D.

A = ACE inhibitors
B = beta-blockers
C = Calcium channel blockers
D = Diuretics

In syndrome X, weight loss alone would be the best target to achieve, but you cannot ignore the hypertension. In choosing between the various options it is unlikely that a thiazide would work sufficiently and beta-blockers are to be avoided if possible in diabetics. Angiotensin II blockers are used where an ACE inhibitor is indicated but not tolerated.

Answer 30

1 (d)

Explanation

Medullary carcinoma of the thyroid may cause diarrhoea, but the mechanism is unknown. Phaeochromocytoma does so presumably due to catecholamine-induced sympathetic activity. Vasoactive intestinal peptide (VIP) production may be a feature of MEN 2 and, as such may be a cause of diarrhoea. Myenteric neuromas are rarely associated with MEN 2b and may cause altered bowel habit. Hyperparathyroidism is a feature of MEN 1 and does not usually cause diarrhoea anyway.

Answer 31

1 (b)

In the original x-ray, although not visible in the reproduction, surgical clips could be seen ligating the stump of the left main bronchus, indicating a previous left pneumonectomy. Even without this information, it is possible to deduce the correct answer. A large left pleural effusion would cause some mediastinal shift away from the effusion. There would be no movement in a complete consolidation. In this case, the shift is toward the side of the pathology, indicating a collapse or a previous pneumonectomy. The latter is the favoured diagnosis given the previous history. Radiotherapy is not curative for lung carcinoma and so he must have had surgery previously to still be alive after 15 years.

Answer 32

1 (d)

An incompetent patient does not have the ability to decide what is or is not in his best interests. However, that right does not devolve to another person. Most relatives in England and Wales do not have the right to make decisions for incompetent adults. Hence you are not bound by the daughter's opinion, although family members will often be able to help you decide what is in the patient's best interest. You could go to the Court, but, under English Common Law, as a doctor you have a duty to act in what you perceive as your patient's best interest. While you would be wise to discuss it with other doctors, you do not need to approach the Courts if you feel the interests of the patient are fairly clear. It may be appropriate to take a patient's quality of life into account in making that decision. However, if you are taking mental incompetence into account in making that decision, you must consider if his mental state is varying and ask if he has a reversible cause of his impaired quality of life. That is why it is inappropriate to withhold treatment on purely the contemporaneous assessment.

Answer 33

1 (b)

This picture shows a jejunal biopsy specimen with villous atrophy due to giardiasis. The organism is seen in the lumen. *Giardia lamblia* is a flagellated protozoan which colonizes and multiplies within the small intestine, often without detriment to the host. The trophozoite is ovoid in shape and contains a central axostyle (rod) and two sucking discs which appear as 'eyes' and give it its characteristic appearance. Symptoms such as anorexia, nausea, borborygmi, dyspepsia and diarrhoea may occur.

Malabsorption and steatorrhoea may occur and are thought to be due to damage to villi. This ranges from mild changes such as partial villous atrophy to total villous atrophy. Cysts and trophozoites may be found in the stool but a negative examination does not exclude the diagnosis. Jejunal aspirates may increase diagnostic yield. Metronidazole or tinidazole are treatments of choice. Mepacrine can also be used but has a lower cure rate. Tinidazole has the advantage of requiring only a single dose.

Answer 34

1 (d)

Explanation

Unfamiliar tests send some candidates into a panic and therefore allow differences to emerge. The usual rule is that unusual tests are usually easy to interpret. Audiograms will be unfamiliar to many candidates, so it is probable they will be fairly easy to interpret. There will be a maximum of four lines plotted on the graph, representing air conduction and bone conduction for each ear. You are less likely to be shown cases of conductive deafness (air conduction lost compared to bone conduction) than sensorineural loss (air and bone conduction both lost), since the former are more in the domain of the ENT surgeon than the physician.

The general format of an audiogram is to place increasing sound frequency on the horizontal axis. The vertical axis shows hearing level in decibels, decreasing towards the top of the axis (in fact, to be accurate, the vertical axis really represents hearing level compared to a representative control group against which the audiometer has been calibrated). In other words, the higher the plot, the better the hearing, as the patient is detecting a given frequency at a lower hearing level.

In this question, you have been told that there is no air–bone gap, i.e. bone conduction is no greater than air conduction. As this would not be the case if the question illustrated a conductive hearing loss, the defect here is sensorineural.

Deterioration in auditory acuity with age is normal. It is usually symmetrical and affects high-tone acuity more severely. Asymmetrical high-tone sensorineural deafness suggests a cerebellopontine angle lesion such as acoustic neuroma or meningioma. Low-tone fluctuating sensorineural hearing loss is suggestive of Ménière's disease.

Noise-induced sensorineural hearing loss secondary to the use of a shotgun only affects the contralateral ear, as the ipsilateral ear is protected by the butt of the gun. The gamekeeper in this case is left handed, so his right ear has been affected by the noise of the gun. By contrast, an explosion next to an individual will affect the ipsilateral ear more. Industrial noise injury is often bilateral, resulting in symmetrical 4 kHz dips.

Answer 35

1 (a)

Felty's syndrome is the association of rheumatoid arthritis and leucopenia, often with splenomegaly. A degree of anaemia, thrombocytopenia and mildly deranged liver function tests may all occur. It usually occurs in the setting of long-standing, severe, seropositive, otherwise stable rheumatoid arthritis, as here. Its pathogenesis is unclear, but complement-fixing antibodies to granulocytes may be important. It is increasingly rare, probably reflecting more widespread and early use of disease-modifying drugs. It predisposes to infection, thrombocytopenic bleeding and skin ulceration and these are indications for treatment, which is itself unsatisfactory – splenectomy is usually only of temporary benefit, and does not reduce the risk of infection, and most rheumatologists cautiously treat with disease-modifying drugs.

There are confounders in the question: methotrexate can cause myelosuppression and abnormal liver function tests, although thrombocytopenia is unusual and the patient has been on a stable dose for some time. It is feasible that reduced renal clearance in an elderly patient following ingestion of a non-steroidal anti-inflammatory drug might raise methotrexate concentration to toxic levels, and non-steroidal anti-inflammatory drugs themselves can cause abnormal liver function and marrow suppression. Viral and cyclical neutropenias are transient and unlikely to predispose to pneumonia.

Causes of neutropenia
- Part of general pancytopenia
- Bone marrow failure
- Splenomegaly (e.g. Felty's syndrome)

- Paroxysmal nocturnal haemoglobinuria (but reticulocytosis often present)
- Drug-induced
- Cyclical
- Inherited
- Viral infections
- Severe bacteria infection
- Autoimmune neutropenia
- SLE
- Hypersensitivity and anaphylaxis

Answer 36

1 (d)

The pulmonary outflow trunk is large. Primary fibrosing alveolitis is the commonest cause of this picture. Unusually, there is no volume loss.

Answer 37

1 (a), (g), (o)
2 (a)

Explanation

The point behind this question is to remind you of (i) 'ECG syndromes' and (ii) the 'non-cardiac' causes of ECG abnormalities – metabolic and drug effects. If you are having difficulty interpreting an ECG it is always worth running through a list of these. Below is a list of those you may meet in the exam and what you should be looking for.

Causes of 'non-cardiac' ECG abnormalities

Calcium effect
Hypercalcaemia
- Shortened QT interval

Hypocalcaemia
- Prolonged QT interval

Potassium effect

Hyperkalaemia
– Peaked, tall T wave
– Widened QRS complex
– Diminution of P-wave amplitude
– Diminution of R-wave amplitude

Hypokalaemia
– Flattened or inverted T wave
– Prominent U wave
– Depressed ST segment
– Prolonged PR interval

Digitalis effects
Downward sloping ST segment depression (reversed tick), particularly in leads V5 and V6
Shortened QT interval
Sinus bradycardia
1st degree AV block
2nd degree AV block
Atrial and nodal tachycardias

Hypothermia
J wave
Sinus bradycardia
Atrial fibrillation
Ventricular fibrillation
Muscle tremor (shivering) artefact
Prolonged QT interval

Answer 38

1   (e)

Answer 39

1   (b)

Explanation

The contraindications for transplantation are always changing. Time was when late middle age was a contraindication, or diabetics were discriminated against. Now most units in the UK will exclude *a priori* only those patients who are likely to reject the kidney for immunological reasons.

Several steps are involved in choosing the most appropriate recipient for a renal transplant. Potential recipients are usually tested regularly for their antibody reactivity to a panel of different HLA antigens. High reactivity against this panel makes it unlikely that a donor kidney will become available which will give a negative cross-match. Unfortunately some patients have persistent high reactivity, usually due to previous multiple blood transfusions, previous pregnancies or previous transplantation. Some units are attempting to deal with these patients by adsorbing out their antibodies in advance of transplantation. Fortunately, recombinant erythropoietin is reducing the need for blood transfusion in end-stage renal failure.

Once a donor kidney becomes available, it is usually matched to the most appropriate recipient. First, the blood group of the donor is compared with those of the potential recipients; ABO incompatibility between donor and recipient is still regarded as an absolute contraindication, although some units are reviewing this. Once a suitable recipient is chosen, a cross-match is performed to detect whether the recipient has antibodies (predominantly anti-HLA antibodies) to donor cells. A positive cross-match is correlated with the antibody-mediated hyperacute rejection and is a contraindication to transplantation.

In the UK we try to match donor and recipient at three loci if possible (HLA-A, HLA-B and HLA-DR). This approach gives a maximum of six out of six exact HLA antigen matches, as most individuals have two alleles at each loci. An additional problem is whether to transplant a kidney into a recipient who has had a previous transplant which shared HLA antigens with the new donor graft. One might expect the patient to have been sensitized to these antigens and therefore have a positive cross-match with the new donor cells. In fact, the cross-match can be negative, but the patient may still develop an antibody response once the second kidney is transplanted. Although this is a potential problem, it may be reasonable to proceed. In fact, this patient lost his first kidney within the first 24 hours (for mechanical reasons).

The final issue is of recurrence in the transplant of the disease that destroyed the native kidneys. This occurs in several conditions, but is not usually considered a contraindication to transplantation. Anti-GBM disease is a special consideration, since, unlike the others, it is self-limiting. Typically, once the acute illness has subsided and the anti-GBM antibody titre has remained low or absent for a suitable period (perhaps 6 months to 1 year), the patient can be considered for transplantation.

Answer 40

1   (a)

The photograph shows rubeosis iridis/neovascularization of the iris, a complication of diabetes mellitus. For discussion of diabetic eye disease, see answer to Exam C, Question 81.

Answer 41

1   (b)

As well as psoriasis, there is joint swelling, which involves the distal interphalangeal joints, and therefore is not rheumatoid.

Answer 42

1   (a)
2   (d)

In any arthritis where there is any suggestion of a possibility of sepsis (e.g. monoarthritis, fever, acute onset, systemic upset), the first investigation must be joint aspiration for microscopy, culture and examination for crystals. The other investigations are all poorly discriminatory (e.g. inflammatory markers will be raised in all of these conditions) or will not alter your immediate management.

The differential lies between (a) and (d); septic arthritis is rare, especially in previously fit young adults, and he would be very sick. There are suggestions of psoriatic arthritis (family history, nail pitting, rash) but fever and conjunctivitis are rare. Gonococcal arthritis may be a true gonococcal arthritis, or a reactive oligoarthritic picture, as here. However, the conjunctivitis, lower limb involvement, keratoderma blenorrhagica on the soles and lack of non-plantar skin lesions or tenosynovitis, point to Reiter's syndrome.

Seronegative arthritides
Reactive arthritis
Ankylosing spondylitis
Psoriatic arthritis
Enteropathic (IBD) arthritides
Seronegative juvenile arthritides

Features of the seronegative arthritides
- Involvement of the sacroiliac joints
- Asymmetrical oligoarthritis
- Enthesopathy (inflammation at the site of tendon insertions into bone), e.g. plantar fasciitis, Achilles tendonitis, costochondritis
- Extra-articular manifestations: uveitis, aortic regurgitation, upper zone pulmonary fibrosis, amyloidosis is rare
- HLA-B27 association

Mucocutaneous lesions in gonorrhoea and Reiter's syndrome

Gonococcal
- Papules with haemorrhagic or pustular centre
- Petechiae (as in meningococcal septicaemia)

Reiter's
- Conjunctivitis (early)
- Uveitis (late)
- Keratoderma blennorrhagica
- Balanitis circinata
- Erythematous lesions on oral mucosa

Causes of hyperlipidaemia

Disorder	Hypercholesterolaemia	Hypertriglyceridaemia
Primary hyperlipidaemias		
Familial hypercholesterolaemia	+++	
Familial combined hyperlipidaemia	+	+
Familial hypertriglyceridaemia	+	+++
Lipoprotein lipase/apoC-11 deficiency	+	+++
Remnant hyperlipoproteinaemia	++	++
Polygenic hypercholesterolaemia	+	
Secondary hyperlipidaemias		
Hypothyroidism	+	
Biliary obstruction	+	
Corticosteroids	+	
Diabetes mellitus		+
Alcohol excess		+
Chronic renal failure		+
Oral contraceptives		+
Thiazide diuretics		+
Nephrotic syndrome	+	+
Myeloma	+	+

Answer 43

1   (e)

Explanation

The examiners are tempting you to think of primary hyperlipidaemias, but the isolated hyper-triglyceridaemia with a normal cholesterol level forces you to consider secondary hyperlipidaemia (see table). The most common cause of secondary hypertriglyceridaemia is alcohol abuse. In most hypertriglyceridaemic states, HDL cholesterol levels are low. The existence of a high triglyceride and raised HDL cholesterol, as in this case, strongly suggests alcohol lipaemia, although it may also be due to oestrogens. Note that HDL cholesterol is not always raised in alcohol-induced lipaemia.

There is no conclusive laboratory test which will definitely demonstrate alcohol abuse. However, γ-glutamyltransferase is often elevated. A spot blood alcohol level may be of use, but will not indicate chronicity. As you are asked for a biochemical test, a raised MCV, which is a haema-tological parameter, would attract no marks.

Answer 44

1   (d), (e)
2   (b)

Essence

A middle-aged, female presents, initially following alcohol abuse, with duodenal ulceration and diarrhoea unresponsive to cimetidine.

Differential diagnosis

Statistically, 20–30 per cent of patients with duodenal ulceration fail to respond to 8 weeks of H_2 receptor antagonist therapy. The other major reason for its failure is non-compliance [answer 1 (g) is a non-existent test to provoke that suggestion]. However, neither of these possibilities explains the diarrhoea. In addition, it is unusual for simple duodenal ulcers to extend beyond the first part of the duodenum. The clinical syndrome of non-responsive deep extensive ulceration with diarrhoea is characteristic of the Zollinger–Ellison (ZE) syndrome, in which there is either a gastrin-secreting pancreatic adenoma or simple islet cell hyperplasia. Because of the latter possibility, ZE syndrome is a better answer than gastrinoma. Fifty to sixty per cent of adenomas causing ZE syndrome are malignant, 10 per cent are multiple and 30 per cent are part of multiple endocrine neoplasia (MEN) type 1.

Diagnosis and treatment

The first requirement is to confirm that the ulcers have not healed, so the first diagnostic test should be a repeat upper GI endoscopy. The diagnosis of ZE syndrome is confirmed by finding a raised fasting serum gastrin level with a raised basal gastric acid output of >15 mmol/h. Fasting gastrin levels should be checked only after the patient has been off H_2-blockers and proton pump inhibitors for at least a week.

An alternative test, not given here as an option, is intravenous secretin, which will raise the level of gastrin in the ZE syndrome but will cause it to fall in normal individuals. Abdominal ultrasound, selective angiography or CT scanning may localize the tumour, but this is a second-line step following confirmation of the diagnosis. Treatment with PPI or high doses of H_2-receptor antagonists to reduce the basal acid secretion may help to heal the ulcers but neither these drugs nor gastrectomy alter the course of the tumour. Excision of tumours after their localization by CT scans or angiography may be of some benefit.

Answer 45

1 (d)

The peripheral blood film shows red blood cells infested with ring trophozoites. The presence of two rings in a single cell, or heavy parasitaemia as in this case, indicates falciparum malaria.

Answer 46

1 (e)

Explanation

The low bicarbonate and high carbon dioxide should generate a respiratory acidosis. In view of the pH, there must be an error.

Such questions are unlikely, but they do provide a test of your understanding by showing that you can recognize inconsistencies. Do not be shy of exposing these, having excluded all other possibilities.

A second trick to watch for is an initial investigation which is inappropriate. For example, in this question a case could be made for giving peak expiratory flow rate as the answer, since in real life this would almost certainly be performed before blood gas analysis. However, repeating the blood gases is a better answer as it shows that you have spotted an error, the results of which need to be explained.

Answer 47

1 (b)

This is a pattern recognition question. It is obvious that there is an ulcer in a young black patient. From its position and nature of the base and edges it is unlikely to be due to leishmaniasis, venous stasis, necrobiosis, pyoderma, syphilis or

> **Causes of leg ulcers**
> - Varicose veins
> - Ischaemic
> - Necrobiosis lipoidica diabeticorum
> - Pyoderma gangrenosum
> - Haemolytic anaemia
> - Sickle cell anaemia
> - Hereditary spherocytosis
> - Syphilitic
> - Leishmaniasis
> - Vasculitis (e.g. Wegener's granulomatosis)

Wegener's granulomatosis. That leaves ischaemia due to degenerative vascular disease (unusual in this age group) or haemolytic anaemia, of which sickle cell disease would be the most common.

An alternative diagnosis would be tropical ulcer. This is a chronic necrotizing lesion which can erode down to bone. Also known as phagedaenic ulcer, it contains a mixed flora including *Borrelia vincenti* and fusiforms.

Answer 48

1 (b)

Explanation

Osteomalacia is suggested by the low calcium and phosphate and the raised alkaline phosphatase. None of the other answers is usually associated with those features. The raised MCV might be concomitantly found if the osteomalacia is due to malabsorption (rather than dietary inadequacy of calcium), the combined dietary inadequacy of calcium and vitamin B_{12} (unlikely) or may be due to the alcohol abuse.

Osteomalacia used to be common in Asian immigrants to Britain due to a combination of factors such as calcium binding by phytate in chapattis (unleavened bread), decreased intake (many Asians are vegans), decreased synthesis of endogenous vitamin D and decreased sunlight exposure. Chapatti flour is now supplemented with calcium and vitamin D. Causes of osteomalacia and rickets are discussed further in Exam B, Answer 93.

Answer 49

1 (b)

Look for loss of the medial aspect of the hemidiaphragm, volume loss in that hemithorax, depression of the inferior pulmonary artery and horizontal fissure, and the loss of the lower right heart border. From a clinical point of view, a monophobic wheeze alerts you to the possibility of a single narrowed bronchus.

Answer 50

1 (d), (e), (h)
2 (d)

These are the three main reasons why patients with rheumatoid deteriorate markedly. Sepsis can be at any site but rheumatoid joints may be infected and aspiration is required to confirm this. Neurological assessment is often difficult because of pre-existing deformities and is often dependent on history (e.g. urinary incontinence) and MR scanning. The peripheral neuropathies seen in rheumatoid may be due to entrapment (usually median at the carpal tunnel, or ulnar nerve at the elbow) or vasculitis affecting the vasa vasorum. A simple flare of disease or loss of drug effect is unlikely to precipitate a dramatic change in functional status.

AA amyloidosis would be the most complete answer of the laboratory abnormalities. As you do not now her full drug history, to attribute the proteinuria (and hence high ESR) and low WCC to a drug would be difficult. Felty's syndrome does not explain the renal disease, but amyloidosis may cause hypersplenism.

However, having been given the option of demonstrating your knowledge of adverse reactions to D-penicillamine, you are being asked to show that you know it has been implicated in a variety of 'autoimmune'-like conditions such as myasthenia and pemphigus, as well as nephropathy and suppression of bone marrow.

Answer 51

1 (a)

Scabies is an allergy to the faeces of the mite *Sarcoptes scabiei*. Papules, vesicles and excoriations are seen and the most affected areas are the finger webs, axillae, nipple areolae, buttock folds, wrist flexures and penis, where it is associated with papules in nine out of ten males.

Answer 52

1 (a)
2 (b)
3 (d)
4 (d)

Explanation

Familial Mediterranean fever (FMF) (relapsing polyserositis) is the most common of the so-called periodic or relapsing fever syndromes; others are hyperimmunoglobulinaemia D and periodic fever syndrome, TRAPS (tumour necrosis factor receptor-associated periodic syndrome), and Muckle Wells syndrome. They are all characterized by recurrent fever associated with an acute phase response, although the other clinical manifestations vary, and the molecular basis of each differs. As most have a persistent acute phase response, even between attacks, affected patients may develop AA amyloidosis. FMF has autosomal recessive inheritance and typically presents with recurrent episodes of joint and/or abdominal pain with fever, with or without family history, and most patients can be controlled with colchicine, a therapeutic trial of which is probably the best diagnostic test. It is commonest in non-Ashkenazi Jewish, Turkish, Armenian and Middle Eastern Arab populations. A large number of mutations have been identified in the so-called 'pyrin' gene on chromosome 16 in affected individuals. In this question, the underlying diagnosis is FMF, and the clinical manifestations in this patient are due to the complication of AA amyloidosis. Rectal biopsy is a useful diagnosis in systemic amyloidosis, but sensitivity is increased by biopsy of an affected organ – kidney or small bowel in this case.

This man has two causes for his hypoalbuminaemia: he has nephrotic syndrome and malabsorption, both due to amyloid deposition.

Malabsorption in Membership

Malabsorption may be defined as a disturbance in the transfer of nutrients from the intestinal lumen into the circulation. This covers a wider spectrum of disease than steatorrhoea. It is important to be able to distinguish the mechanisms of malabsorption on the basis of diagnostic tests which you should know for the examination.

General tests
These are fairly routine tests which would suggest malabsorption, e.g. macrocytic anaemia associated with low red cell folate and, later, low serum B_{12}, low serum albumin, calcium and potassium.

Three-day stool fat excretion
This should be performed whilst the patient is on a defined fat diet (100 g/day). The documentation of steatorrhoea suggests at least one of:

- intraluminal hydrolysis due to lack of lipase activity (e.g. pancreatic disease, Zollinger–Ellison syndrome)
- fat solubilization due to bile salt deficiency (e.g. biliary obstruction, interrupted enterohepatic circulation, bacterial overgrowth)
- decreased reabsorption due to resection of small bowel, damage to mucosal cells or increased transit
- impaired transport of chylomicrons. In other words, it is a rather non-specific investigation (which most labs hate doing!).

Jejunal or duodenal biopsy
This allows examination of the mucosa for characteristic lesions (Whipple's disease, amyloidosis, lymphoma) or for pathogens (e.g. *Giardia, Cryptosporidium*). Serial biopsies may be necessary to document a response to therapy as a diagnostic test (coeliac disease). In practice, anti-endomysial antibodies have replaced biopsy to diagnose coeliac disease, but it is still used to monitor therapy. The procedure also allows jejunal aspiration for the diagnosis of bacterial overgrowth.

Smooth muscle endomysial IgA antibodies
This serological test has a sensitivity and

specificity of the order of 90 per cent in coeliac disease; the antigen is tissue transglut-aminase. Coeliac disease has a serological prevalence of around 0.2 per cent in Western populations. IgA deficiency, more than 10 times as common in coeliacs than the general population, renders the test useless, and IgG antibodies can be helpful. A few more cases can be detected by measuring antibodies to gluten or reticulin.

D-Xylose excretion
Failure to absorb xylose and excrete it in the urine is an indicator of loss of absorptive surface in the gut. A normal test may suggest pancreatic rather than jejunal disease, but there is a high false-negative rate. In addition D-xylose excretion is abnormal in renal disease, hypothyroidism, ascites, after gastric surgery, with diarrhoea (which may be pro-voked by the xylose!) and in the elderly, as well as in malabsorptive states. In short, many gastroenterologists find it of limited value.

Bile acid breath test
In bacterial overgrowth, deconjugation of bile acids occurs early in the small intestine, rather than in the large bowel. Hence if a test dose of $[^{14}C]$glycocholic acid is given by mouth, the $^{14}CO_2$ level in expired air is high and peaks early when there is bacterial overgrowth. Measuring the amount of hydrogen in expired air following a dose of lactulose works on a similar principle. If transit time is fast, the breath test will give false positives.

Schilling test
Where absorption (and hence urinary excre-tion) of $[^{57}Co]$cyanocobalamin is impaired, its failure to significantly improve when given with intrinsic factor suggests malabsorption due to ileal disease. However, it also occurs in bacterial overgrowth and pancreatic disease. In the latter case this is due to the requirement for pancreatic proteolysis to release B_{12} for binding to intrinsic factor.

Tests of pancreatic exocrine function
- Endoscopic retrograde cholangiopancreatography (ERCP) allows visualization of the pancreatic duct, biopsy and aspiration of duodenal contents following stimulation with secretin and/or cholecystokinin.
- Para-aminobenzoic acid (PABA)/bentiromide test: $[^{14}C]$PABA conjugate is ingested and ^{14}C measured in the urine over a 6-hour period. This conjugate is hydrolysed by pancreatic chymotrypsin.
- Pancreolauryl (fluorescein dilaurate) test: this is a substrate for pancreatic aryl esterase, releasing the fluorescein which can then be measured in the urine.

As we have discussed, all these tests have sig-nificant problems and several in combination are often needed to make a diagnosis.

Answer 53

1   (d)

The blood film shows a complete spectrum of myeloid cells, with a few blasts. The levels of neutrophils and myelocytes exceeds those of blast cells and promyelocytes. The presence of splenomegaly helps distinguish CML from a severe leukaemoid reaction in marrow infiltration.

Answer 54

1   (a)

Essence
A South American presenting with chronic cardiac failure, abnormal oesophageal motility, constipa-tion and pulmonary embolism.

Differential diagnosis

The most prominent feature of this condition is cardiac failure. Most of the clinical features, including the hepatomegaly, are part of the syndrome of cardiac failure. The dysphagia could also have been part of that syndrome, but for the marked abnormality of the barium swallow which demonstrates that it is an independent phenomenon.

The echocardiogram demonstrates that the cause of the cardiac failure is a global myopathy, thus all but excluding an ischaemic cause. The differential includes causes of cardiac myopathy with disordered oesophageal motility.

The most likely diagnosis is Chagas' disease or chronic infection with *Trypanosoma cruzi*. No other diagnosis takes advantages of all the information, and it the only explanation which makes his geographical origins significant. The fact that he has been away from Argentina is of no relevance since Chagas' disease is the end point of a chronic infection, usually acquired in childhood.

(Pan)systemic sclerosis or scleroderma (a less appropriate term) would explain the combination of cardiac myopathy and oesophageal abnormality. However, it would be relatively rare to have such a severe systemic presentation in the absence of any cutaneous lesions. A primary cardiomyopathy is occasionally associated with skeletal muscle abnormalities, but clinical oesophageal disease is not a recognized feature. In this case the echocardiographic abnormalities are compatible only with a dilated (congestive) cardiomyopathy which does not explain the oesophageal abnormality.

AL amyloidosis is another possible explanation, but it more usually causes a constrictive cardiac picture, with dilatation being a pre-terminal feature.

Megacolon in this case is due to destruction of ganglion cells, leading to a neuropathic colon, the same process occurring in the upper GI tract. Megacolon may be congenital (Hirschsprung's disease) or acquired. Other causes of the latter include schizophrenia and depression (mechanism unclear), systemic sclerosis, amyloidosis, myxoedema, parkinsonism, cerebral atrophy and spinal cord injury.

Answer 55

1   (e)
2   (a), (c)

Strictly speaking, (a) (mononeuritis multiplex) cannot be excluded on the basis of the data, and indeed it may be axonal. However, the symmetry and chronicity of the symptoms suggests chronic peripheral neuropathy. His occupation implies that this is not alcohol related and there is nothing in the history to suggest previous medication. He is a little young to have an idiopathic neuropathy.

Causes of peripheral neuropathy
- Acute symmetrical peripheral neuropathy: commonest cause Guillain–Barré (demyelinating)
- Multiple mononeuropathy: commonest cause vasculitis (primary or secondary)
- Chronic symmetrical demyelinating peripheral neuropathy: relatively uncommon, e.g. HSMN type 1 (Charcot–Marie–Tooth type I), hereditary liability to pressure palsies, Refsum's disease, chronic inflammatory demyelinating polyneuropathy, paraproteinaemic demyelinating neuropathy
- Chronic symmetrical axonal peripheral neuropathy: commonest causes alcohol and diabetes; vasculitis; HSMN type 2; B_{12} deficiency; no cause found in 25 per cent

---

The approach to this question involves the classification of neuropathies into demyelinating and axonal. Demyelinating neuropathies cause a marked reduction in nerve conduction velocity, commonly measured at the median and/or common peroneal nerves, as well as a reduction in action potentials. In axonal neuropathies, conduction velocities are well preserved.

Important causes of axonal neuropathy include HSMN-2, diabetes, B_{12} and folate deficiency, renal failure, carcinomatous neuropathy and most drug-related neuropathies (e.g. vincristine, isoniazid).

Important demyelinating neuropathies include HSMN-1, diabetes, Guillain–Barré syndrome and the 'acquired demyelinating neuropathies'.

Answer 56

1   (e)

Explanation

A massively raised AST in excess of 25 000 IU/L is characteristic of liver necrosis secondary to carbon tetrachloride toxicity. Although carbon tetrachloride was once used as a dry cleaning agent, it is now limited to industrial use. Exposure to low concentrations may cause fatty degeneration of the liver; higher concentrations will cause centrilobular necrosis and necrosis of renal tubules.

Acute exposure is followed by nausea, vomiting, diarrhoea and abdominal pain. High concentrations can lead to confusion and coma; death may result if exposure is not terminated. Typically, liver damage is maximal 2 days after exposure and may progress to fulminant hepatic failure and encephalopathy. Acute tubular necrosis is the result of direct toxicity and may occur in the absence of hepatic dysfunction. Hepatic enzyme levels rise in advance of jaundice.

Individuals appear to differ in their sensitivity to carbon tetrachloride. Previous hepatic or renal disease or high alcohol consumption, as in this case, may increase susceptibility.

Early administration of *N*-acetylcysteine may be of benefit, but otherwise management is that of liver and renal failure, including dialysis when appropriate.

Answer 57

1   (b), (f)
2   (b), (c)

Essence

A young man presents with a moderately long history of intermittent arthritis, skin lesions, dyspnoea and chest signs, itchy eyes, polyuria and polydipsia, hepatomegaly and anaemia.

Differential diagnosis

The clinical syndrome suggests a chronic systemic illness. Systemic lupus erythematosus could explain some of the features, but other features make it a less likely diagnosis: the patient is male, and the chest x-ray appearance would be rather unusual, as would be polyuria and polydipsia. It certainly should be addressed in the investigations. The most likely clinical diagnosis is sarcoidosis. The skin lesion is typical of lupus pernio and this picture of extrathoracic sarcoidosis is common in West Indians. Tuberculosis is not excluded by the negative stain for AFB, but this clinical picture with tuberculosis would be unusual. Furthermore, one would predict that a patient with disseminated tuberculosis would be much less well and would have more florid abnormalities on his chest x-ray. Malignant disease such as lymphoma and lung carcinoma with secondaries ought to be considered, but again this constellation of extrathoracic features would be very unusual. Although the syndrome of inappropriate ADH secretion associated with lung carcinoma could explain the polyuria, this neoplasm is very rare in a man of this age.

Sarcoidosis is commonly associated with hypercalciuria and less frequently with hypercalcaemia. This can be sufficiently severe to cause nephrocalcinosis and polyuria. Hypercalcaemia alone can cause polyuria. Alternatively, involvement of the CNS with sarcoidosis may cause central diabetes insipidus.

Note that the second question asks for the initial management. Hence the need to correct any basic electrolyte abnormality. The answer would have been different if asked for a diagnostic test – gallium scans are a useful research investigation but are not routinely available outside of teaching centres. Before such an investigation it would be better to measure serum ACE (helpful in diagnosis and in monitoring response to treatment) and to obtain a biopsy. In this case it may be tempting to biopsy the skin lesion (a less invasive test), but this would still leave the nature of the lung lesion unconfirmed and it appears on the chest x-ray to be within easy reach of the bronchoscope.

Answer 58

1   (c)

Explanation

The examiners like to test your understanding of thyroid function tests by giving results in situations where they can be misleading. These include:

- T3 thyrotoxicosis, as here. Relapse of hyperthyroidism while on carbimazole may be due to T3 thyrotoxicosis.
- Subclinical thyroid disease. TSH is elevated but T4 is within the normal range. Currently accepted practice is to treat these patients with thyroxine to suppress TSH into the normal range.
- Pregnancy. Thyroxine-binding globulin levels (TBG) increase during pregnancy so total thyroxine levels rise. TSH is still a reliable indicator of thyroid status, except in the first trimester, where it is often suppressed due to the thyrotrophic action of human chorionic gonadotrophin.
- Coincident disease. In acute illness, TSH is often suppressed, probably through several mechanisms. In chronic illness, the tests are often difficult to interpret; in chronic renal failure thyroid hormone levels are often diminished but TSH maintained.

The oral contraceptive stimulates TBG production in much the same way as pregnancy. Iodine-containing drugs, such as amiodarone, can inhibit thyroid hormone secretion, leading to a rise in TSH. Corticosteroids and dopaminergic drugs cause suppression of TSH secretion.

The important overall message is that TSH is a reliable indicator of thyroid status except when the hypothalamic–pituitary axis is manipulated, as in pregnancy, dopamine agonists, etc.

The diagnosis in this question must be T3 thyrotoxicosis as either of the other possibilities

would cause a rise in T4. Relapse of thyrotoxicosis while on carbimazole is a relative indication for definitive treatment (radioiodine or thyroidectomy). It is now more usual to treat women of childbearing age with radioiodine, as there is no evidence of any risk from gonadal irradiation providing pregnancy is avoided for the following 4 months.

It is useful to remember a list of causes of hyperthyroidism: The following account for over 90 per cent of cases:

- Graves' disease
- Toxic multinodular goitre
- Toxic solitary nodule

The 'common' rare causes that may crop up are:

- TSH-driven hyperthyroidism
- Factitious hyperthyroidism
- Exogenous iodide (Jod–Basedow phenomenon), e.g. drugs, x-ray contrast
- Thyroiditis
- McCune–Albright syndrome, as one of many possible endocrinopathies.

Answer 59

1   (c)

There should not be much difficulty with this. The danger is in overdiagnosing optic atrophy, so ensure you have looked thoroughly around the field and excluded other pathology. In this case, there is none.

Answer 60

1   (c)

Essence

A 66-year-old woman presents with sinus pain, breathlessness, haemoptysis, and other chest signs, haematuria and renal failure.

Differential diagnosis

Your initial approach to this question should centre on the renal failure, as this is the major 'hard fact' contained in the question. As well as renal failure, the patient has lung disease. She has a history of dyspnoea and a small haemoptysis, signs in the chest, and an abnormal chest x-ray. These signs are not very specific and should be interpreted in the light of the known renal disease. The differential diagnosis of interest here is that of the pulmonary-renal syndromes.

What is the nature of the lung pathology? Pulmonary oedema is a frequent finding in renal failure. However, the patient does not appear to be fluid overloaded as the jugular venous pressure is not raised, she has no dependent oedema, and the heart size is normal on chest x-ray. This makes pulmonary oedema unlikely to be the sole explanation of the chest problem. She is unlikely to have pneumonia as she is afebrile, although this remains a possibility; and although *Legionella* infection would be possible, it is ruled out by the length of the history. Finally, one comes to pulmonary haemorrhage. Everything is in keeping with this explanation of her chest problem, and although it is an uncommon diagnosis in the general population, pulmonary haemorrhage is not uncommon in patients with renal failure.

The differential diagnosis is now that of renal failure and pulmonary haemorrhage. In the absence of any other major feature, the three conditions that this association should alert you to are Goodpasture's disease, vasculitis and, less commonly, SLE. (There are a few other associations but these are much rarer.) Are there any further clues in the information provided? The history of nasal involvement suggests the clinical diagnosis of Wegener's granulomatosis, one of the vasculitides commonly associated with renal failure. Taken together with previous information, it is reasonable to use this 'softer data' to establish a diagnosis of Wegener's granulomatosis.

Bacterial endocarditis does cause rapidly progressive glomerulonephritis and cardiac failure. Right-sided endocarditis may cause embolic pulmonary lesions but they would not present a diffuse radiographic picture. It is very rare for sarcoidosis to present with renal failure, and then it is usually due to interstitial nephritis, acute tubular necrosis or the complications of hypercalcaemia. Finally, Churg–Strauss syndrome does not fit as it is usually associated with asthma and it is much less commonly associated with renal involvement than other vasculitides.

Answer 61

1 (a), (c)

Explanation

You may be tempted by tuberculous meningitis (but would then have to omit diabetes) but it is a poorer answer because of the relatively low proportion of lymphocytes in the CSF. The information that there is no growth on culture is less helpful, as in the context one may reasonably assume that the cultures are negative only up to a few days.

Ambiguous results may suggest interference by doctors, and should alert you to partially treated conditions or their recovery phase. Similarly, relatively unusual conditions may produce unusual CSF pictures, such as fungal meningitis.

Always be aware of the probably clinically irrelevant information – in this case the elevated blood glucose level. However, by definition she is diabetic and therefore this needs to be included.

Answer 62

1 (b)

The coarseness of features in hypothyroidism is sometimes mistaken for acromegaly. This lady has the puffy features and dry skin typical of hypothyroidism. The degree of facial hair (which attracted the distractor, polycystic ovary syndrome) and periorbital swelling (which attracted the distractor, acute nephritis) are both within the range of normal.

Answer 63

1   (e)

This depends on having two pieces of knowledge: that the dense region in the centre of the image is pathological and that at this level it is visualizing the pons. With those two pieces of information plus the sudden onset, this is likely to be pontine haemorrhage. Central pontine myelinosis could adopt this appearance, but is excluded by the history.

Answer 64

1   (d)

Explanation

Allopurinol inhibits the enzyme xanthine oxidase which is involved in the production of uric acid from purines.

$$\text{Hypoxanthine} \xrightarrow[\text{oxidase}]{\text{Xanthine}} \text{Xanthine} \xrightarrow[\text{oxidase}]{\text{Xanthine}} \text{Uric acid}$$

Azathioprine has some therapeutic value itself, but is almost completely converted to 6-mercaptopurine. 6-Mercaptopurine is in turn metabolized to 6-thiouric acid by xanthine oxidase. For this reason, azathioprine requirements are drastically reduced in the presence of allopurinol.

In this case, it is probable that the GP unwittingly introduced allopurinol as a treatment for gout without altering the dose of azathioprine.

The bone marrow depression caused by azathioprine increased and white blood cell count dropped. The patient does not need treatment for neutropenic sepsis as although at risk, he is currently well enough to be a routine outpatient. The allopurinol needs to be stopped.

Answer 65

1   (a)

The cutaneous features of Reiter's syndrome affecting palms and soles, known as keratoderma blenorrhagica, resemble pustular psoriasis, with which it is anyway associated, both being linked to HLA-B27. Macules, papules, vesicles and pustules occur as do thickening, hyperkeratosis and crusting. This man actually had pustular psoriasis.

Answer 66

1   (b)

Back pain may be considered mechanical (worse with activity, variable intensity, no systemic features or long tract symptoms/signs), inflammatory (better with activity, sacroiliac pain usually radiates into the buttocks) and 'nasty' (tumour or infection). The elevated ESR and steady progression puts this case in the latter category. In the absence of other clues (e.g. abnormal chest x-ray, known primary) the diagnosis must be reached by analysis of the x-rays. There are several features favouring TB in this case; the long history, involvement of the thoracolumbar junction, preserved pedicles. The MR scan reproduced here shows the extension into T12 and the epidural space.

Extra-articular manifestations of the arthritides

Seropositive rheumatoid	Seronegative group (AS, PsA, reactive)	SLE	Systemic sclerosis
Scleritis	Uveitis	Retinal vasculitis	
Nodules		Cytoid bodies	
Episcleritis		Episcleritis	
Lower zone fibrosis	Upper zone fibrosis	Pleuritis/effusion	Pulmonary hypertension
Nodules		(Pulmonary hypertension)	Lower zone fibrosis
Pleuritis/effusion			
Pericarditis	Aortitis (AV block)	Pericarditis	Restrictive cardiomyopathy
		Myocarditis/valve lesions	Conduction abnormalities
–	Asymptomatic	–	Hypomotility
		Glomerulonephritis	Hypertension
Small vessel vasculitis++	–	Immune complex vasculitis	Digital ischaemia
Peripheral neuropathy	Cauda equina syndrome	Organic brain syndromes	Trigeminal neuralgia
Compressive neuropathy		Transverse myelitis	Autonomic neuropathy
Mononeuritis		(Peripheral neuropathy)	Hypertensive
Sicca/Sjögren's			
Improves in pregnancy	Men don't get pregnant	Worse in pregnancy	Pregnancy is risky
ESR/CRP++	ESR/CRP+	ESR+/CRP–	ESR/CRP–
Chronic disease/Felty's	–	Chronic disease/haemolysis	–
AA amyloid++	AA amyloid+	Amyloid–	Amyloid–

Radiological features of spinal infection versus tumour

	Pyogenic infection	Tuberculosis	Neoplastic disease
No. of vertebrae involved	1	Often 2 or more contiguous	Often 2 or more non-contiguous
Rate of progression	Rapid	Slow	Rapid
Site	Lower lumbar	Thoracolumbar	Any
Initial lesion	Disc space	Subchondral bone	Body and pedicles
Bone destruction	Limited	Extensive (collapse/wedging-gibbus)	Extensive (collapse)
Paraspinal abscess	Rare	Yes	No

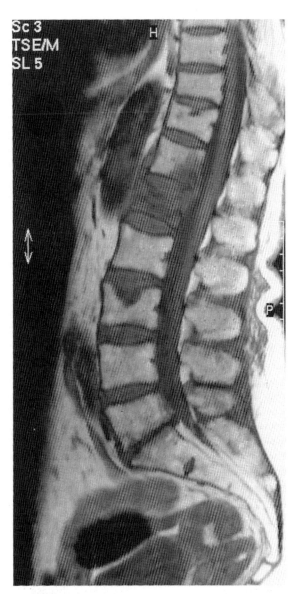

Sagittal T1 weighted MR lumbar spine demonstrating paraspinal tuberculous abscess.

Answer 67

1 (c)

Essence

A young obese woman develops raised intracranial pressure after treatment for acne.

Discussion

This woman was prescribed isotretinoin for her acne. The clues lie in the fact that the GP offered contraceptive advice (isotretinoin is teratogenic and has a long half-life) and that the acne was severe but resolved on therapy: isotretinoin is the most effective drug for acne. A dermatologist must prescribe it. One of the side effects of isotretinoin is benign intracranial hypertension (BIH). Steroids and nitrofurantoin can both cause BIH but are not used for acne, whilst erythromycin is used for acne but does not cause BIH. Tetracyclines are used for acne and cause BIH but are not as potent as isotretinoin in both treatment and side effect, making isotretinoin the preferred answer.

BIH (or pseudotumour cerebri) is a syndrome of raised intracranial pressure in the absence of a space-occupying lesion. The cause is unknown. In 98 per cent it occurs in the absence of any other pathology, usually in obese young women. In 2 per cent a number of drugs appear to be capable of inducing the condition, including vitamin A and the retinoids, tetracyclines, lithium nitrofurantoin nalidixic acid. Although corticosteroids are used in the initial treatment of BIH, their withdrawal after long-term treatment for any condition may induce BIH. The condition may also occur in deficiency of vitamin A and after dural sinus thrombosis. BIH presents with the symptoms and signs of raised intracranial pressure, which may be severe enough to cause progressive visual loss through compression of the optic nerve. Diagnosis requires exclusion of a tumour. The condition resolves rapidly with correction of any endocrine abnormality or removal of an offending drug. Otherwise treatment involves weight loss, repeated lumbar puncture, acetazolamide, frusemide and, paradoxically, corticosteroids. Lumbar–peritoneal shunting is a last resort.

Answer 68

1 (e)

The history is obviously of amaurosis fugax (differential includes migraine or acute glaucoma) and so you are expecting a lesion in the carotid territory. The internal carotid is easily distinguished from the external carotid by the lack of branching. The internal carotid also has a sigmoid angulation at the carotid siphon in its intracavernous portion.

Answer 69

1   (c)
2   (c), (g)
3   (d)

Essence

A 58-year-old man presents with a severe systemic febrile illness associated with chess signs and chest x-ray changes, diarrhoea, haematuria and proteinuria, hyponatraemia and a raised plasma aspartate aminotransferase (AST).

Differential diagnosis

This patient has a prodromal illness with systemic symptoms, meningism and a pneumonia unresponsive to several antibiotics. Atypical pneumonias should be suspected when a systemic illness has a chest x-ray much worse than the symptoms (although this is not always true) and is not responsive to conventional antibiotics. This man's relative lymphopenia, abnormal liver function tests, hyponatraemia, with protein and blood in his urine, are all supportive of an atypical pneumonia.

Legionella pneumophila causes severe systemic symptoms often with nausea, vomiting and diarrhoea and even delirium or renal failure. Neutrophilia and lymphopenia may be present. The liver function tests are usually deranged, the plasma sodium is low and there is protein and blood in the urine. Treatment is with erythromycin and rifampicin is added in severe cases.

Mycoplasma pneumonia is the most common of the 'atypical pneumonias' and accounts for a considerable proportion of pneumonias presenting to hospital. The cough is often dry and there are several extrapulmonary features. Over half the patients have GIT symptoms, 25 per cent have

skin involvement (sometimes erythema multiforme), arthralgia, myalgia and 6 per cent have CNS signs. About half of all patients have cold agglutinins and some have a haemolytic crisis. *Mycoplasma* usually causes unilateral consolidation although bilateral involvement may occur. Treatment is with erythromycin or tetracycline.

Chlamydia psittaci pneumonia (psittacosis if contracted from parrots, ornithosis if contracted from turkeys or pigeons) is a systemic illness with mild pneumonia or severe pneumonia. The chest x-ray shows bilateral patchy consolidation. Treatment is with tetracycline. Relapses are frequent and the bird source must be taken to a vet. (Pigeon fancier's lung is something entirely different. It is an extrinsic allergic alveolitis, and is not infection.)

Despite the association with a parrot, the clinical features in this case are better explained by Legionnaires' disease than by psittacosis or *Mycoplasma* infection.

Answer 70

1   (d)

The large cobblestone defects with a smooth outline in parts of the oesophagus suggest varices. Varices are often confused with candidiasis; the latter gives a diffuse, small cobblestone outline to the whole of the barium-filled oesophagus. Carcinoma shows up as an irregular narrowing in part of the oesophagus. Compare with Exam B, Question 83.

Answer 71

1   (c)

Explanation

The diagnosis of pre-eclampsia can be difficult, as other disorders, including malignant hypertension, produce similar clinical pictures. The final proof that the diagnosis of pre-eclampsia is correct comes following delivery, at which point it disappears, while other conditions persist. This alone is evidence that pre-eclampsia is a distinct condition associated with the gravid uterus, different from other causes of hypertension in pregnancy.

Pre-eclampsia is the most common cause of nephrotic syndrome during pregnancy. One of its earliest signs is an increase in plasma urate. Proteinuria is a relatively late sign, as is an increase in plasma urea and creatinine. Hypertension is also an early feature and, of course, must be present for the diagnosis to be made. Although 85 per cent of pre-eclamptics have oedema, this is not necessary for a positive diagnosis. Headaches, abdominal pain and vomiting suggest that progression to eclampsia is imminent.

The major differential in this case is SLE, which can be difficult to distinguish from pre-eclampsia. A positive VDRL would favour the diagnosis of SLE, as antiphospholipid antibodies (lupus anticoagulant), which give a false-positive VDRL, are commonly found in SLE. Afro-Caribbeans also have a higher risk of developing SLE. However, yaws may be an alternative cause of the positive VDRL. Pre-eclampsia is not associated with the skin, joint and pleuritic symptoms of SLE. High titres of antinuclear factor and anti-double-stranded DNA antibody, and low serum complement levels further support the diagnosis of SLE. Although renal biopsy would distinguish between the two conditions, it is not indicated as delivery of the child will treat the putative pre-eclampsia.

Other forms of glomerulonephritis occasionally present for the first time during pregnancy and can be difficult to distinguish from pre-eclampsia. Once again, delivery of the child will aid diagnosis and, of course, treatment.

Causes of a positive VDRL are discussed in the answer to Exam A, Question 81.

Answer 72

1 (d)

Essence

An elderly man develops mild hypokalaemia and confusion after starting antihypertensive medication. He has high serum lithium levels.

Discussion

Thiazides can cause confusion in the elderly, which may be related to the hyponatraemia and hypokalaemia that can develop. They inhibit the renal conservation of sodium and lithium may be retained in its place resulting in lithium toxicity. It therefore is compatible with all the features of this case. Note that calcium channel blockers can also increase lithium levels – but these would not explain the electrolyte abnormalities in this case.

Thiazide diuretics

Uses

Effects	Implications
Hypokalaemia	Arrhythmias; digoxin toxicity Routine use of potassium supplements is not indicated
Hypomagnesaemia Hyponatraemia Hyperuricaemia Hyperlipidaemia Impaired glucose tolerance (by inhibiting insulin release) Impotence (mechanism unknown)	None – usually minor

- First-line drug for uncomplicated hypertension
- Treatment of hypercalcuria (causes renal calcium resorption)

Note

Ineffective in renal failure as their action depends on excretion by the renal tubule.

Answer 73

1 (a)

The most striking feature is this man's ascites. Are there any clues as to the cause? His face shows marked pigmentation. The pigmentation is not jaundice, otherwise any cause of cirrhosis could explain the picture.

> **Hint**
> If you cannot see anything unusual in a picture, go back and ask yourself about generalized disorders of pigmentation. They are easy to miss.

Answer 74

1 (d)
2 (b), (e)

Essence

A young man presents with severe abdominal pain, a predominantly motor peripheral neuropathy affecting the proximal upper limbs, tachycardia, hypertension, papilloedema, hyponatraemia and proteinuria.

Differential diagnosis

The coexistence of abdominal pain and peripheral neuropathy has a short differential. Diabetics may uncommonly develop a motor peripheral neuropathy and autonomic neuropathy may be associated with abdominal pain; the same may be said of lead poisoning. Arsenic poisoning may also be associated with neuropathy and GI symptoms. Alcohol may cause a peripheral neuropathy and is associated with pancreatitis. However, there are no other features to support these diagnoses and they would leave other features unexplained. Guillain–Barré syndrome may be associated with peripheral motor neuropathy, hypertension and papilloedema, but the severity and dominance of

the abdominal pain make it unlikely. Peripheral neuropathy may complicate GI malignancy, but the patient is very young and it requires a metastatic complication to explain the papilloedema (the peripheral neuropathy of malignancy is usually a non-metastatic complication). The best explanation of these clinical features is acute intermittent porphyria (AIP). AIP usually presents with abdominal crises and a peripheral neuropathy with hypertension and tachycardia. Papilloedema may also occur and hyponatraemia may be a feature of the syndrome of inappropriate ADH secretion. Similarly, about 10 per cent develop proteinuria.

> **Causes of the syndrome of inappropriate ADH secretion**
> Malignancy
> – Small cell carcinoma of the lung
> – Pancreas
> – Prostate
> – Leukaemia
> – Lymphoma
>
> CNS disorders
> – Meningoencephalitis
> – Abscess
> – Stroke
> – Head injury
> – Vasculitis
> – CNS sarcoid
>
> Metabolic
> – Porphyria
>
> Chest diseases
> – Tuberculosis
> – Pneumonia
> – Abscess
> – Aspergilloma
> – Malignancy
>
> Drugs
> – Opiates
> – Chlorpropamide
> – Cytotoxics
> – Chlorpromazine

The diagnosis of the syndrome of inappropriate ADH secretion is made by finding a concentrated urine (sodium >20 mmol/L) in the presence of hyponatraemia (sodium <125 mmol/L) or low plasma osmolality (<260 mmol/kg) and the absence of hypovolaemia.

Answer 75

1   (a)

Leprosy is the most common cause of peripheral neuropathy on a worldwide basis. It is a chronic granulomatous disease caused by *Mycobacterium leprae* and causes a spectrum of illnesses in humans. At one end of the spectrum is the high-resistance form, tuberculoid leprosy, which is characterized by a few hypopigmented lesions with thickened superficial nerves. The centres of these lesions are often anaesthetic. Lepromatous leprosy is the low-resistance form with extensive, bilaterally symmetrical, diffuse skin involvement. Loss of eyebrows (madarosis), leonine facies, thickened skin, nasal collapse and saddle nose, and keratitis and iridocyclitis make good examination material.

Answer 76

1   (c), (h)

Choroidal metastases are the most common intraocular malignancy. They are often indistinct with minimal retinal elevation, and have a mottled appearance due to overlying pigment epithelium. While often painful, vision is usually unaffected. They are often bilateral and there is usually a history of malignant disease. Treatment of choice is local radiotherapy. Blurring of disc margins with engorged veins and haemorrhage at and around the disc are the characteristic findings of papilloedema.

Answer 77

1   (c)

While any of the answers could explain the new fit, head trauma, pregnancy and space-occupying lesion are relatively uncommon. Had the fit been compatible with the normal inter-fit frequency of the patient, then it would have been most likely that it was not due to any precipitant. However, after such a period of stability, that seems unlikely and the commonest such cause is introduction of an additional medication.

Answer 78

1   (d)

The clue is in the history; few pulmonary lesions produce such dramatic radiological changes (hilar lymphadenopathy, diffuse shadowing) with relatively little respiratory compromise. In addition, relatively few diseases cause problems with hands and lungs and not much else. The x-rays of the hands are typical, with well defined lucencies and soft tissue swelling (dactylitis). Other changes that may be seen in the hands include coarse trabeculation, periarticular calcification, resorption of distal phalanges. As with most lists, other than normal, there are essentially three patterns of pulmonary involvement:

- Bilateral hilar lymphadenopathy (up to 50 per cent; associated with erythema nodosum)
- Pulmonary infiltrate, often with small nodules, as here (or hilar lymphadenopathy + pulmonary infiltrate). The nodules can be of almost any size
- Pulmonary infiltrate + fibrosis (as here).

This chest x-ray shows diffuse infiltrates, particularly in upper zones, with small nodules and mid/upper zone fibrosis associated with upper zone volume loss, the typical sarcoid distribution.

Answer 79

1 (d)
2 (c), (e)

Essence

A young diabetic develops cardiac failure associated with non-specific ECG changes following a 'flu-like' illness.

Differential diagnosis

The classical differential diagnosis of cardiac versus respiratory causes for dyspnoea is relatively easy in this case. The clinical features are suggestive of myocardial disease. This diagnosis hinges on the differential of subacute cardiac failure in such a patient. Her diabetes makes her susceptible to myocardial infarction, and although infarcts in diabetics are often painless (i.e. silent), she is young even for a diabetic to have major vessel disease of sufficient severity to cause an infarction. In addition, the ECG changes are non-specific, against ischaemic disease and in favour of myocarditis. Also in favour of myocarditis is the relationship to a 'flu-like' illness. Having said that, the possibility of an acute presentation of cardiomyopathy remains, as this often presents during an acute viral illness. However, it is said that exertion during a 'flu-like' illness (she was on a 'strenuous' walking holiday) makes the development of myocarditis more likely. The troponin measurement may be raised in a myocarditis and is therefore not useful in excluding ischaemia in this case.

The urea is raised as a consequence of cardiac failure and not intrinsic renal damage. Arterial blood gas will just show hypoxia and will not lead to any change in management as the patient will be on oxygen regardless. D-dimers are positive in the case of pulmonary embolism, but also positive in a variety of inflammatory conditions and will not provide differentiating information. A negative D-dimer would not negate the importance of excluding PE in this patient.

The key investigation is an echocardiogram that will usually show little, as most patients with viral myocarditis do not have demonstrable wall motion or dilated chamber abnormalities on echocardiography. Those with abnormalities need to be monitored clinically and radiologically for the rare complication of fulminant cardiac failure. Arrhythmia may occur independently of echo abnormalities and needs to be considered.

Multiple small PE could give this picture and this would be the principal differential diagnosis in this case. Given that the echocardiogram is likely to be normal, the next investigation to do would be a VQ scan.

Answer 80

1 (d)

See fuller discussion of hyperlipidaemia in Exam B, Question 43. The Fredrickson/WHO classification was based on the electrophoretic patterns of lipoprotein levels that occur in patients with hyperlipidaemia. The limitation of this system is that genetic understanding has revealed a large and diverse group of diseases. Nevertheless it does provide a basis for understanding. (See table on the next page.)

Answer 81

1 (a)

On the chest x-ray the normal left-sided aortic knuckle is absent; it is not clearly visible on the right but the trachea is slightly deviated to the left, which is characteristic. The right-sided descending aorta is clearly visible on the CT scan. This may be associated with a variety of congenital heart lesions.

Answer 82

1 (c)

Explanation

With the exception of the sodium and potassium (which remain essentially unchanged), all the

Type	Elevated lipoprotein	Elevated lipid	Typical lesion
I	Chylomicrons	Triglycerides	Eruptive Xanthoma
IIa	LDL	Cholesterol	Tendinous Xanthoma, Tuberous Xanthoma, Xanthelasma
IIb	LDL and VLDL	Cholesterol and triglycerides	Tendinous Xanthoma, Tuberous Xanthoma, Xanthelasma
III	IDL+chylomicron remnants	Cholesterol and triglycerides	Any Xanthoma, Palmar Xanthoma almost pathognomonic
IV	VLDL	Triglycerides	Eruptive Xanthoma
V	Chylomicrons and VLDL	Cholesterol and triglycerides	Eruptive Xanthoma

Type of Xanthoma	Description	Typically seen in
Xanthelasma palpebrarum	Flat, polygonal yellow patches around eyes	1° Any primary hyperlipoproteinaemia 2° Some secondary eg cholestasis
Tuberous xanthoma	Red-yellow nodules at pressure points	1° Type II & III 2° Nephrotic syn. & hypothyroidism
Tendinous xanthoma	Subcutaneous nodules on figures and Achilles tendon	1° Type II & III 2° Any esp. cholestasis
Eruptive xanthoma	Crops of yellow papules on buttocks and extensor surfaces	1° Types I, IV & V 2° Any esp. diabetes
Plane xanthoma	Macular lesions on palmar crease Can be generalised	Palmar pathognomonic for type III Generalised = type I, IV or MGUS

values have increased. It is unlikely that random biological or laboratory variation would push all results in the same direction. In fact there is mild haemoconcentration. This is the result of the increased venous pressure that occurs on standing up. Cells, proteins and protein-bound substances are retained while solutes leach out with the fluid.

An alternative cause of venous hypertension might be local venous stasis. However, if this occurs for any period of time hypoxia results in loss of potassium from within the cells.

An alternative to haemoconcentration of the second sample might be haemodilution of the first. However, if there is a drip running into the arm, one can expect a rise in one or more of the glucose, sodium or albumin.

Answers (b) or (c) are correct. The more likely is (c) given that the patient is in a nursing home; she is more likely to have a cuffed then a standing sample.

Answer 83

1   (b)

The x-ray shows fine ulceration extending throughout the oesophagus. Oesophageal candidiasis is the likely diagnosis, but a similar appearance could occur following cytomegalovirus or herpes simplex infection.

Oesophageal candidiasis may occur following immunosuppression of any kind (AIDS, transplant recipients, chemotherapy, etc.).

Diagnosis to look out for in barium swallows
- Oesophageal/pharyngeal pouch
- Oesophageal diverticulum
- Achalasia
- Carcinoma
- Benign stricture
- Oesophageal web
- Varices
- Oesophageal candidiasis/oesophagitis
- Hiatus hernia
- Extrinsic pressure (nodes/aneurysms/left atrium)
- May be normal with other pathology, e.g. bamboo spine, cervical rib, soft tissue calcification

---

Answer 84

1 (a)

Essence

A young man with a 3-year history of increasing sensorineural deafness and tinnitus has lost his ipsilateral corneal reflex.

Differential diagnosis

The coexistence of the lost corneal reflex with sensorineural deafness and tinnitus means either there is a single lesion in the cerebellopontine angle or there are multiple lesions. No single central lesion will cause these two features alone and it is highly unlikely that two lesions in the brainstem would cause these features alone with loss of only the corneal reflex. Do not succumb to the temptation to discount the corneal reflex just because you may find it a difficult sign of which to be sure.

By far the most common lesion in the cerebellopontine angle is an acoustic neuroma.

Although it usually arises from the vestibular division of the eighth nerve, deafness and tinnitus are the earliest clinical features. Similarly, the most vulnerable of the other cranial nerves in the region are those fibres of the fifth carrying corneal sensation. Later on, a more extensive area of hemianaesthesia, hemifacial spasm, attacks of vertigo, ataxia, and spastic paraparesis may occur. Indeed, limb signs usually come to overshadow relatively trivial cranial nerve features.

The differential diagnosis is with other lesions in the cerebellopontine angle. Lesions arising within the pons which could produce these clinical features, such as multiple sclerosis, pontine glioma (usually in young boys) and astrocytoma, are likely to present with more complex neurological signs. Extrinsic lesions, such as meningioma, haemangioblastoma, cholesteatoma, basilar artery aneurysm, neuroma of other cranial nerves, medulloblastoma, nasopharyngeal carcinoma, metastatic carcinoma and lymphoma, are more likely to pick off isolated cranial nerves. However, most of these are likely to present first with other clinical features, are made more or less likely by the age of the patient, and the history is too long for any malignant process.

Weber versus Rinne's

Air conduction should be better than bone conduction; therefore, in Rinne's test, a tuning fork should be heard better if held in front of the external auditory meatus than if the base is held against the mastoid process; if not, the test is negative and implies a problem with air conduction. In Weber's test a tuning fork with its base held against the forehead will be heard better on the side where air conduction is impaired, but will not be heard if there is sensorineural deafness. In the presence of incomplete deafness, if these tests are abnormal they suggest a problem with air conduction; if normal they point to the inner ear or eighth nerve.

Answer 85

1 (c)

In an immunocompromised patient, the cause is most likely to be infective. Infective causes of papulovesicular eruptions are chickenpox, herpes simplex, smallpox, orf, and hand, foot and mouth disease. The occurrence of crops of lesions of varying ages is typical of chickenpox. Chickenpox and shingles, in their various clinical forms, are common questions in the Membership examination. Remember to consider the systemic complications of chickenpox. For example, although relatively uncommon, acute chickenpox pneumonia is one differential diagnosis for a 'snowstorm' appearance on a chest x-ray.

Answer 86

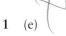

1 (e)

Explanation

Another illustration of 'non-cardiac' causes of electrocardiographic abnormalities, discussed in the answer to Exam B, Question 37. The main ECG manifestations of low serum potassium are flattening or inversion of the T waves, depression of the ST segment, prolongation of the PR interval and prominent U waves. The relative loss of the T wave, and the loss of the P wave in the U wave as the PR interval is prolonged, may result in a U wave being mistaken for a T wave. Other non-specific manifestations of hypokalaemia include an increased frequency of ventricular extrasystoles and enhanced sensitivity to digoxin.

Answer 87

1 (b)

Explanation

The key points in this case are: a raised MCV, which is often seen in acquired (but not hereditary) sideroblastic anaemia; a raised serum iron and ferritin; and a mixed normochromic/hypochromic blood film, characteristic of sideroblastic anaemia.

The hereditary form usually occurs in males. Splenomegaly is unusual in the acquired form, but can occur. Platelet levels are reduced in 30 per cent of patients with acquired disease, but may occasionally be raised. Bone marrow examination

will reveal ring sideroblasts to confirm the diagnosis. The question may have been interpreted as being the 'likely diagnosis of the acquired sideroblastic anaemia'. If so, myeloproliferative disorder is the most likely, which would also be confirmed by a bone marrow biopsy.

> **Causes of acquired sideroblastic anaemia**
> - Primary
> - Myeloproliferative disease
> - Drugs (e.g. antituberculous drugs)
> - Lead
> - Alcohol

Answer 88

1 (a), (b)

The malaise is due to hypoaldosteronism. These areas of calcification must be adrenal – they are suprarenal and the asymmetry in shape is characteristic. Calcification may be seen (on plain films as well) in Addison's, chronic infections, adrenal cystic disease (after previous haemorrhage), or in primary adrenal carcinoma, although bilateral disease would be unusual in this case.

Answer 89

1 (d)

The absence of a structural lesion makes one think of a metabolic abnormality. However, other symptoms are likely to be present if any answer other than gastroparesis due to autonomic neuropathy were correct. The intractable nature also makes hypoglycaemia, ketoacidosis and hyperosmolarity less likely since they would have been diagnosed before the vomiting could be described as intractable. One would hope that this would also be true of renal failure, although it may present subacutely and not be as rapidly life-threatening. However, it is highly likely that some other clue would have become obvious.

Answer 90

1 (a)

Essence

A young man with recurrent non-bloody diarrhoea and bronchitis has splenomegaly, anaemia,
lymphopenia, thrombocytopenia, hypoalbuminaemia, hypogammaglobulinaemia, gastritis,
jejunal villous atrophy and mild colitis.

Differential diagnosis

You will probably choose the jejunal problem first.
Does the patient have primary coeliac disease? Malabsorption might explain the hypoalbuminaemia
and anaemia, but to explain the low immunoglobulin levels you would have to postulate either a
protein-losing enteropathy, which is rare in coeliac
disease, or malignant transformation, for which he
is young. (Continue to look for a unifying diagnosis; it is better than a disease plus a complication.)
Other causes of jejunal villous atrophy include
infectious enteritis, lymphoma, Whipple's disease,
chronic ulcerative enteritis, kwashiorkor, tropical
sprue, food allergy and primary hypogammaglobulinaemia. The splenomegaly would make lymphoma high on your list, but you might have
expected something more from the biopsy.
Common variable hypogammaglobulinaemia is
compatible with all the features of this case: presentation as a young adult (unlike other hypogam-
maglobulinaemias), recurrent chest infections, a
coeliac-like picture and features suggestive of
inflammatory bowel disease, gastritis, splenomegaly, anaemia, lymphopenia, thrombocytopenia,
hypoalbuminaemia, and hypogammaglobulinaemia. Intestinal lymphangiectasia would cause
hypogammaglobulinaemia, hypoalbuminaemia
and lymphopenia, but is likely to have different
jejunal histology. It may complicate lymphomas
(which could explain his splenomegaly and
anaemia) or inflammatory bowel disease (which
would explain his colitis), but this would be a more
complex answer. Lymphoma alone may be associated with hypogammaglobulinaemia, but the colitis
and long history are strongly against it.

Classification of immunodeficiency*
UNLF:Primary
– Antibody deficiency
    X-linked agammaglobulinaemia
    (Bruton)
    Non-familial hypogammaglobulinaemia
    Selective class/subclass deficiencies
    Thymoma with hypogamma-
    globulinaemia
    Transient hypogammaglobulinaemia
    (infancy)
    Transcobalamin II deficiency

– T cells
    Thymic aplasia
    Purine nucleoside phosphorylase
    deficiency

– Mixed T- and B-cell defects
    Severe
        Severe combined immunodeficiency
        (SCID)
        (a) unknown aetiology
        (b) adenosine deaminase deficiency
        Reticular dysgenesis

        Biotin-dependent carboxylase
        deficiencies

    Moderate
        Short limbed dwarfism and
        immunodeficiency
        Orotic aciduria
        Bloom's syndrome

    Mild
        Ataxia telangiectasia
        Wiskott–Aldrich syndrome
        X-linked lymphoproliferative
        syndrome
        Secondary

– Antibody
    CLL
    Myeloma
    Drugs (e.g. methotrexate, phenytoin,
    penicillamine, gold)
    Nephrotic syndrome
    Protein-losing enteropathy
    Dystrophia myotonica

- T cell
  AIDS
  Hodgkin's disease and other lymphomas
  Malnutrition
  Zinc deficiency
  Drugs (e.g. steroids, cyclophosphamide, cyclosporin)

*After Webster, ADB (1987), in Weatherall DJ, Ledingham JGG, Warrell DA (eds), *Oxford Textbook of Medicine*, second edition. Oxford: OUP.

Answer 91

1   (e)

There is peribronchial thickening on the plain chest film; the CT shows this clearly with cystic spaces and a coarse honeycomb pattern. Causes include childhood measles/pertussis, bronchial obstruction (mucus, tumour), chronic aspiration and hypogammaglobulinaemia (Kartagener's would show dextrocardia).

Answer 92

1   (a)

The most striking feature is the muscle wasting. However, as in clinical practice, psoriasis may be an incidental finding in the examination, both in this section and the clinical examination, so do not be tempted to the more dramatic diseases to explain why the patient is bed-bound.

The classical descriptions of psoriatic plaques are:

- non-itchy (according to the text books, but often pruritic in practice)
- well circumscribed
- slightly raised
- silvery scales on a red background.
- extensor surfaces, sacrum, scalp and genitalia affected.

Other features include:

- nail changes
- arthropathy.

The differential diagnosis for muscle wasting is wide, the most important causes in Membership being nerve disease such as motor neurone disease (fasciculation, upper motor neurone signs and bulbar involvement) and peripheral neuropathy – a particular favourite being diabetic amyotrophy, which is essentially a mononeuropathy of the femoral nerve giving wasting of the quadriceps. In everyday practice, the most common cause is probably disuse in arthritides, trauma and prolonged illness.

Answer 93

1   (c)
2   (c)

Explanation

Rickets (osteomalacia in adults) is a disease of inadequate bone mineralization. This is usually due to vitamin D deficiency or abnormalities of its metabolism, but it also occurs as a result of increased renal clearance of phosphate and hence hypophosphataemia.

Causes of rickets and osteomalacia
Vitamin D disorders
- Dietary deficiency
- Inadequate absorption
- Disorders of metabolism
- Hereditary (vitamin D-dependent rickets)
- Anticonvulsants
- Renal failure

Renal loss of phosphate
- Chronic acidosis (e.g. renal tubular acidosis, acetazolamide)
- Hereditary renal phosphate leak
- Vitamin D-resistant rickets
- Neurofibromatosis

Generalized tubular disorders (Fanconi's syndrome, e.g. Wilson's disease, myeloma)
- Primary mineralization defects (rare)
- Hereditary hypophosphatasia
- Etidronate treatment

If the patient has one of the vitamin D disorders you are likely to be given a clue to abnormal vitamin D metabolism, e.g. the patient is vegan or on anticonvulsants. In addition, it is often possible to distinguish vitamin D disorders from hypophosphataemic states biochemically: serum calcium is normally depressed in the vitamin D group, and normal in the phosphate-losing group. However, this is not invariably true. Hypophosphataemia occurs in both groups: in the vitamin D group, secondary hyperparathyroidism enhances renal phosphate loss.

Vitamin D-resistant rickets is an X-linked hereditary disorder of renal phosphate handling with no other renal abnormality except an increase in urinary glycine. There is an associated inappropriately low level of 1,25-dihydroxyvitamin D [1,25(OH)$_2$-vitamin D], and patients respond to combined phosphorus and vitamin D supplementation. Calcification or ossification of tendon insertions, ligaments and joint capsules is a unique feature of this disorder.

Vitamin D-dependent rickets is another rare form useful for the examination as it tests your understanding of vitamin D metabolism.

In type 1, there is a low level of 1,25(OH)$_2$-vitamin D due to a defect in renal hydroxylation, so that the biochemistry is difficult to distinguish from dietary rickets unless the 25-hydroxyvitamin D level is known. This is the metabolite measured in most 'vitamin D' assays. The disease has an autosomal recessive inheritance.

In type 2 vitamin D-dependent rickets, there is resistance to the effects of 1,25(OH)$_2$-vitamin D, the levels of which are therefore elevated. At a molecular level, this is a spectrum of disorders with several different mechanisms of resistance. Alopecia may be associated with the bony abnormalities. High doses of vitamin D are required for treatment.

Answer 94

1   (a)

Eosinophilia usually means parasites, drugs or Churg–Strauss vasculitis. Subcutaneous nodules are seen on the chest wall; while the other parasitic infections listed in the differential may have cutaneous and CNS manifestations, nodules and fits are only common in cysticercosis. Vasculitis may of course present with palpable purpura, but these lesions are not purpuric. Paragonimiasis can also sometimes present with subcutaneous (and indeed brain) cysts, but have you heard of it?!

Answer 95

1   (d)

Explanation
The logic underlying this answer is as follows:

- The probability of the patient being a heterozygous carrier is 2/3.
- The probability that her fiancé has the abnormal gene is 1/25.
- If both carry the gene, the probability of having a homozygous child is 1/4.

The overall chance of the patient having an affected child is thus: $2/3 \times 1/25 \times 1/4 = 1/150$.

The difficult part of the question is working out the patient's chance of being a carrier. Cystic fibrosis has a recessive pattern of inheritance, thus the patient's parents must both be carriers. Hence, each of their children has a 1 in 4 chance of being homozygous and developing the disease, a 1 in 2 chance of being a heterozygous carrier, and a 1 in 4 chance of having two normal genes. However, because of her age, our patient knows she cannot by homozygous and that chance is removed. The probability that she is heterozygous then becomes 2 in 3.

This can be illustrated by a simple analogy. If a bag contains one black ball (representing the homozygous state), two red balls (the heterozygous state), and one white ball (normal), the chance of picking a red ball is 1 in 2. If the black ball is then removed, corresponding to our patient knowing she cannot be homozygous, the chance of picking a red ball becomes 2 in 3.

Note that you are given no information about the health of the fiancé's family, but it is reasonable to assume there is no history of cystic fibrosis and that he has a 1 in 25 chance of carrying the gene.

Answer 96

1   (a)

These lesions show the classical well-defined margins and can occur anywhere in the body.

Answer 97

1   (e)

Explanation

Inherited in an autosomal dominant mode, Gilbert's syndrome (disease) is a common congenital hyperbilirubinaemia found in 2–5 per cent of the population. Fasting, stress, intercurrent illness and intravenous nicotinic acid produce a rise in plasma bilirubin and icterus may be noticeable. The prognosis of this condition without treatment is excellent.

Answer 98

1   (a)

The clue is in the question; you would not be told he was of normal size unless you expected him not to be. The differential diagnosis of the radiological appearances (upper zone fibrosis, bronchial wall thickening) includes chronic extrinsic allergic alveolitis and aspergillosis. Other features of cystic fibrosis are large volume lungs, fluid levels, honeycomb lungs and pneumothoraces.

Answer 99

1   (b)

Explanation

This patient has the characteristic laboratory findings of paroxysmal nocturnal haemoglobinuria (PNH); neutropenia, anaemia, thrombocytopenia and reticulocytosis. The diagnosis can be based upon the differential diagnosis of neutropenia, discussed in the answer to Exam B, Question 35. PNH is an acquired clonal disease, thought to arise from a somatic mutation affecting the cell membrane. It affects leucocytes, platelets and red cells. The abnormality of the red cell membrane renders it sensitive to lysis by complement, resulting in a chronic intravascular haemolysis.

PNH typically presents between the ages of 20 and 40 in both males and females. Patients often present with gradual onset of exertional dyspnoea and malaise, and occasionally slight jaundice. Characteristically, this is accompanied by the intermittent passage of dark urine due to haemoglobinuria. This often occurs mostly at night resulting in discoloration of the urine passed first thing in the morning. It is possible, however, for the haemoglobinuria to go unnoticed during the course of the disease.

The degree of the haematological abnormalities may vary. Anaemia may be severe enough to warrant transfusion. Reticulocyte counts vary from less than 1 per cent to 40 per cent, and neutrophil and platelet counts can also vary widely. The blood film appearance may be unremarkable, and the MCV may be high, reflecting the reticulocytosis. The plasma contains free haemoglobin. Haptoglobins are typically absent and Hb electrophoresis normal.

The classic diagnostic laboratory test is the Ham test which involves suspending red cells in fresh normal ABO-compatible serum acidified to pH 6.5. The acidification activates the alternative complement pathway. It has, however, been replaced by flow cytometry.

Answer 100

1 (a)

This lesion has numerous small papules, typically on the trunk and arms with fine scaling. They may be brown, pink or depigmented and are especially obvious after tanning. Pityriasis rosea appears in rows roughly parallel to the ribs and you are likely to be shown a typical herald patch with it.

▌Examination C▌

Questions

Question 1

A 24-year-old man with progressive low back pain and weakness finally sees his doctor on account of an episode of left loin pain. Investigations show haematuria and a urinary pH of 7.
Other investigations show:

Plasma sodium	135 mmol/L
Plasma potassium	2.8 mmol/L
Plasma urea	5.7 mmol/L
Plasma creatinine	107 µmol/L
Plasma chloride	115 mmol/L
Plasma bicarbonate	16 mmol/L

1   What is the diagnosis?
   (a) Type I (distal) renal tubular acidosis
   (b) Type II (proximal) renal tubular acidosis
   (c) Type IV renal tubular acidosis
   (d) Bartter's syndrome
   (e) Gittleman's syndrome

2   Suggest two abnormalities which might be seen on a plain radiology:
   (a) Small renal outlines
   (b) Horseshoe kidney
   (c) Renal calculi
   (d) Sloughed renal medullary papillae
   (e) Brown tumours
   (f) Greenstick fractures
   (g) Looser's zones
   (h) Subchondral erosions
   (i) Osteitis fibrosa et cystica
   (j) Erosion of subendostial bone on ulnar aspect of hand bones

Question 2

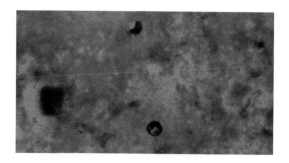

A Ziehl–Neelsen stain of a stool sample from a patient with chronic diarrhoea.

1   What is the diagnosis?
   (a) *Isospora*
   (b) *Mycobacterium avium-intracellulare*
   (c) *Mycobacterium tuberculosis*
   (d) *Cryptosporidium*
   (e) *Giardia*

Question 3

A 72-year-old man presents with a history of pain in his right leg. Investigations show:

Plasma sodium	141 mmol/L
Plasma potassium	4.2 mmol/L
Plasma bicarbonate	24 mmol/L
Plasma urea	6 mmol/L
Plasma creatinine	90 µmol/L
Plasma calcium	2.45 mmol/L
Plasma phosphate	1.3 mmol/L
Serum bilirubin	12 µmol/L
Serum albumin	50 g/L
Plasma alkaline phosphatase	1364 IU/L *(normal range 30–100)*
Plasma aspartate aminotransferase	18 IU/L *(normal range 5–35)*

1   What is the initial treatment?
   (a) Simple analgesia
   (b) Vitamin D
   (c) Vitamin D and calcium
   (d) Bisphosphonate
   (e) Calcitonin

Question 4

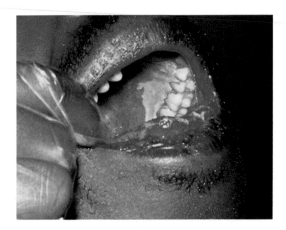

This man also has a painful swollen knee.

1   Which of the following is least likely in the differential?
    (a) Reiter's syndrome
    (b) Crohn's disease
    (c) Coeliac disease
    (d) Gonorrhoea
    (e) Behçet's syndrome

Question 5

A 52-year-old patient is found to have an MCV of 103 fL.

1   Which of the following is not a recognized cause:
    (a) Alcohol abuse
    (b) Haemolysis
    (c) Azathioprine therapy
    (d) Cyclosporin therapy
    (e) Folate deficiency

Question 6

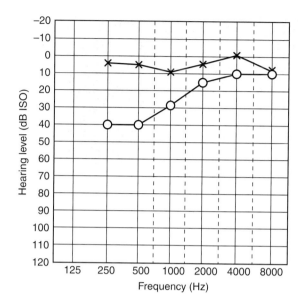

This 69-year-old man complains of fluctuating tinnitus, vertigo and a feeling of fullness in his right ear. There is no air–bone gap.

1   What is the likely diagnosis?
   (a) Cerebellopontine angle tumour
   (b) Ear wax
   (c) Ménière's disease
   (d) Noise-induced hearing loss
   (e) Age-related hearing loss

Question 7

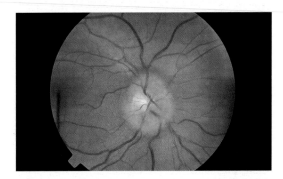

This woman had an uncomplicated pregnancy but developed severe headache 1 week after delivery.

1 What can you see on fundoscopy?
  (a) Optic neuritis
  (b) Acute retinal necrosis
  (c) Papilloedema
  (d) Central retinal artery occlusion
  (e) Central retinal vein occlusion

2 Suggest the likely two differential diagnoses:
  (a) Central venous thrombosis
  (b) Diabetes mellitus
  (c) Eclampsia
  (d) Cerebral tumour
  (e) Pituitary ischaemia
  (f) Cerebral arteritis
  (g) Hypertensive encephalopathy
  (h) Demyelination
  (i) Amniotic fluid embolism
  (j) Subarachnoid haemorrhage

3   She had this investigation; what is it and what does it show?

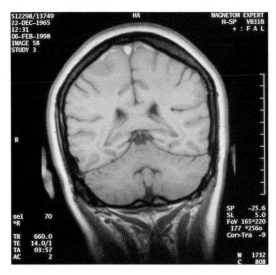

(a) T1-weighted coronal brain MR; sagittal sinus thrombosis
(b) Contract enhanced coronal CT scan; sagittal tumour
(c) T2-weighted sagittal brain MR; sagittal sinus thrombosis
(d) T1-weighted coronal MR; pituitary necrosis
(e) T2-weighted sagittal brain MR; cerebral arteritis

Question 8

A 55-year-old man was referred by his GP with an 18-month history of increasing tiredness, weight loss, dyspnoea, and dry cough. There was no history of musculoskeletal or skin abnormalities. He was a lifelong non-smoker who had worked in a factory for the past 20 years. He was on no medication. He had travelled abroad three times in the past 10 years, to Italy, Spain and Greece.

On examination he was dyspnoeic on moderate exertion. He was not clubbed and had no lymphadenopathy. There were a few inspiratory crepitations on chest auscultation and the blood pressure was 165/95 mmHg. The rest of the examination was within normal limits. He was unable to produce sputum for examination. Urinalysis was normal.

His chest radiograph showed reticular shadowing sparing the lower zones, being more marked on the left. His lung function tests (expressed as percentages of predicted values) were as follows: FEV, 77, FVC 60, TLC 62, RV 70, Kco 50. Full blood count (including differential count) and routine biochemistry screen (including calcium) were normal. Bronchoalveolar lavage showed an increased number of neutrophils. Serum angiotensin-converting enzyme (SACE) was normal.

1   Which two of the following are possible diagnoses?
(a) Cryptogenic fibrosing alveolitis
(b) Sarcoidosis
(c) Mild left ventricular failure
(d) Tuberculosis

(e) Obstructive sleep apnoea
(f) Chronic extrinsic allergic alveolitis
(g) *Mycoplasma* pneumonia
(h) *Legionella* pneumonia
(i) Berylliosis
(j) Alveolar cell carcinoma

2 What are your first two management strategies?
(a) Search for and eliminate any precipitating antigen
(b) Open lung biopsy
(c) Trial of diuretic
(d) Trial of corticosteroids
(e) Induced sputum for microscopy and culture
(f) Autoimmune serology
(g) *Mycoplasma* serology
(h) Mantoux test
(i) Echocardiogram
(j) *Legionella* urinary antigen test

Question 9

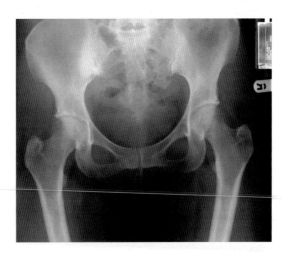

1 This woman has back pain after having borne three children. What is the radiological diagnosis?
(a) Unilateral sacroiliitis
(b) Ankylosing spondylitis
(c) Disruption of symphysis pubis
(d) Osteitis condensans ileii
(e) Transient osteoporosis of pregnancy

Question 10

A 27-year-old female patient approaches you for advice. Her only child, a 10-year-old boy, has a disease inherited in an autosomal recessive manner. The boy's father died several years ago, but your patient has since married a cousin on her mother's side of the family. She wishes to know whether a child resulting from her new marriage will also have the disease.

1   What is the probability of this occurring?
  (a) 1/4
  (b) 1/16
  (c) 1/32
  (d) 1/64
  (e) 1/128

Question 11

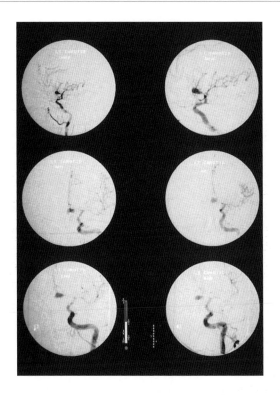

1   What is the diagnosis?
  (a) Polyarteritis nodosa
  (b) Carotid stenosis
  (c) Aneurysm of the anterior communicating artery
  (d) Aneurysm of the posterior communicating artery
  (e) Ventricular aneurysm

Question 12

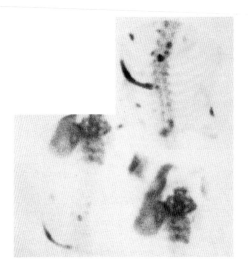

1   What is the most likely diagnosis?
     (a) Metastatic carcinoma of the prostate
     (b) Metastatic carcinoma of the colon
     (c) Paget's disease
     (d) Osteomalacia
     (e) Hyperparathyroidism

Question 13

An 18-year-old unmarried female presents with heavy bleeding per vagina. She is febrile and admits to 2 months of amenorrhoea prior to this episode.
     Investigations show:

Hb	6.2 g/dL
WBC	24 × 10⁹/L
Platelets	30 × 10⁹/L
Prothrombin time	31 s *(control 12)*
Activated partial thromboplastin time	60 s *(control 32)*
Fibrinogen degradation products	400 mg/L *(normal <100)*

1   What important additional haematological information would you request next?
     (a) Differential white count
     (b) Red cell indices (MCV, MCH and MCHC)
     (c) The microscopic appearance of the blood film
     (d) Bone marrow aspirate and trephine
     (e) Coombs test

2   What is the most likely aetiology?
   (a) Septic abortion
   (b) Anaemia secondary to PV haemorrhage
   (c) Septic bone marrow failure
   (d) Amniotic fluid embolus
   (e) Pre-eclampsia

Question 14

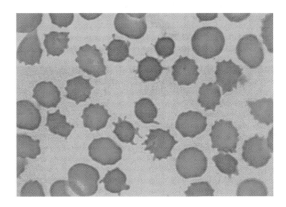

1   What is the underlying diagnosis?
   (a) Abetalipoproteinaemia
   (b) Hereditary spherocytosis
   (c) Uraemia
   (d) Pyruvate kinase deficiency
   (e) Hereditary elliptocytosis

Question 15

A 21-year-old male history student developed jaundice. For the past 2 weeks he had felt unwell with anorexia, lethargy, muscle pains and a sore throat. He had not improved after a course of erythromycin. There had been no change in colour of urine or stool. He had never been abroad. He did not smoke but drank one bottle of vodka at weekends. He had had several female sexual contacts with in the past 6 months. His brother had Gilbert's syndrome. He did not keep any pets and had no allergies. He was on no medications and did not abuse narcotics.

On examination he was pyrexial (38.2°C), icteric, with several enlarged slightly tender cervical and axilliary lymph nodes. There was a 3 cm hepatomegaly and the splenic tip was palpable. He had a small tattoo on his left forearm. Urinalysis was normal.

The results of investigations performed were as follows:

Hb	12.6 g/dL
MCV	90 fL
MCHC	34 g/L
WBC	11.8×10^9/L
Neutrophils	42 per cent
Lymphocytes	56 per cent
Eosinophils	2 per cent
Platelets	56×10^9/L
Blood film	autoagglutination of red cells
ESR	42 mm in the first hour
Monospot	negative
Serum albumin	38 g/L
Plasma aspartate aminotransferase	120 IU/L *(normal range 4–20)*
Plasma alanine aminotransferase	80 IU/L *(normal range 2–17)*
Plasma bilirubin	106 μmol/L
Plasma alkaline phosphatase	140 IU/L
Chest x-ray	normal

1   What is the likely diagnosis:
    (a) Epstein–Barr virus
    (b) Cytomegalovirus
    (c) Toxoplasmosis
    (d) Hepatitis B
    (e) Hepatitis C

Question 16

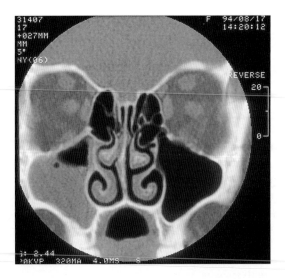

This woman presented with discharge from one ear and a unilateral facial nerve palsy.

1 What is the likely diagnosis?
  (a) Otitis media
  (b) Acoustic neuroma
  (c) Sjögren's syndrome
  (d) HIV infection
  (e) Wegener's granulomatosis

Question 17

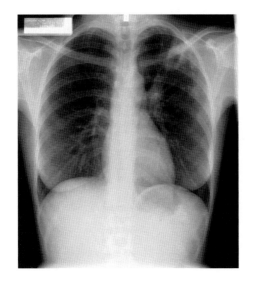

1 What is the likely diagnosis?
  (a) Staphylococcal pneumonia
  (b) Bronchogenic carcinoma
  (c) Secondary lung tumour
  (d) Wegener's granulomatosis
  (e) Tuberculosis

Question 18

A 26-year-old woman is seen in outpatients with her carer. She has been well since her deep venous thrombosis 4 months ago, and had never been seen in a hospital previously. She is very tall with a high arched palate, together with a soft ejection systolic murmur. Her cranial and peripheral nerve examination is normal.

1   This patient should be:
   (a) Prescribed calcium and vitamin D_3
   (b) Prescribed pyridoxine
   (c) Referred for echocardiography
   (d) Prescribed oestrogen and progesterone
   (e) Discharged

Question 19

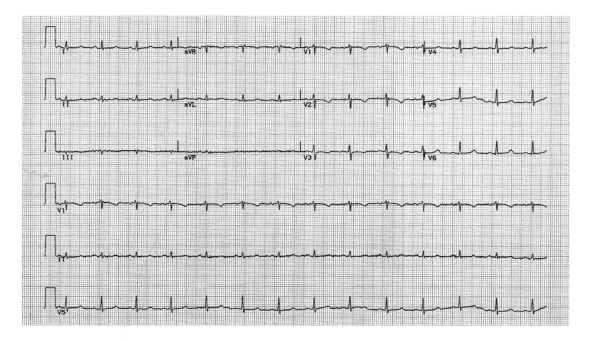

An elderly lady is found on a long-stay rehabilitation ward to be more confused than usual. This is her ECG.

1   What is the most appropriate investigation?
   (a) Serum potassium
   (b) Thyroid function
   (c) Measure temperature with low reading thermometer
   (d) Chest x-ray
   (e) Cardiac enzymes

Question 20

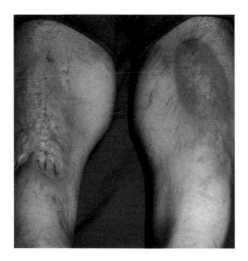

1   What is this?
   (a) Diabetic amyotrophy
   (b) Psoriasis
   (c) Necrobiosis lipoidica diabeticorum
   (d) Partial thickness burn
   (e) Livedo reticularis

Question 21

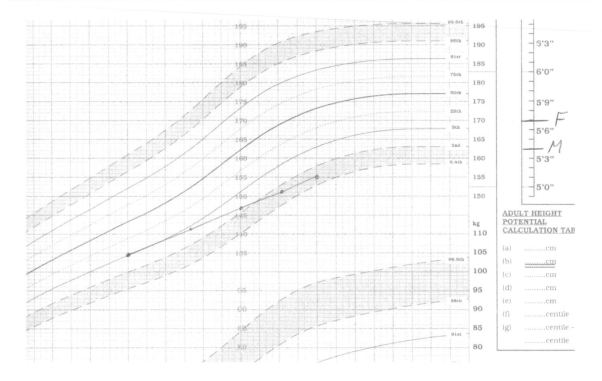

Parents of a 16-year-old boy are concerned that he is being bullied at school. He is not unwell although has been avoiding sports and PE at school. His growth chart is attached.

FSH	1.7 U/L *(normal range 1.8–3.2)*
LH	0.1 U/L *(normal range 0.2–4.9)*
TSH	5 mU/L *(normal range 2–10)*

1 What is the diagnosis?
  (a) Pubertal delay
  (b) Hypogonadotrophic hypogonadism
  (c) Hypergonadotrophic hypogonadism
  (d) Sporadic constitutional delay
  (e) Familial constitutional delay

Question 22

A previously healthy 52-year-old telephonist went to her GP because of intermittent epigastric pain radiating to the back, and weight loss over the past 5 months. Unresponsive to cimetidine and antispasmodics she returned to her GP with a 6-day history of itchiness. She had noticed over the preceding 3 weeks that her eyes and urine had turned yellow. She gave a history of polydipsia. There was no history of travel abroad, transfusions, or contact with jaundiced persons. Her last sexual contact was 4 years previously. Her weight had dropped from 78 to 69 kg. She did not drink alcohol.

On examination she was pale, jaundiced and afebrile. There was mild epigastric tenderness, hepatomegaly (3 cm below the costal margin), and her gallbladder was palpable. The remainder of the examination was normal.

The results of investigations were as follows:

Hb	10.8 g/dL
MCV	80 fL
WBC	9.7×10^9/L
ESR	77 mm in first hour
Plasma aspartate aminotransferase	48 IU/L *(normal range 4–20)*
Plasma bilirubin	172 µmol/L
Plasma alkaline phosphatase	474 IU/L *(normal range 30–100)*
Plasma glucose (random)	11 mmol/L
Urine analysis	bilirubin ++
	urobilinogen –
	glucose ++
Chest and plain abdominal x-rays	normal

1   Which investigation is most likely to provide the diagnosis?
   (a) Anti-mitochondrial antibody
   (b) Hepatitis C serology
   (c) Endoscopic retrograde cholangiopancreatogram (ERCP)
   (d) CT scan upper abdomen
   (e) Abdominal ultrasound

Question 23

A 26-year-old man was brought to A and E from the local mainline station where he had been found drunk, unable to give a history. On examination, he had gross erythema and oedema of his left conjunctiva, was covered in tattoos and smelled of alcohol. The rest of the examination and all initial investigations revealed no further abnormality. The following morning, he admitted to being under the outpatient care of a psychiatrist on account of his desire to 'scratch the back of his eyeball'. He could not explain why he wanted to do this. He denied any other problems. He was by now fully orientated, had no cognitive defect and displayed no evidence of delusions or hallucinations, which he denied ever having. His conversation was laced with expletives which were introduced explosively into the interview without warning and following which he would resume as if uninterrupted. He tended to wink and nudge the doctor during the interview. Subsequent thyroid function tests were normal.

1   What is the diagnosis?
   (a) Acute relapsing schizophrenia
   (b) Gilles de la Tourette's syndrome
   (c) Lesch–Nyhan syndrome
   (d) Alcohol intoxication
   (e) Side effect of chronic neuroleptic medication

Question 24

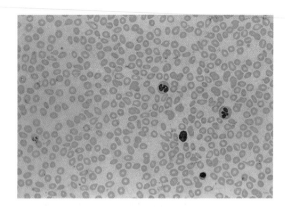

This is the peripheral blood film of a 72-year-old man with splenomegaly and anaemia.

1   What is the diagnosis?
  (a) Lymphoma
  (b) Acute lymphoblastic leukaemia
  (c) Iron deficiency
  (d) Myelofibrosis
  (e) Microangiopathic haemolytic anaemia

Question 25

A 48-year-old pilot becomes acutely short of breath. Arterial blood gas analysis shows:

pH	7.38
Pa_{O_2}	8.0 kPa
Pa_{CO_2}	3.6 kPa

1   Give two possible diagnoses:
  (a) Pneumothorax
  (b) Opiate overdose
  (c) Emphysema
  (d) Acute pulmonary embolism
  (e) Pneumonia
  (f) Brainstem cerebrovascular accident
  (g) Panic attack
  (h) Recurrent thromboembolism
  (i) Pulmonary fibrosis
  (j) Acclimatization

Question 26

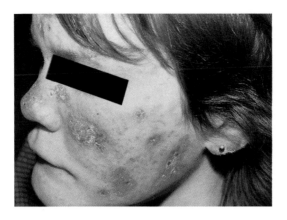

1   What is the diagnosis?
    (a) Lupus vulgaris
    (b) Lupus pernio
    (c) Scrofula
    (d) Discoid lupus
    (e) Systemic lupus erythematosus

Question 27

A 78-year-old woman is admitted to the gynaecological ward with problems associated with her inoperable ovarian tumour. She is vomiting and her CT scan shows her to have compression of her large bowel.

1   The first-line treatment for her vomiting would be:
    (a) Metoclopramide
    (b) Cyclizine
    (c) Ondansetron
    (d) Dexamethasone
    (e) Levomepromazine

Question 28

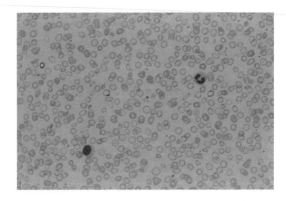

This is the peripheral blood film of a 72-year-old man who has become anaemic.

1   What is the likely diagnosis?
     (a) Megaloblastic anaemia
     (b) Iron deficiency anaemia
     (c) Myelofibrosis
     (d) Chronic lymphocytic leukaemia
     (e) Multiple myeloma

Question 29

A 65-year-old man presented as an emergency with an 8-hour history of moderate pain of sudden onset in the nape of the neck. He gave a history of chronic moderate low back pain for many years for which he had been seeing an osteopath. He had also been told that he had 'too many fats in his blood'. On admission his blood pressure was 150/94 mmHg. There were no abnormal physical signs.

His ECG was normal as were radiographs of his cervical, thoracic and lumbar spine and chest.

Two hours after admission, the pain in his neck became suddenly much worse. He became pale and his blood pressure fell to 120/60 mmHg. The blood pressure was the same in both arms. Physical examination was still normal as were the ECG and chest radiograph repeated at this time.

1   What are the two most likely diagnoses?
     (a) Acute myocardial infarction
     (b) Acute aortic dissection
     (c) Pneumonia
     (d) Acute pulmonary embolism
     (e) Oesophageal rupture

Hint
Uncommon presentations of common conditions may be more common than common presentations of uncommon conditions.

(f) Vertebral collapse
(g) Disc prolapse
(h) Oesophageal carcinoma
(i) Mesothelioma
(j) Acute pneumothorax

Question 30

A 15-year-old Asian girl presents with increasing malaise and vomiting. She has recently emigrated to the UK.
   Investigations show:

Plasma sodium	127 mmol/L
Plasma potassium	4.7 mmol/L
Plasma urea	14 mmol/L
Plasma creatinine	135 µmol/L
Plasma bicarbonate	13 mmol/L
Plasma glucose	1.7 mmol/L

1 What is the diagnosis?
   (a) Hypopituitarism
   (b) Addison's disease
   (c) Malaria
   (d) Meningitis
   (e) Anorexia nervosa

Question 31

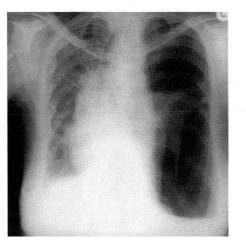

1 What is the diagnosis?
   (a) Rotated radiograph
   (b) Left tension pneumothorax

(c) Dextrocardia
(d) Consolidation/collapse central regions of right lung
(e) Massive bullous disease of left hemithorax

Question 32

A young man complains of shoulder pain for several days and thereafter felt as if something was out of place. The only abnormality is winging of the right scapula. Routine investigations are normal.
    Neurophysiological studies show normal nerve conduction, but the EMG report reads:

    Right serratus anterior: fasciculation and occasional fibrillations, low recruitment pattern with high firing rate. Maximum size of motor units 5.0 mV
    Right supraspinatus: occasional fasciculation and full recruitment pattern with low firing rate. Maximum size of motor units 4.0 mV
    Right biceps: no spontaneous activity, full recruitment pattern with low firing rate. Maximum size of motor units 3.5 mV
    Right extensor digitorum communis: occasional fasciculation and full recruitment pattern with low firing rate. Maximum size of motor units 5.0 mV
    Right dorsal interosseous: no spontaneous activity, full recruitment pattern with normal firing rate. Maximum size of motor units 3.0 mV.

1   Which muscle(s) is(are) normal?
    (a) Right serratus anterior
    (b) Right biceps
    (c) Right extensor digitorum communis
    (d) Right dorsal interosseous
    (e) Right trapezius

2   What is the neurophysiological diagnosis?
    (a) Axonal peripheral neuropathy
    (b) Demyelinating neuropathy
    (c) Mononeuritis multiplex
    (d) Partial denervation
    (e) Myositis

3   What is the likely underlying diagnosis?
    (a) Multiple sclerosis
    (b) Treponemal disease
    (c) Diabetes
    (d) B_{12} deficiency
    (e) Neuralgic amyotrophy

Question 33

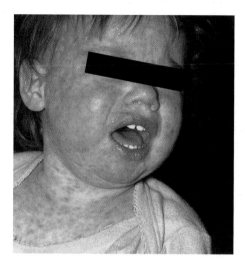

This patient also had coryza and his 5-year-old brother had a similar illness 2 weeks ago.

1   What is the diagnosis?
(a) Rubella
(b) Exanthem subitum
(c) Fifth disease
(d) Measles
(e) Roseola infantum

Question 34

A 46-year-old asthmatic, managed with systemic steroids, complains of muscle aches and weakness. On examination telangiectasia are present on her face.
Investigations show:

Plasma sodium	141 mmol/L
Plasma potassium	4.1 mmol/L
Plasma urea	5.0 mmol/L
Plasma calcium	2.60 mmol/L
Plasma aspartate aminotransferase	15 IU/L *(normal range 5–35)*
Plasma creatine phosphokinase	820 IU/L *(normal range 25–170)*
Hb	10.9 g/dL
WBC	6.0×10^9/L
ESR	46 mm in 1st hour

1   What is your differential diagnosis?
    (a) Muscular dystrophy
    (b) Dermato/polymyositis
    (c) Steroid-induced myopathy
    (d) Inclusion body myositis
    (e) Acute vasculitic neuropathy
    (f) Myasthenia gravis
    (g) Hypercalcaemia
    (h) Hypothyroidism
    (i) Cushing's syndrome
    (j) Periodic hypokalaemic paralysis

2   What is the most useful investigation?
    (a) Electromyography
    (b) Autoantibody screen
    (c) Muscle biopsy
    (d) Nerve conduction studies
    (e) Chest x-ray

Question 35

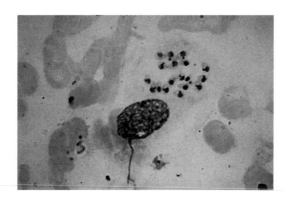

This bone marrow is taken from a patient with a pyrexia of unknown origin and hepatomegaly.

1   What is the diagnosis?
    (a) Leishmaniasis
    (b) Schistosomiasis
    (c) Onchocerciasis
    (d) Loa Loa
    (e) Gnathostomiasis

Question 36

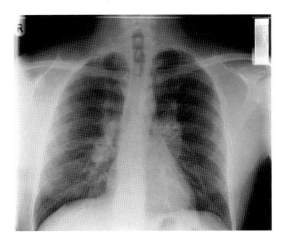

A 25-year-old male presents with painful lesions on the shins and ankle arthritis, following a sore throat.

1   What is the diagnosis?
   (a) Tubercular arthritis
   (b) Post-adenovirus reactive arthritis
   (c) Non-Hodgkin's lymphoma
   (d) Parvovirus infection
   (e) Sarcoidosis

Question 37

Following an acute myocardial infarction, a 55-year-old man presents with mild dyspnoea and ankle swelling. When there is no response to diuretics, a pulmonary flotation catheter is used to obtain the following pressures:

Site	Pressure (mmHg)
Right atrium (mean)	6
Right ventricle	22/10
Pulmonary artery	19/8
Pulmonary wedge (mean)	4

1   What is the diagnosis?
   (a) Pulmonary embolism
   (b) Pulmonary hypertension
   (c) Acquired ventricular septal defect
   (d) Right ventricular infarction
   (e) Cardiac tamponade

Question 38

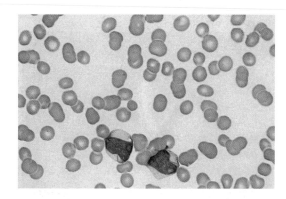

This is the peripheral blood film of a 53-year-old woman with purpura of the lower limbs.

1   What is the diagnosis?
   (a) Acute myeloblastic leukaemia
   (b) Chronic lymphocytic leukaemia
   (c) Acute lymphoblastic leukaemia
   (d) Chronic myeloid leukaemia
   (e) Atypical lymphocytosis

Question 39

A dialysis patient is offered a cadaveric kidney through the national sharing scheme, but it has to be declined because the patient has a positive direct cross-match with the donor.

1   This means that:
   (a) The donor has preformed antibodies specific for recipient cells
   (b) The recipient has preformed antibodies specific for donor cells
   (c) The donor has T lymphocytes cytotoxic to recipient cells
   (d) The recipient has T lymphocytes cytotoxic to donor cells
   (e) The recipient and donor have incompatible blood groups

Question 40

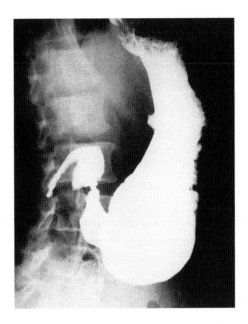

1   This patient complained of dysphagia. What is the diagnosis?
   (a) Carcinoma of the stomach
   (b) Carcinoma of the oesophagus
   (c) Achalasia of the cardia
   (d) Lesser curvature peptic ulcer
   (e) Acquired pyloric stenosis

Question 41

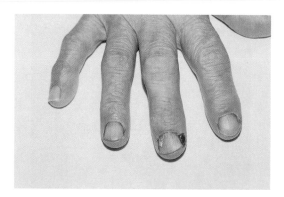

1 What is the likely diagnosis?
  (a) Psoriasis
  (b) Sarcoidosis
  (c) Herpetic whitlow
  (d) Henoch–Schonlein vasculitis
  (e) Rheumatoid vasculitis

Question 42

A 67-year-old man who had suffered from rheumatoid arthritis for many years was referred for further investigation. He complained of 4 months' increasing tiredness and lethargy and was now experiencing nausea and abdominal discomfort.

His rheumatoid arthritis had initially been controlled with non-steroidal anti-inflammatory drugs and several years previously he had received a course of penicillamine. His medication now consisted of prednisolone 6 mg daily and indomethacin.

He had no other medical problems and was reasonably self-sufficient considering the deformities of his hands. He had continued to work as a civil servant until 2 years ago.

On examination there was no evidence of active arthritis. His cardiovascular and respiratory systems were normal. He had mild hepatomegaly and moderate splenomegaly.

Urinalysis revealed proteinuria (++).

Results of investigations performed were as follows:

Hb	9.9 g/dL
WBC	9.2×10^9/L
Platelets	101×10^9/L
Plasma sodium	144 mmol/L
Plasma potassium	5.1 mmol/L
Plasma urea	31.2 mmol/L
Plasma creatinine	499 μmol/L
Creatinine clearance	21 ml/min
Renal ultrasound	kidney size at upper limit of normal; no evidence of obstruction

A renal biopsy was abandoned after several attempts to obtain tissue. Following the procedure he had a life-threatening haemorrhage but is now stable.

1   To guide further management what procedure what would you arrange next?
  (a) OGD ± biopsy
  (b) Colonoscopy ± biopsy
  (c) Sigmoidoscopy ± biopsy
  (d) Proctoscopy ± biopsy
  (e) Bronchoscopy ± biopsy

Question 43

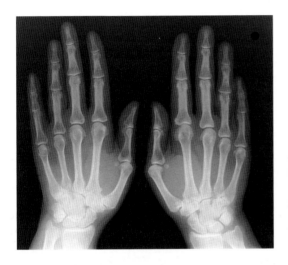 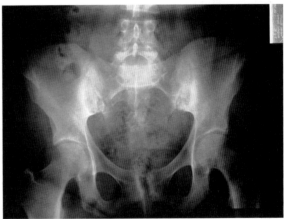

This man feels non-specifically unwell and rather depressed about it, and in the course of his investigations these x-rays of his hands and pelvis are taken.

1   Which of the following would you check next?
  (a) Sedimentation rate
  (b) Serum protein electrophoresis
  (c) Serum calcium level
  (d) Chest x-ray
  (e) Bone biopsy

2   What is the diagnosis?
  (a) Hyperparathyroidism
  (b) Multiple myeloma
  (c) Sarcoidosis
  (d) Gout
  (e) Tuberculosis

Question 44

A 27-year-old married woman with amenorrhoea of 7 months' duration is found to have mild jaundice, hepatosplenomegaly, lymphadenopathy and palmar erythema.
Investigations show:

Hb	10.4 g/dL
WBC	2.8×10^9/L
Platelets	72×10^9/L
ESR	29 mm in first hour
Plasma bilirubin	58 μmol/L
Plasma aspartate aminotransferase	190 IU/L *(normal range 5–35)*
Plasma alanine aminotransferase	105 IU/L *(normal range 2–17)*
Plasma alkaline phosphatase	65 IU/L *(normal range 30–100)*
Serum albumin	35 g/L
Serum globulin	68 g/L
Hepatitis B surface antigen	negative
Antinuclear factor	positive at titre of 1/512
Anti-smooth muscle antibodies	positive
Anti-mitochondrial antibodies	positive at titre of 1/64

1   What is the diagnosis?
   (a) Primary biliary cirrhosis
   (b) Chronic active hepatitis
   (c) Wilson's disease
   (d) Hepatitis C infection
   (e) Drug toxicity

Question 45

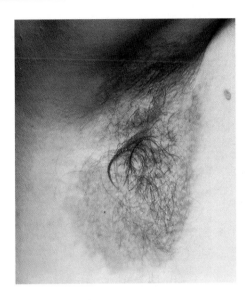

1   What is this physical sign?
    (a) Chicken skin
    (b) Acanthosis nigricans
    (c) Melanoma
    (d) Topical dermatitis
    (e) Necrobiosis lipoidica

Question 46

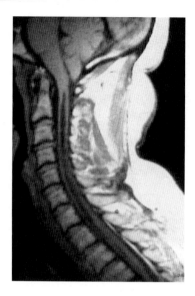

A cleaner presented to the rheumatological clinic complaining of burning her left hand. She was referred for this investigation with diagnosis of cervical spondylosis.

1   What is the radiological diagnosis?
 (a) Prolapsed vertebral disc
 (b) Syringomyelia
 (c) Arnold–Chiari malformation
 (d) Cerebellar haemorrhage
 (e) Cervical spondylosis

Question 47

A 22-year-old woman develops dyspnoea and chest pain after an argument with her husband's mistress. She has tachypnoea and tetany on admission and is given 35 per cent oxygen in A and E. Investigations show:

Plasma sodium	139 mmol/L
Plasma potassium	4.2 mmol/L
Plasma calcium	2.22 mmol/L
Plasma glucose	4.6 mmol/L
Hb	12.8 g/dL
WBC	$6.1 \times 10^9/L$

Arterial blood gases
    pH   7.58
    $Pa\text{CO}_2$ 2.9 kPa
    $Pa\text{O}_2$ 18 kPa
Plasma bicarbonate   19 mmol/L
Base excess   12 mmol/L
Chest x-ray   normal

1   What is your immediate management?
    (a) Salicylate levels
    (b) Reassurance
    (c) Serum glucose
    (d) Oxygen
    (e) Sedation

Question 48

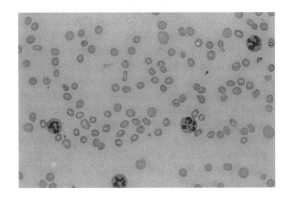

This is the peripheral blood film of a 35-year-old woman who is pale.

1   What is the diagnosis?
    (a) Megaloblastic anaemia
    (b) Sideroblastic anaemia
    (c) Spherocytosis
    (d) Iron deficiency anaemia
    (e) Folate deficiency

Question 49

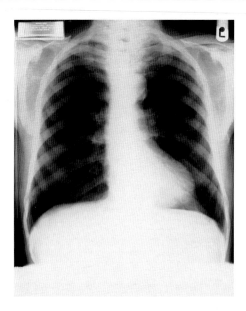

1 What does this chest x-ray show?
   (a) Renal osteodystrophy
   (b) Primary hyperparathyroidism
   (c) Myelosclerosis
   (d) Disseminated prostatic carcinoma
   (e) Disseminated carcinoma of the breast

Question 50

A 28-year-old man complained of abdominal cramps, weight loss and dyspnoea. On examination he looked unwell. Other than the development of asthma 5 years ago, there was no history of note. There was no dyspnoea at rest and general examination was unremarkable.

The following investigations were performed:

Hb	12.4 g/dL
WBC	9×10^9/L
Neutrophils	2.9×10^9/L
Lymphocytes	0.9×10^9/L
Eosinophils	4.8×10^9/L
Basophils	0.1×10^9/L
Na	142 mmol/L
K	4.3 mmol/L
Platelets	368×10^9/L
Creatinine	91 μmol/L

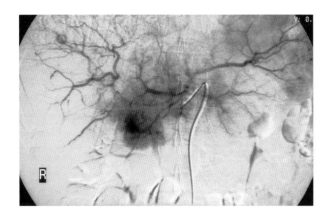

1   What is the likely diagnosis?
    (a) Churg–Strauss syndrome
    (b) Microscopic polyarteritis
    (c) Takayasu's arteritis
    (d) Wegener's granulomatosis
    (e) Polyarteritis nodosa

2   What treatment would you initiate?
    (a) Prednisolone
    (b) Co-trimoxazole
    (c) Prednisolone and cyclophosphamide
    (d) Cyclophosphamide
    (e) Azathioprine

Question 51

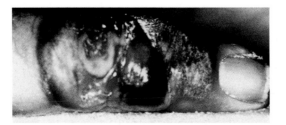

This lesion developed on the finger of a sheep farmer.

1   What treatment would you give?
    (a) Tetracycline
    (b) Erythromycin
    (c) Suramin
    (d) Chloramphenicol
    (e) Penicillin

Question 52

An 18-year-old girl is investigated because of recurrent warts, resistant to conventional treatment. Investigations show:

Plasma sodium	139 mmol/L
Plasma potassium	4.7 mmol/L
Plasma urea	6.3 mmol/L
Plasma creatinine	87 µmol/L
Serum bilirubin	18 µmol/L
Plasma aspartate aminotransferase	19 IU/L *(normal range 5–35)*
Plasma alkaline phosphatase	89 IU/L *(normal range 30–100)*
Serum albumin	28 g/L
Serum IgG	3.95 g/L *(normal range 7.2–19)*
Serum IgA	1.1 g/L *(normal range 0.85–5)*
Serum IgM	0.49 g/L *(normal range 0.5–2)*
Hb	12.8 g/dL
Platelets	187×10^9/L
WBC	4.8×10^9/L
Neutrophils	3.5×10^9/L
Lymphocytes	0.9×10^9/L
Urinalysis	no abnormality
Clotting screen	normal

1   What is the most likely diagnosis?
(a) Protein-losing enteropathy
(b) Small intestinal lymphangiectasia
(c) Malnutrition
(d) Liver failure
(e) Nephrotic syndrome

Question 53

A 43 year-old Asian male, non-smoker and teetotaller, was admitted with a 2-day history of lethargy, sore throat, runny nose and headache. He developed vomiting and became confused a few hours before admission. Three days prior to admission he had returned to London with his family from a visit to Tunisia. His son was recovering from a bout of *Shigella* diarrhoea. He had no history of allergies. A splenectomy had been performed on him a year previously after a road accident. He was on no medication.

On examination he was disorientated, confused, febrile (39.7°C) and photophobic. The blood pressure was 98/56 mmHg and the pulse was 110 beats/min, regular but of low volume. There was a petechial rash on the left arm and right thigh. He had mild neck stiffness, a positive Kernig's sign but the optic discs were normal. Urinalysis was normal.

1   What is the diagnosis?
    (a) *Shigella* meningitis
    (b) *Klebsiella* meningitis
    (c) Pneumococcal meningitis
    (d) Tuberculous meningitis
    (e) Meningococcal meningitis

Question 54

A 29-year-old Iraqi postgraduate student gives a 3-month history of weight loss, malaise and night sweats. He has pallor, abdominal distention and hepatosplenomegaly.
    Investigations:

Hb	7.8 g/dL
MCV	80 fL
WBC	2.1×10^9/L (68 per cent lymphocytes)
Platelets	82×10^9/L
Blood film	normocytic normochromic anaemia
ESR	72 mm in first hour
Plasma calcium	2.48 mmol/L *(corrected)*
Plasma AST	72 IU/L *(normal range 5–35)*
Plasma alkaline phosphatase	112 IU/L *(normal range 30–100)*
Serum albumin	24 g/L
Serum globulin	64 g/L
Chest x-ray	normal

1   What two tests are most likely to elucidate the cause?
    (a) Liver biopsy
    (b) Bone marrow biopsy
    (c) Blood culture
    (d) Mantoux test
    (e) Thick and thin blood film
    (f) Clotting studies
    (g) Haemoglobin electrophoresis
    (h) CT chest
    (i) HIV test
    (j) Upper GI tract endoscopy

Question 55

A 29-year-old Asian newsagent was referred with a 4-week history of recurrent headaches, backache, fever and lethargy. He had developed tingling and weakness in the right foot and leg. On the morning of admission he experienced difficulty in passing urine and retrospectively admitted to two episodes of blurring of vision over the preceding few months. He had received treatment for a slipped disc 2 years previously and had received steroid eye drops for itchiness 1 year previously. He drank 6 pints of beer a week and smoked 10 cigarettes a day. He had several social problems following the break-up of his marriage. He was taking paracetamol for headaches. His last trip abroad was 3 months previously to Kenya, where he kept very well.

On examination, he was fully conscious and had unimpaired higher mental function. Examination of his optic discs and cranial nerves was unremarkable. Apart from a full bladder, the remainder of the examination was unremarkable.

He was catheterized and admitted for investigations. Later that day he developed paraesthesiae and weakness in both legs and feet. The findings were now of impaired hip and knee flexion (power grade 4/5), increased knee and ankle jerks, extensor plantar response in the right foot, and impairment of all modalities of sensation up to level T4.

The results of investigations were as follows:

Hb	13.3 g/dL
MCV	88 fL
MCHC	33 g/L
WBC	12.7×10^9/L
Neutrophils	40 per cent
Lymphocytes	58 per cent
Eosinophils	2 per cent
Platelets	156×10^9/L
ESR	62 mm in first hour
Serum albumin	40 g/L
Plasma aspartate aminotransferase	20 IU/L *(normal range 4–20)*
Plasma alanine aminotransferase	70 IU/L *(normal range 2–17)*
Plasma bilirubin	6 μmol/L
Plasma alkaline phosphatase	80 IU/L
Serum vitamin B_{12}	200 pmol/L *(normal range 150–750)*
Urinalysis	normal

1 Select the two most likely diagnoses:
   (a) Traumatic disc prolapse
   (b) Spinal column tumour
   (c) Pyogenic abscess
   (d) Tuberculosis of the spine
   (e) Paget's disease
   (f) Myeloma
   (g) Multiple sclerosis
   (h) Vitamin B_{12} deficiency
   (i) Syphilis HTLV-1 infection
   (j) Dissection of aortic aneurysm

Question 56

A man 2 weeks into treatment for presumed tuberculosis was found to have a newly elevated aspartate transaminase.

1   Which of the following would be your first course of action?
    (a) To discontinue all his anti-tuberculous chemotherapy and then reintroduce agents one by one
    (b) Discontinue isoniazid and wait to see if liver enzymes fall
    (c) Ignore the abnormality unless the patient became jaundiced
    (d) Review the initial diagnosis of tuberculosis, as TB rarely causes hepatitis
    (e) Perform an ECG to exclude a silent myocardial infarction

Question 57

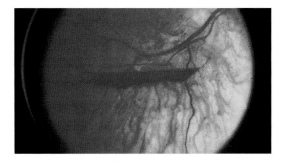

1   What is this lesion?
    (a) Intraretinal haemorrhage
    (b) Subretinal haemorrhage
    (c) Subchoroidal haemorrhage
    (d) Preretinal haemorrhage
    (e) Subconjunctival haemorrhage

Question 58

A 72-year-old woman is admitted to A and E because of increasing drowsiness.
    Investigations show:

Plasma sodium	158 mmol/L
Plasma potassium	3.9 mmol/L
Plasma urea	28 mmol/L
Plasma creatinine	158 µmol/L
Plasma glucose	62 mmol/L
Arterial blood gases	
pH	7.32
Pao_2	11.8 kPa
$Paco_2$	5.3 kPa
Plasma bicarbonate	19 mmol/L

1   What is the diagnosis?
  (a) Diabetic ketoacidosis
  (b) Hyperosmolar non-ketotic diabetic coma
  (c) Acute renal failure
  (d) Hypernatraemic coma
  (e) Hyperlactataemia

Question 59

You are called by the SHO in psychogeriatrics for some advice over the telephone. Six weeks ago they admitted a 79-year-old gentleman as the community psychiatric nurse was having difficulty managing his dementia in the community on account of persistent visual hallucinations. Three months previously the patient had been seen at a domestic visit by the consultant psychogeriatrician. A diagnosis of multi-infarct dementia was made. His past medical history was unremarkable except for a myocardial infarction 6 months previously.

He takes aspirin 75 mg o.d. and sulpiride 50 mg b.d.

Since admission the patient has been seen to be very slow in initiating movement. He shakes most of the time and is difficult to feed because of drooling.

1   What would you recommend?
  (a) Commence Sinemet tablets three times daily
  (b) Commence entacapone tablets three times daily
  (c) Reduce sulpiride dose
  (d) Stop sulpiride
  (e) Commence Aricept (donepezil)

Question 60

A 33-year-old male accounts executive with a 15-year history of insulin-dependent diabetes was admitted complaining of shortness of breath. He had never been properly followed for his diabetes because of poor compliance. He was known to have proliferative diabetic retinopathy which had been treated on two occasions with photocoagulation. His renal function had been slightly impaired when last seen 10 months before the current admission.

He had been reasonably well until 6 weeks previously when he had developed increasing weakness. Over the last week, he had become increasingly short of breath. He was a non-smoker and a 'social drinker'. His only medication was twice daily subcutaneous insulin. The only past history of note was a Ramstedt's procedure for pyloric stenosis as a neonate.

On admission, he had bilateral basal crepitations and had marked ankle oedema. His JVP was raised 4 cm. He was producing no urine.

His creatinine was 1133 μmol/L and he had small scarred echogenic kidneys on ultrasound. Chest x-ray was compatible with mild pulmonary oedema.

Four hours after admission a left subclavian double lumen catheter was inserted and he was commenced on haemodialysis. One hour later his shortness of breath deteriorated very markedly and he was now *in extremis*.

1   What are the two most likely causes for his acute deterioration?
   (a) Pulmonary oedema due to acute fluid overload
   (b) Pulmonary oedema due to acute myocardial infarction
   (c) Haemothorax
   (d) Pericardial haemorrhage
   (e) Pulmonary haemorrhage
   (f) Pulmonary embolism
   (g) Dialysis related allergic reaction
   (h) Septicaemia
   (i) Intracerebral bleed
   (j) Air embolism

Question 61

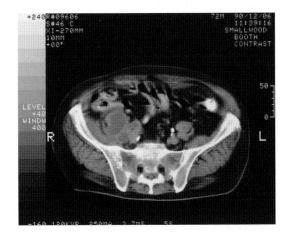

This woman is unwell, with weight loss, night sweats and back pain.

1   What would be the most likely cause of the CT scan abnormalities?
   (a) Inflammatory bowel disease
   (b) Renal cell tumour
   (c) Tuberculosis
   (d) Retroperitoneal fibrosis
   (e) Bladder tumour

Question 62

A 40-year-old advertising executive was alarmed to be told by friends that her eyes were turning yellow. She had been diagnosed as having rheumatoid arthritis 2 years previously and this had been symptomatically controlled with paracetamol. Apart from pruritus, which had been diagnosed as skin sensitivity to soap, she had been well. She gave no history of foreign travel, visits to dockyards, tattooing, recent sexual contact, or blood transfusions.

On examination, she was icteric, afebrile and had scratch marks all over her thighs and back. Her liver was enlarged 3 cm below the costal margin. The remainder of the examination, including urinalysis, was normal.

The results of investigations performed were as follows:

Hb	13.4 g/dL
WBC	6.7×10^9/L (59 per cent neutrophils, 36 per cent lymphocytes)
Platelets	182×10^9/L
ESR	20 mm in first hour
Plasma sodium	136 mmol/L
Plasma potassium	4.5 mmol/L
Plasma calcium	2.45 mmol/L
Plasma phosphate	0.84 mmol/L
Plasma urea	5.4 mmol/L
Plasma glucose	6.5 mmol/L
Serum albumin	40 g/L
Serum total protein	95 g/L
Plasma aspartate aminotransferase	134 IU/L *(normal range 4–20)*
Plasma alanine aminotransferase	108 IU/L *(normal range 2–17)*
Plasma alkaline phosphatase	780 IU/L
Plasma bilirubin	96 μmol/L
Plasma thyroxine	120 nmol/L *(normal range 70–140)*
Chest x-ray	normal
ECG	normal
Serum paracetamol	not detected
Hepatitis A, B and C screen	negative
EBV and CMV serology	negative

1   What is the most likely diagnosis?
   (a) Chronic active hepatitis
   (b) Primary biliary cirrhosis
   (c) Chronic paracetamol poisoning
   (d) Chronic alcohol abuse
   (e) Chronic viral hepatitis

Question 63

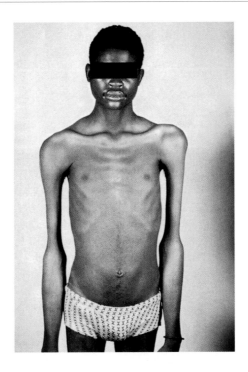

1   What is the diagnosis?
   (a) Marfan's syndrome
   (b) Syringomyelia
   (c) Facioscapulohumeral dystrophy
   (d) Malaria
   (e) Yaws

Question 64

A 52-year-old man presents with recurrent transient ischaemic attacks which have persisted despite aspirin prophylaxis. The decision is made to anticoagulate him with warfarin. The following haematological results are obtained prior to his first dose:

Hb	13.8 g/dL
WBC	8.9×10^9/L
Platelets	172×10^9/L
Prothrombin time	14 s *(control 12)*
Activated partial thromboplastin time	62 s *(control 35)*
Thrombin time	12 s *(control 12)*
Bleeding time	8 min *(control 5)*

1 What investigation would help confirm the diagnosis?
   (a) MRI brain
   (b) Bone marrow biopsy
   (c) Repeat clotting using 50:50 mix with control serum
   (d) Factor VIII levels
   (e) Factor IX levels

Question 65

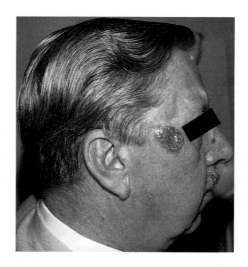

1 What is the likely diagnosis?
   (a) Basal cell carcinoma
   (b) Squamous cell carcinoma
   (c) Keratoacanthoma
   (d) Malignant melanoma
   (e) Carbuncle

Question 66

Two weeks following an episode of diarrhoea, a 27-year-old man presents acutely unwell. Investigations show:

Plasma sodium	143 mmol/L
Plasma potassium	8.5 mmol/L
Plasma bicarbonate	12 mmol/L
Plasma urea	53 mmol/I
Plasma creatinine	1231 μmol/L
Hb	7 g/dL
WBC	7.6×10^9/L
Platelets	15×10^9/L

1 What is the most likely diagnosis?
  (a) Rhabdomyolysis
  (b) Thrombotic thrombocytopenic purpura
  (c) Disseminated intravascular coagulation
  (d) Haemolytic-uraemic syndrome
  (e) Prerenal failure due to dehydration

Question 67

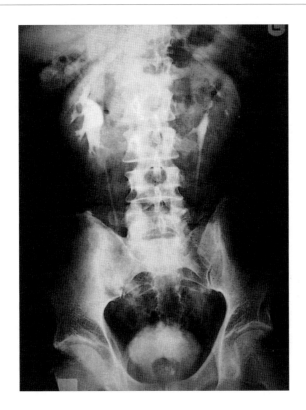

1 What is the abnormality on this intravenous urogram?
  (a) Nephrocalcinosis
  (b) Retroperitoneal fibrosis
  (c) Duplex ureters
  (d) Polycystic kidney disease
  (e) Horseshoe kidney

Question 68

A 55-year-old man complains of chest pain. His blood pressure is 100/70 mmHg. His ECG on admission is shown.

1   Where is the most likely site of the coronary lesion?
    (a) Left anterior descending artery
    (b) Right coronary artery
    (c) Left main stem
    (d) Left circumflex artery
    (e) Second obtuse marginal artery

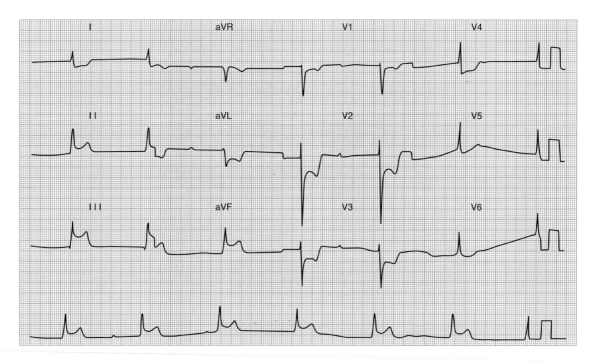

2   What treatment is indicated?
    (a) Intraventricular temporary pacing
    (b) Intraventricular permanent pacing
    (c) Monitoring
    (d) Treatment with intravenous atropine
    (e) Treatment with isoprenaline

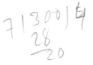

Question 69

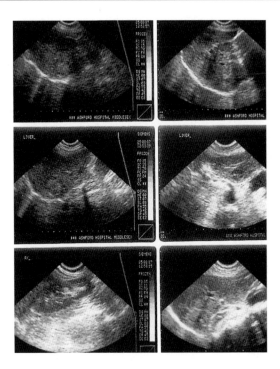

1 What abnormality does this ultrasound scan of the abdomen show?
(a) Pancreatic pseudocyst
(b) Transplanted kidney
(c) Multiple liver metastases
(d) Cholecystectomy
(e) Aortic aneurysm

Question 70

A previously healthy, 36-year-old lawyer was admitted with a 4-day history of fever, lethargy, anorexia and vomiting. Rigors, an erythematous rash over the legs, arms and chest, and pain in the right hypochondrium had developed the day before admission. He had returned 4 days previously from a holiday in Tanzania and Zambia. Before departure he had consulted the travel clinic, received all appropriate immunizations and had taken chloroquine and proguanil prophylaxis which he had continued upon his return. He had been bitten by several flying insects. His homosexual partner was apparently well. He did not smoke or drink alcohol.

He was fully conscious, febrile (39.2°C) and mildly jaundiced. He had a blood pressure of 130/90 mmHg and pulse of 102/min, regular. There was no neck stiffness and the Kernig's sign was absent. He had a macular, erythematous, blanching rash on the thighs, arms and anterior chest wall. There were two healing insect bite wounds on the right forearm but no eschar. He had oral herpes simplex, pharyngitis and injected conjunctiva. There was a 3 cm hepatomegaly, non-tender axillary lymphadenopathy and the tip of the spleen was palpable. Urinalysis was normal.

Results of investigations performed were as follows:

Hb	14.6 g/dL
WBC	8.8×10^9/L
Neutrophils	46 per cent
Lymphocytes	50 per cent
Eosinophils	4 per cent
Platelets	82×10^9/L
ESR	28 mm in first hour
Plasma sodium	130 mmol/L
Plasma potassium	4.6 mmol/L
Plasma urea	10.4 mmol/L
Plasma glucose	4.2 mmol/L
Serum albumin	38 g/L
Plasma aspartate aminotransferase	180 IU/L *(normal range 4–20)*
Plasma alanine aminotransferase	110 IU/L *(normal range 2–17)*
Plasma bilirubin	94 µmol/L
Plasma alkaline phosphatase	94 IU/L *(normal range 30–100)*
Chest x-ray	normal

1   Which of the following is the least likely diagnosis?
  (a) African tick typhus fever
  (b) Malaria
  (c) Relapsing fever
  (d) Typhoid fever
  (e) Trypanosomiasis

2   Which of the following is the most urgent investigation?
  (a) Blood film for spirochaetes
  (b) Blood film for buffy coat
  (c) Thick and thin blood film
  (d) Blood film for atypical lymphocytes
  (e) Blood culture

Question 71

A 65-year-old woman complains of proximal muscle weakness. Investigations show the following:

Plasma sodium	130 mmol/L
Plasma potassium	4.2 mmol/L
Serum creatine phosphokinase	740 IU/L *(normal range 25–170)*
Hb	12.1 g/dL
MCV	102 fL

1   What is the diagnosis?
     (a) Hypothyroidism
     (b) Polymyositis
     (c) Inclusion body myositis
     (d) Osteomalacia
     (e) Treatment for hypercholesterolaemia

Question 72

You are called urgently to see a diabetic patient who has become very unwell minutes after being given intravenous ampicillin for a chest infection. She started to wheeze and complain of chest tightness and abdominal pain. Her pulse is 125/min, her blood pressure 95/60 mmHg and she is cyanosed.

1   What is the first medication you would prescribe?
     (a) Adrenaline 0.5–1.0 mL 1:10 000 intramuscularly
     (b) Adrenaline 0.5–1.0 mL 1:10 000 intravenously
     (c) Adrenaline 0.5–1.0 mL 1:1000 intramuscularly
     (d) Adrenaline 0.5–1.0 mL 1:1000 intravenously
     (e) Adrenaline 0.5–1.0 mL 1:100 intramuscularly

Question 73

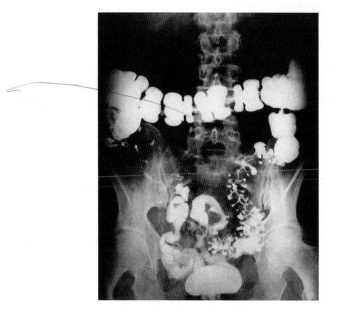

1   What is the diagnosis?
     (a) Ischaemic colitis

(b) Diverticular disease
(c) Pneumocystoides
(d) Ulcerative colitis
(e) 'Apple core' tumour

Question 74

You suspect a patient has Wegener's granulomatosis.

1   What serological investigation would help confirm this?
    (a) Antiglomerular basement membrane antibody
    (b) Anti-double-stranded DNA antibody
    (c) Antinuclear factor
    (d) Antineutrophil cytoplasmic antibody (cytoplasmic staining pattern)
    (e) Antineutrophil cytoplasmic antibody (perinuclear staining pattern)

Question 75

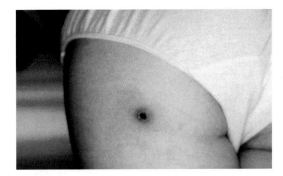

This patient had recently returned from Africa and had a fever and generalized rash.

1   What is the cause of this lesion?
    (a) Rickettsial infection
    (b) Typhoid fever
    (c) American trypanosomiasis
    (d) Tarantula bite
    (e) *Plasmodium falciparum*

Question 76

A 68-year-old lady was admitted following an episode of haemoptysis. She had been unwell for some days with cough productive of green sputum occasionally flecked with blood. On direct questioning she admitted to episodes of diarrhoea over several months. She smoked heavily, although this could not be quantified accurately, and drank a glass of stout per night.

On examination she was thin and cachectic. Her temperature was 38.0°C, pulse 88/min and blood pressure 150/85 mmHg. She had cv (systolic) waves visible in the JVP and a rough pansystolic murmur, audible in the precordium. There were widespread coarse crepitations to auscultation throughout the chest, and mild hepatic enlargement (1 cm), but no other abnormalities in her abdomen. There were no neurological features.

Her chest radiograph showed cardiac enlargement and multiple rounded opacities in both lung fields. These opacities were of differing sizes and had borders that were poorly defined. Hepatic ultrasound showed numerous rounded regions which were relatively poor in echoes.

Full blood count was as follows:

Hb	9.6 g/dL
WBC	15.3×10^9/L
Platelets	431×10^9/L

Biochemistry was within normal limits.

1 What is the diagnosis?
   (a) Staphylococcal pneumonia
   (b) Carcinoid syndrome
   (c) Right heart endocarditis with mycotic emboli
   (d) Metastatic disease from unknown primary
   (e) Wegener's granulomatosis

2 What two investigations should be performed?
   (a) 2D echocardiography
   (b) Urinary 5-hydoxyindoleacetic acid levels
   (c) ESR
   (d) Multiple blood cultures
   (e) CT chest and abdomen
   (f) cANCA
   (g) Open lung biopsy
   (h) Q fever serology
   (i) Staphylococcal serology
   (j) Ultrasound of abdomen

Question 77

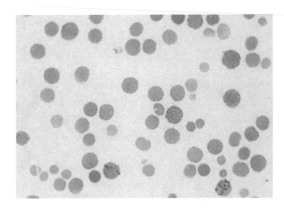

A 16-year-old boy has anaemia and splenomegaly. This is his peripheral blood film stained with cresyl blue.

1 What is the diagnosis?
   (a) Acute myeloid leukaemia
   (b) α-Thalassaemia
   (c) Sickle cell disease
   (d) Malaria
   (e) β-Thalassaemia

Question 78

A 62-year-old woman deteriorates following emergency abdominal surgery for a perforated bowel. She is confused, hypotensive and dyspnoeic. She is transferred to the intensive therapy unit, where the following results are obtained:

Radial artery pressure	80/40 mmHg
Right atrial pressure (mean)	6 mmHg
Pulmonary artery pressure	20/8 mmHg
Pulmonary capillary wedge pressure (mean)	10 mmHg
Cardiac index	8.7 L/min/m² *(normal range 2.6–4.2)*
Chest x-ray	no abnormality

1 What is the most likely diagnosis?
   (a) Acute myocardial infarction
   (b) Acute pneumonia
   (c) Adult respiratory distress syndrome
   (d) Gram-negative septic shock
   (e) Pulmonary embolism

2   What is the cause of her dyspnoea?
    (a) Pericardial effusion
    (b) Metabolic acidosis
    (c) Pulmonary oedema
    (d) Metabolic alkalosis
    (e) Abnormality of central respiratory centre

Question 79

A 69-year-old retired bank manager presented complaining of tripping up while walking. This seemed to be due to weakness of his left leg. However, this was an intermittent problem with episodes lasting for up to 2 days over a period of 2 months and with no apparent factor precipitating each exacerbation. Talking to his wife, it appeared that he had been intermittently mildly confused for several months, on some days uncharacteristically forgetting his grandchildren's names, while on others he would be entirely normal. There was no history of trauma. He was otherwise healthy apart from symptoms of prostatic hypertrophy. On examination, he had upper motor neurone signs of a left hemiparesis, affecting his left leg more than the arm. He was fully orientated and there was no evidence of cognitive impairment. One week later, the symptoms and signs had completely resolved.

1   What are the two most likely possible diagnoses?
    (a) Multi-infarct dementia
    (b) Subdural haematoma
    (c) Parasagittal glioma
    (d) Extradural haematoma
    (e) Recurrent transient ischaemic attacks
    (f) Demyelination
    (g) Alcoholism
    (h) Korsakoff's syndrome
    (i) Hypoglycaemia
    (j) Lead toxicity

Question 80

A patient develops anaphylactic shock and becomes cyanosed. You administer adrenaline, as is appropriate.

1   Name the most important next three management procedures you would initiate:
    (a) Oxygen by nasal cannula
    (b) Oxygen by face mask
    (c) H_1 antagonist intravenously
    (d) H_2 antagonist intravenously
    (e) Dextrose and insulin infusion
    (f) Sodium bicarbonate infusion
    (g) Analgesia

(h) Noradrenaline infusion to avoid dangerous hypotension
(i) Fluids by central venous line to maintain venous pressure
(j) Fluids by peripheral venous line to maintain venous pressure
(k) Infusion of nitrate to maintain blood pressure
(l) Aminophylline infusion
(m) Intravenous hydrocortisone
(n) Insertion of endotracheal tube
(o) Administration of alcohol to counter shock

Question 81

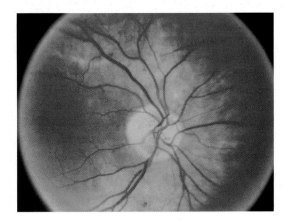

1   What is the diagnosis?
   (a) Proliferative diabetic retinopathy
   (b) Preproliferative diabetic retinopathy
   (c) Hypertensive retinopathy
   (d) Background diabetic retinopathy
   (e) Diabetic maculopathy

Question 82

A 43-year-old woman presents with a 2-month history of nausea and pruritis. The following investigations are performed:

Plasma sodium	142 mmol/L
Plasma potassium	5.9 mmol/L
Plasma urea	36.9 mmol/L
Plasma creatinine	1152 µmol/L
Hb	7.9 g/dL
MCV	58 fL
Serum ferritin	120 µg/L *(normal range 15–300)*

1   What additional test would you request to confirm the more chronic cause of the anaemia?
    (a) Autoimmune screen
    (b) Renal biopsy
    (c) Iron studies
    (d) Chromosomal analysis
    (e) Haemoglobin electrophoresis

Question 83

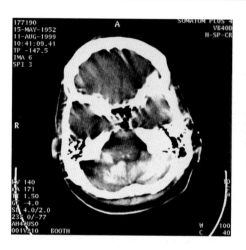 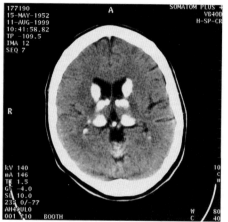

1   Give the most likely diagnosis:
    (a) Hyperparathyroidism
    (b) Multiple intracranial metastases
    (c) Hypoparathyroidism
    (d) Histoplasmosis
    (e) Cysticercosis

Question 84

A 74-year-old woman with a long history of rheumatoid arthritis was admitted with a 2-week history of increasing anorexia, nausea and vomiting. Three weeks previously she had developed an itchy, erythematous rash predominantly over her trunk. This had then faded over a period of 6 days. She had stopped passing urine.

Her rheumatoid arthritis had been treated in the past with gold, but for the past 5 years her only medication had been various non-steroidal inflammatory drugs. She did not drink alcohol, but had smoked 20 cigarettes/day until 5 years ago.

She was confined to a wheelchair by immobility resulting from her arthritis. She was unable to feed herself because of severe deformities of the small joints of the hand. She lived at home with her husband who had given up his job in order to care for her.

On examination, she was slightly confused, but otherwise had no abnormal neurological signs. She had numerous excoriations over her trunk and limbs. Her pulse was 88/min and regular, and her blood pressure was 185/105 mmHg. Her jugular venous pressure was elevated 4 cm and she had slight dependent oedema. The urine contained protein (+) and blood (++), and on microscopy there were 1–2 red blood cells per high power field (hpf), 16 white cells/hpf and 6 granular and white cell casts/hpf. It was sterile on culture. The rest of the physical examination was normal apart from evidence of inactive rheumatoid arthritis.

The results of investigations performed were as follows:

Hb	10.2 g/dL
WBC	11.6×10^9/L *(normal differential count)*
Platelets	223×10^9/L
Plasma sodium	132 mmol/L
Plasma potassium	8.1 mmol/L
Plasma bicarbonate	12 mmol/L
Plasma urea	45 mmol/L
Plasma creatinine	873 µmol/L
Abdominal ultrasound	no evidence of obstruction; renal size within normal limits

1   What is the diagnosis?
   (a) Pyelonephritis
   (b) Interstitial nephritis
   (c) Nephritic syndrome
   (d) Proximal renal tubular acidosis
   (e) Obstructive nephropathy

2   What are your first two management measures?
   (a) Administer an intravenous infusion of bicarbonate
   (b) Attempt to establish a diuresis with high dose furosemide
   (c) Administer an intravenous infusion of salbutamol
   (d) Administer a fluid challenge
   (e) Establish a central venous line
   (f) Administer an intravenous infusion of calcium gluconate (or chloride)
   (g) Administer renal doses of dopamine
   (h) Administer an intravenous infusion of dextrose and insulin
   (i) Commence (or refer for) dialysis
   (j) Administer an ion exchange resin such as Calcium Resonium

Question 85

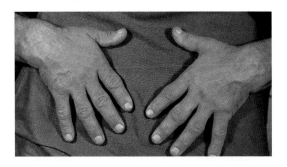

1   What is the diagnosis?
    (a) Achondroplasia
    (b) Acromegaly
    (c) Osteoarthritis
    (d) Gout
    (e) Pseudoachondroplasia

Question 86

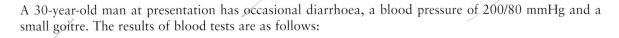

A 30-year-old man at presentation has occasional diarrhoea, a blood pressure of 200/80 mmHg and a small goitre. The results of blood tests are as follows:

Plasma sodium	139 mmol/L
Plasma potassium	4.8 mmol/L
Plasma urea	5.3 mmol/L
Plasma calcium	2.8 mmol/L
Plasma thyroxine	105 nmol/L *(normal range 50–150)*
Plasma TSH	4 mU/L *(normal range 0.5–5)*

1   What is the diagnosis?
    (a) Multiple endocrine neoplasia type I
    (b) Multiple endocrine neoplasia type II
    (c) Isolated VIP-oma
    (d) Isolated phaeochromocytoma
    (e) T4-thyrotoxicosis

Question 87

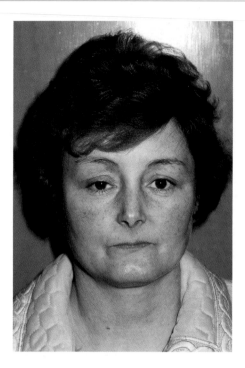

This woman has had a procedure to treat one of the symptoms of her scleroderma.

1   What was it?
    (a) Stellate ganglion block
    (b) Digital sympathectomy
    (c) Lung transplant
    (d) Prostacyclin infusion
    (e) Cyclosporin treatment

Question 88

An A and E SHO asks for your advice over the telephone as to whether a patient can be discharged from A and E. He has made a diagnosis of community-acquired pneumonia. Apart from the following features, the patient is otherwise well.

1   Which of these features is an adverse prognostic feature?
    (a) Age of 51 years
    (b) Oxygen saturation of 95 per cent
    (c) Urea of 6.9 per cent on air
    (d) Respiratory rate of 26/min
    (e) Inability to name the years of the second world war

2   What would you recommend to the A and E SHO?
   (a) Discharge the patient home with oral amoxicillin
   (b) Discharge the patient home with oral erythromycin
   (c) Discharge the patient home with oral amoxicillin and oral erythromycin
   (d) Bleep your house officer and arrange admission
   (e) Tell the A and E SHO that you will come and admit the patient

Question 89

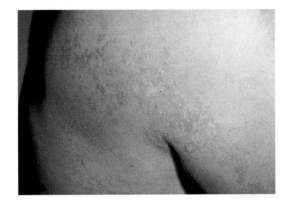

1   What is this papular eruption?
   (a) Herpes zoster
   (b) Psoriasis
   (c) Eczema
   (d) Lichen planus
   (e) Gottron's papules

Question 90

A 35-year-old British chartered surveyor first presented to his GP in 1988 with a 3-week history of sweats, myalgia and lethargy. No diagnosis was made and the symptoms subsided. He presented again in 1992 with similar symptoms and with a single episode of minor haemoptysis. He was a non-smoker and took no medication. He had had no other previous illnesses.

Examination, including urinalysis, revealed no abnormalities.

His chest radiograph showed widespread nodular shadows. No acid-fast bacilli were seen in or grown from numerous sputum samples. A Mantoux test was negative at a dilution of 1:1000 and a Kveim test was negative. Serum angiotensin-converting enzyme activity was 58 (normal range <42).

He was given a complete course of antituberculous chemotherapy and simultaneously a reducing course of prednisolone. Neither produced any change in his radiographic abnormalities although he felt slightly better.

He is now readmitted for further investigations. Serum sodium, potassium, calcium, urea and creatinine are all normal. Repeat Mantoux test is still negative. During this admission he had a generalized tonic–clonic seizure which was witnessed by the house physician.

1   What two investigations would you perform ?
   (a) EEG
   (b) Repeat bronchoscopy with biopsy
   (c) Open lung biopsy
   (d) CT brain
   (e) Repeat serum ACE
   (f) Repeat Kveim test
   (g) Lumbar puncture
   (h) High resolution CT chest
   (i) Induced sputum for AFB
   (j) Autoimmune screen

Question 91

A 45-year-old Kuwaiti was being treated for urinary tract tuberculosis on the basis of a positive urine culture for mycobacteria. Six weeks into his course of antituberculous chemotherapy, he presented feeling nauseated and itchy.

1   The most likely explanation for these symptoms is:
   (a) Allergic reaction to antituberculous drugs
   (b) Emergence of mycobacterial resistance
   (c) Incorrect original diagnosis
   (d) Systemic reaction to the killing of bacteria
   (e) Renal failure

Question 92

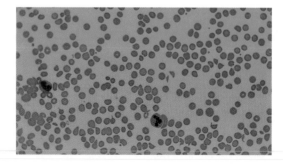

This is the peripheral blood film of an acutely unwell boy 2 weeks following a diarrhoeal illness.

1 What is the likely diagnosis?
   (a) Haemolytic-uraemic syndrome
   (b) Microangiopathic haemolytic anaemia
   (c) Disseminated intravascular coagulopathy
   (d) Thrombotic thrombocytopenic purpura
   (e) Sickle cell disease

Question 93

1 In small intestinal lymphangiectasia, which of the following investigations are unlikely to be diagnostic?
   (a) Small intestinal biopsy
   (b) Barium studies of the small bowel
   (c) Faecal excretion of intravenously administered $^{51}CrCl_3$
   (d) Hydrogen breath test
   (e) Serum immunoglobulin levels

Question 94

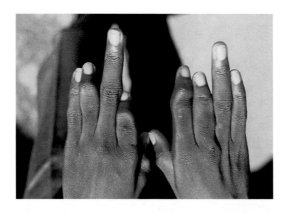

This patient was born with normal sized fingers.

1 What is the likely diagnosis?
   (a) Trauma
   (b) Iron deficiency
   (c) Hyperparathyroidism
   (d) Sickle cell disease
   (e) Osteomyelitis

Question 95

A 23-year-old medical student complains of lethargy, cough and intermittent headache of 4 weeks' duration. He has mild neck stiffness but no focal neurological signs.

CSF findings are:

Opening pressure	270 mm
Appearance	straw-coloured fluid
WBC	$205 \times 10^6/L$ ($205/mm^3$)
Lymphocytes	88 per cent
Neutrophils	8 per cent
Eosinophils	4 per cent
Protein	1.2 g/L
Glucose	1.4 mmol/L
Indian ink stain	negative
Plasma glucose	5.4 mmol/L
VDRL	negative

1 What diagnosis should you first attempt to exclude?
(a) Herpes simplex encephalitis
(b) Tuberculous meningitis
(c) Cerebral abscess
(d) Cerebral toxoplasmosis
(e) Fungal meningitis

Question 96

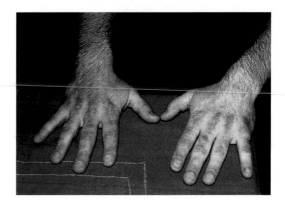

1 What is the diagnosis?
(a) Polymyositis
(b) Dermatomyositis
(c) Addison's disease
(d) Dermatitis artefacta
(e) Bulimia nervosa

Question 97

A 38-year-old secretary gives a several month history of non-specific headaches, fatigue and pruritis. She is on an antihypertensive and painkillers for her headaches. Investigations show:

Hb	11.6 g/dL
WBC	8.0×10^9/L
Plasma bilirubin	40 μmol/L
Plasma aspartate aminotransferase	90 IU/L *(normal range 5–35)*
Plasma alkaline phosphatase	350 IU/L *(normal range 30–100)*
Serum albumin	34 g/L
Serum globulin	48 g/L
Plasma cholesterol	9.0 mmol/L
Hepatitis B surface antigen	negative
Antinuclear factor	1/160
Anti-Sm antibodies	positive

1   What would you include in your differential?
   (a) Hepatitis C
   (b) Resolving hepatitis A
   (c) Analgesia abuse
   (d) Primary biliary cirrhosis
   (e) Autoimmune hepatitis

2   Which two investigations would you request?
   (a) Viral hepatitis serology
   (b) Anti-mitochondrial antibodies
   (c) Bone-specific alkaline phosphatase
   (d) Liver biopsy
   (e) Anti-dsDNA antibodies
   (f) Paracetamol level
   (g) Salicylate level
   (h) Fasting lipid profile
   (i) Protein electrophoresis
   (j) Abdominal ultrasound

Question 98

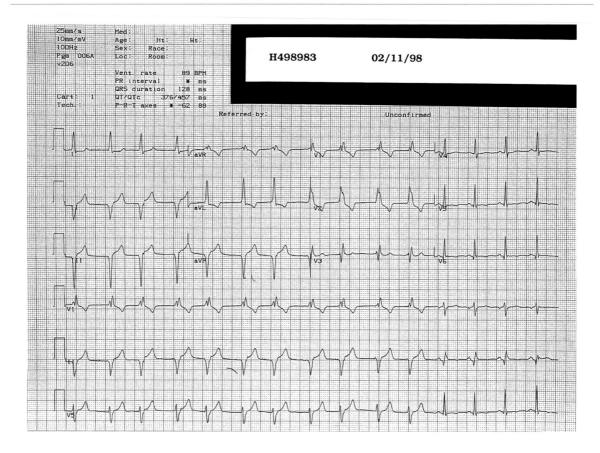

1   This ECG shows:
  (a) Anterior ischaemia
  (b) Complete left bundle branch block
  (c) Partial left bundle branch block
  (d) Fluctuating right bundle branch block
  (e) Left anterior hemiblock

Question 99

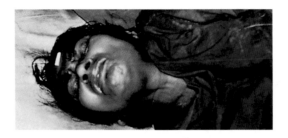

1   What is the diagnosis?
   (a) Thyroid storm
   (b) Tetanus
   (c) Strychnine poisoning
   (d) Cushing's syndrome
   (e) Bilateral orbital cellulitis

Question 100

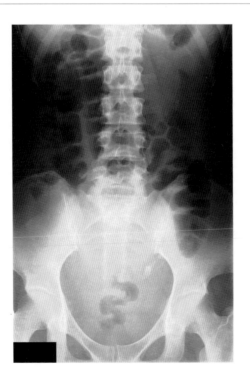

This young woman had an abdominal film after developing constipation. She had recently been to the dentist and been taking analgesics following extraction of wisdom teeth.

1 The x-ray shows:
   (a) Nephrocalcinosis
   (b) Swallowed teeth
   (c) Benign tumour
   (d) Malignant tumour
   (e) Ectopic pregnancy

Answers

Answer 1

1 (a)
2 (c), (g)

Explanation

In renal tubular acidosis (RTA) there is a failure to acidify urine to a level appropriate for blood pH; systemic acidosis is therefore not corrected. Unlike renal failure, anions such as sulphate and phosphate are filtered normally and are therefore unavailable to balance the loss of bicarbonate; electrical neutrality is instead maintained by renal chloride absorption, resulting in a hyperchloraemic metabolic acidosis with a normal anion gap.

In proximal (type II) RTA, there is a diminished renal bicarbonate threshold because bicarbonate reabsorption in the proximal tubules is incomplete. The increased urinary bicarbonate excretion lowers the plasma bicarbonate concentration until a new steady state is reached. At this stage the urine is free of bicarbonate and has an acid pH to match the systemic acidosis. Proximal RTA in its primary form usually presents in infants with failure to thrive, polyuria and growth retardation. Secondary forms may occur in patients with generalized proximal tubular damage due to cystinosis, Wilson's disease or myeloma, and after renal transplantation. There is no metabolic bone disease and nephrocalcinosis is unusual.

The pathophysiology of distal (type I) RTA is complex, but can be thought of in simple terms as a failure of hydrogen ion secretion in the distal tubules. The urine is therefore never acid, even in the presence of systemic acidosis.

The systemic acidosis reduces tubular reabsorption of calcium, resulting in hypercalciuria and secondary hyperparathyroidism: nephrocalcinosis and bone disease are therefore characteristic. Distal RTA is most commonly a dominantly inherited condition.

In both disorders acidosis provokes potassium loss and hypokalaemia, and patients often complain of weakness as a result.

The diagnosis of distal RTA can be made in a patient with a hyperchloraemic metabolic acidosis and a urinary pH above 5.5. If acidosis is mild or absent, an ammonium chloride loading test may be necessary. Normal individuals should lower their urinary pH to below 5.5; patients with distal RTA will not.

Proximal tubular acidosis should be considered especially in patients with hyperchloraemic acidosis and associated features such as glycosuria and aminoaciduria. If the metabolic acidosis is severe enough, an early morning urine of pH 5.5 or less supports the diagnosis. If a low urinary pH is not found, an ammonium chloride test should be performed to exclude the diagnosis of distal RTA. A definitive diagnosis can be made by bicarbonate titration. The characteristic finding is an elevated urinary excretion of bicarbonate in the face of a normal plasma bicarbonate.

This patient has distal RTA as the urine pH is high despite systemic acidosis, and because there is clinical evidence of bone disease and nephrocalcinosis.

Answer 2

1 (d)

Ziehl–Neelsen staining on stool samples is used for detection of mycobacteria or cryptosporidia. The latter are easily identified by red staining of the ovoid or circular oocyst.

Answer 3

1 (d)

Explanation

The differential is that of a very high alkaline phosphatase with a normal calcium in an elderly gentleman. The likely diagnosis is Paget's disease of bone. Rarely it may be confused with osteomalacia, but the calcium is usually low in this condition. Patients with Paget's who are symptomatic should be started on a course of bisphosphonate.

The causes of an elevated alkaline phosphatase are discussed in the answer to Exam A, Question 3.

Answer 4

1 (c)

All the answers bar one are differential diagnoses of mouth ulceration and acute monoarthritis of a large joint. (Those of you tempted to ascribe the oral lesion to leukoplakia should have been put off by the knee pain.) Do not expect any features of the mouth ulcer itself to give any clues as to the diagnoses. It is simply a matter of going through the differential of these two features. It is particularly 'grey' because there is likely to be at least one other important clinical feature that has been omitted. While other answers are possible, these are the best and would attract highest marks.

Answer 5

1 (d)

Explanation

This is probably one of those 'either you know it or you don't' questions and it makes a point that would be disguised in much history and data in the exam.

Causes of mouth ulcers	
Idiopathic aphthous ulcers	Primary skin disorders
Gastrointestinal disorders	Lichen planus
Crohn's disease	Benign mucosal pemphigoid
Ulcerative colitis	Bullous pemphigoid
Coeliac disease	Pemphigus
Behçet's syndrome	Erythema bullosa
Reiter's syndrome	Erythema multiforme
Vasculitis	Dietary deficiencies
Viral infections	Iron
Herpes simplex	Folic acid
Coxsackie	Vitamin B_{12} (pernicious anaemia)
Chickenpox	Pyridoxine
Trigeminal zoster	Riboflavin
HIV	Zinc
Bacterial infections	Haematological disorders
Secondary syphilis	Acute leukaemia
Yersinia	Neutropenia
Tuberculosis	Malignancy
Gonorrhoea	Trauma
Vincent's angina	False teeth
Other infections	Burns
	Candida

Answer 6

1 (c)

Explanation

The diagnosis of Ménière's disease is based on a classical history of fluctuation of the characteristic features: sensorineural deafness, tinnitus, vertigo (typically lasting hours) and a feeling of fullness in the affected ear. The approach to audiograms is discussed in the answer to Exam B, question 34.

Answer 7

1 (c)
2 (a), (c)
3 (a)

As the pregnancy was uncomplicated and the headache occurred 7 days post-delivery, amniotic/fluid embolus is excluded (and does not usually present with headache), and eclampsia is less likely but not impossible. Cerebral venous thrombosis is the commonest cause of cerebrovascular disease in the puerperium and presents with worsening headache, seizures, weakness or numbness.

Answer 8

1 (b), (f)
2 (a), (d)

Essence

A middle-aged man presents with chronic cough, dyspnoea and weight loss, reticular shadowing on chest x-ray and restrictive pattern abnormality on lung function testing.

Differential diagnosis

As discussed previously, the primary question about dyspnoea is whether it is primarily a cardiac or respiratory problem. One may lead to the other, so it is important to sort out as much of the primary problem as possible. In addition, there are causes of dyspnoea that resist categorization as either cardiac or respiratory, such as severe anaemia or hyperventilation.

Here, the absence of any cardiac signs and a plethora of abnormalities related to the lungs points to a pulmonary problem.

Always consider lung disease under a number of categories:

- bronchial
- interstitial
- vascular
- pleural
- chest wall
- neuromuscular.

From the chest x-ray and lung function tests this is clearly an interstitial disease and the rele-

---

Differential diagnosis of interstitial pulmonary fibrosis
- Pneumoconiosis
- Berylliosis
- Extrinsic allergic alveolitis
- Drugs, e.g. nitrofurantoin, busulphan, bleomycin, amiodarone, methotrexate (even low dose)
- Radiation
- Uraemia
- Chronic pulmonary venous hypertension
- Sarcoidosis
- Histiocytosis X
- Autoimmune disease
    - Rheumatoid arthritis
    - SLE
    - Progressive systemic sclerosis
    - MCTD (mixed connective tissue disease)
    - Sjögren's disease
    - Polymyositis/dermatomyositis
    - Chronic active hepatitis
    - Autoimmune thyroid disease
    - Ulcerative colitis
    - Pernicious anaemia
- Cryptogenic

vant differential diagnosis is that of interstitial pulmonary fibrosis.

Since there are no clues from the history suggesting that the pulmonary fibrosis is part of a multisystem disorder, or secondary to another specific cause such as one of the above drugs, we are left with purely pulmonary causes. While it is true that certain of the autoimmune diseases may present with pulmonary fibrosis before extrathoracic manifestations appear, this is rare and these would be classified as cryptogenic fibrosing alveolitis at this stage. In practice, you would of course arrange autoimmune serology, but all the 'connective tissue diseases' require features other than pulmonary fibrosis and positive serology for diagnosis, so this is actually an unhelpful investigation.

This whittles down the differential to extrinsic allergic alveolitis (EAA), sarcoidosis, histiocytosis X, and cryptogenic fibrosing alveolitis (CFA). CFA is associated with inspiratory crepitations and basal fibrosis and is less likely in their absence. Clubbing occurs in 50 per cent so this is a less discriminatory feature. Patients with histiocytosis X usually have no abnormalities on examination but have a characteristic bronchoalveolar lavage with 'histiocytosis X' cells. EAA may present as either chronic or acute disease, and in a significant percentage of the chronic disease, no precipitating cause is ever found. In acute disease the bronchoalveolar lavage is typically neutrophilic. Respiratory crepitations and clubbing are uncommon in chronic EAA, and fibrosis usually spares the lung bases. Chronic EAA is the most likely diagnosis; although normal SACE does not formally exclude lone thoracic sarcoidosis, it is less likely. Kveim tests are no longer done because of the risk of new variant CJD. In practice, high resolution CT and possibly transbronchial biopsy might be undertaken as alternatives to a trial of steroid therapy. Beryllium was used in the manufacture of ceramics and is still used in the nuclear industry and in the manufacture of x-ray tubes. Chronic berylliosis presents as the result of a chronic exposure to beryllium, or years after an acute toxic exposure. It presents in an identical way to sarcoidosis and the pathological lesion is similar. Only 50 cases have ever been reported in the UK and so it is much less likely an answer than sarcoidosis.

Management

The two management strategies available with chronic EAA are an exhaustive search for and elimination of the precipitating antigen, and steroid therapy. For lone thoracic sarcoidosis, the only option is steroid therapy.

While further information is occasionally obtained from lung biopsy, this is an invasive procedure with a significant complication rate. It is worth noting that secondary fibrotic lung disease (EAA and in association with autoimmune disease) is generally more steroid responsive and of better prognosis than CFA.

The disease course is clearly too indolent for carcinoma or infection.

Pulmonary fibrosis and the idiopathic interstitial pneumonias (IIPs)

There are a number of known aetiologies for pulmonary fibrosis which are diverse, including physical (e.g. radiation), drug-related (e.g. bleomycin) and infective causes (e.g. tuberculosis). However, a great proportion of the disease burden remains of unknown aetiology and there has been much controversy over the classification of this condition. For many years, cases where the aetiology of pulmonary fibrosis was unknown were referred to as cryptogenic fibrosing alveolitis (CFA), or idiopathic pulmonary fibrosis (IPF). However, nowadays, where the cause of pulmonary fibrosis is unknown the disease is referred to as idiopathic interstitial pneumonia.

The American Thoracic Society/European Thoracic Society have recently devised a schema to emphasize the importance of an integrated clinical and pathological approach to the diagnosis of idiopathic interstitial pneumonia (see table on next page). Seven idiopathic interstitial pneumoniae have now been characterized as separate disease entities. The most important of these conditions is called idiopathic pulmonary fibrosis or cryptogenic fibrosing alveolitis (IPF/CFA). Whereas this diagnosis was previously ascribed to all cases of pulmonary fibrosis of unknown aetiol-

The diagnosis of idiopathic interstitial pneumonia

Histological pattern	Clinicopathological diagnosis
Usual interstitial pneumonia (UIP)	Cryptogenic fibrosing alveolitis (CFA)/idiopathic pulmonary fibrosis (IPF)
Non-specific interstitial pneumonia (NSIP)	Non-specific interstitial pneumonia
Organizing pneumonia (OP)	Cryptogenic organizing pneumonia/bronchiolitis obliterans-organizing pneumonia (BOOP)
Diffuse alveolar damage (DAD)	Acute interstitial pneumonia (AIP)
Desquamative interstitial pneumonia (DIP)	Desquamative interstitial pneumonia (DIP)
Respiratory bronchiolitis (RB)	Respiratory bronchiolitis-associated interstitial lung disease (RBILD)
Lymphocytic interstitial pneumonia (LIP)	Lymphocytic interstitial pneumonia (LIP)

Common clinicopathological features of fibrosing interstitial lung diseases

Clinical	Pathological
Progressive dyspnoea on exertion	Fibrosis of the interstitium involving collagen, smooth muscle and elastic elements
Non-productive cough	Architectural remodelling of the interstitium
Abnormal breath sounds on auscultation	Chronic inflammation of the interstitium
Abnormal chest x-ray or HRCT scan	Hyperplasia of type II cells
Restrictive pattern and reduced capacity of the lung for carbon monoxide (DLCO) on lung function tests	Hyperplasia of endothelial cells

ogy, it is now a very specific condition where the histological pattern seen on biopsy is termed usual interstitial pneumonia (UIP). It is now realized that it is very important to distinguish this condition from the six other IIPs since the clinical course of UIP is very different. Median survival for IPF/CFA is only 2.9 years following diagnosis, which is considerably worse than any of the other IIPs. In addition, IPF/CFA appears to be far more resistant to conventional anti-inflammatory therapies, which are the main therapeutic approach available for the treatment of this disease.

Answer 9

1   (d)

The triangular sclerotic area at the inferior aspect on the iliac side of the left sacroiliac joint (osteitis

condensans ileii) is of no relevance to her back pain; it is commonly seen in multiparous woman. Osteoporosis cannot be diagnosed with plain films. The cause of her back pain is not apparent from these x-rays.

Answer 10

1   (c)

The answer is best explained using the following pedigree.

In order to have an affected child with an autosomal recessive disease, the mother must be a carrier, i.e. heterozygous. If her cousin is also heterozygous, the probability of them having an affected child is 1 in $(2 \times 2) = 1/4$. As shown in the pedigree, the probability that her cousin is also heterozygous for the abnormal gene is 1/8. Thus the overall probability that a child will be affected is 1 in $2 \times (2 \times 8) = 1/32$.

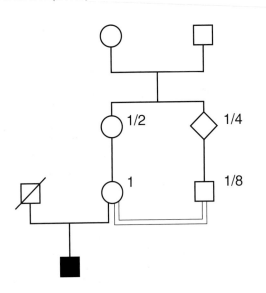

Answer 11

1 (c)

An arteriogram is likely to show coronary artery disease or an aneurysm at some site; the shape of the internal carotid should be recognizable and allow sufficient orientation to point towards the anterior communicating artery, which is also the commonest site of a cerebral aneurysm (30 per cent), with 25 per cent on the PCA and 20 per cent at the middle cerebral bifurcation.

Answer 12

1 (c)

Radiologically, this is more likely to be Paget's disease because of the asymmetrical distribution of the lesions and also their hemipelvic distribution. However, multiple sclerotic bony metastases cannot be excluded.

Answer 13

1 (c)
2 (a)

Explanation

Microangiopathic haemolytic anaemia (MAHA) and disseminated intravascular coagulation (DIC) are two popular conditions which often come up in the Membership. They may present similarly, i.e. bleeding and with similar aetiologies.

In MAHA, damage to small vessel vascular endothelium causes adherence of fibrin fragments which trap and fragment erythrocytes and platelets. In pure MAHA, clotting is therefore normal. The blood film is characteristic, with red cell fragments and fibrin strands, and nucleated red cells due to the reticulocytosis.

DIC results when a variety of insults cause simultaneous thrombosis and fibrinolysis within the circulation. This may be low grade and compensated and therefore clinically unapparent, or may be unbalanced with consumption of clotting factors and haemorrhage. In pure DIC, any anaemia is due to bleeding and clotting is deranged due to consumption of coagulation factors. FDPs are elevated as fibrinolysis is also occurring. The trauma to red cells from deposits of fibrin in small vessels may itself be sufficient to cause a MAHA.

The common causes of both these disorders are a variety of obstetric disasters, sepsis and carcinoma. Less common causes of MAHA which may occur in Membership type questions are:

- haemolytic uraemic syndrome and thrombocytopenic purpura (discussed further in Exam C, Answer 66)
- accelerated hypertension
- scleroderma crisis
- drugs: oral contraceptive, cyclosporin A, mitomycin.

In the case presented here, a white cell differential count will not contribute to the diagnosis. Similarly, various indicators of haemolysis (e.g.

elevated methaemalbumin, unconjugated bilirubin, reduced haptoglobins) will not establish the type of haemolysis. The mean corpuscular volume could theoretically help to distinguish anaemia due to bleeding from that due to haemolysis. However, the anaemia is too acute to be reflected by a real fall in MCV, and this parameter may be elevated by the reticulocytosis. The presence of leucocytosis argues against a diagnosis of bone marrow failure secondary to sepsis. Finally, whilst pre-eclampsia and amniotic fluid embolus are causes of MAHA in pregnancy, they are diseases of the second and third trimesters.

Answer 14

1 (a)

Acanthocytes are abnormal red blood cells which can be recognized by their spicules. If you see them in Membership, the likely diagnosis is abetalipoproteinaemia, although they may be seen in fewer numbers in severe liver disease and haemolytic anaemia (Zieve's syndrome).

Interpreting blood films in Membership

For many candidates (and at least one of the authors of this book), the prospect of interpreting blood films produces an acute feeling of nausea! The reason is simple – candidates have a reason-able chance of having come across most Membership cases in real life, but most physicians rarely, if ever, have to look at blood films.

Once again, a little focused pre-examination groundwork can pay dividends. First, try to remember what different red cell abnormalities look like. The differential diagnosis for each abnormality is often quite limited. Sometimes you are asked to understand the red cell abnormalities in addition to, or even instead of, providing a diagnosis. Cynics might say that if you can describe the appearance of the cell in Greek, you might stand a chance of getting the right answer! This may not be entirely correct, but there is some truth in it. For instance, remember that a description ending in -cytosis refers to the size of the cell whereas -chromia (or -chromasia) refers to haemoglobinization. It then does not take a genius to work out that microcytosis means small cells, elliptocytosis means elliptical cell or hypochromasia means pale-staining.

All this might sound patronizingly straightforward, but simple logic often deserts candidates in the examination room. If you are asked to describe the abnormalities in a blood film with red cells of variable shape and staining, you should be able to work out that they show poikilocytosis (variable shape, not to be confused with anisocytosis which is variable size) and polychromasia.

We have provided several examples of red cell abnormalities in questions in this book, but below is a diagrammatical representation of some of the abnormalities:

Abnormality	Significance
Acanthocytes	Occur in genetic disorders of lipid metabolism
Anisocytosis	Simply means variation in size
Basophilic stippling	Represents RNA and reflects defective haemoglobin synthesis. Seen in the dyserythropoietic anaemias, such as lead poisoning and thalassaemia
Burr cells	Irregularly shaped cells which occur in uraemia, Ca stomach, pyruvate kinase deficiency and hypokalaemia
Elliptocytes	Ovoid cells which occur in abundance in hereditary elliptocytosis
Howell–Jolly bodies	Nuclear remnants seen most often following splenectomy
Hypochromia	Pale-staining because of defective haemoglobinization; usually due to iron deficiency or defective haemoglobin synthesis (thalassaemia, sideroblastic anaemia)
Microcytosis	Small cells due to defective haemoglobinization. In iron deficiency, the lack of haemoglobin in the developing cell leads to an extra cell division, the result being smaller mature cells
Macrocytosis	Large cells due to dyserythropoiesis or premature release. May indicate a megaloblastic anaemia (low vitamin B_{12} or folate – look for hypersegmented polymorphs) when there is one less cell division during red blood cell division. Causes of simple macrocytosis include alcohol, liver disease, myelosuppressive drugs, reticulocytosis and myxoedema
Poikilocytosis	Variable shaped cells (this general description includes Burr cells, tear-drops and schistocytes)
Polychromasia	Also called anisochromasia. Variation in haemoglobinization or presence in film of red blood cells of different ages (e.g. in response to bleeding, haemolysis or dyserythropoiesis)
Reticulocytes	Young, often large, red cells signify active erythropoiesis (e.g. in haemolysis)
Schistocytes	Fragmented red cells. Seen in intravascular haemolysis
Sickle cells	Characteristic of sickle cell disease
Spherocytes	Spherical cells. Indicates damage to the cell membrane; may be genetic (hereditary spherocytosis) or acquired (following red cell damage, e.g. haemolysis)
Target cells	Red cells with central staining, a ring of pallor and a thin outer ring of staining. Seen in deficient haemoglobinization (e.g. thalassaemia, liver disease, iron deficiency anaemia and hyposplenism). In liver disease it is thought to be due to altered lipid components in the cell membrane
Tear-drop poikilocyte	A prominent feature of myelofibrosis

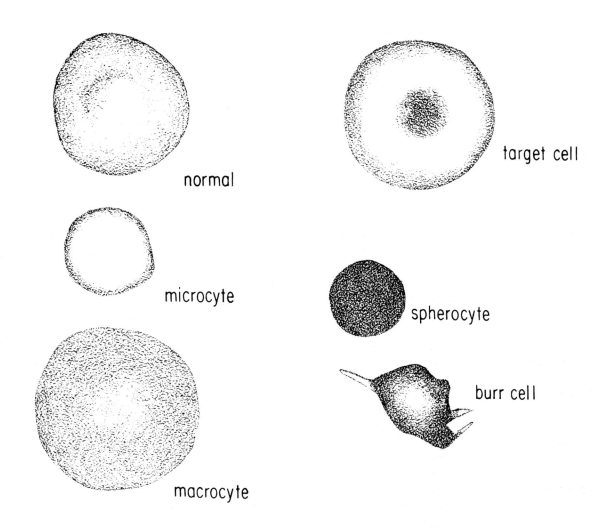

normal

target cell

microcyte

spherocyte

macrocyte

burr cell

Answer 15

1 (a)

Essence

A young man, whose brother has Gilbert's syndrome, develops hepatocellular jaundice, hepatosplenomegaly and lymphadenopathy after a 'flu-like' illness.

Differential diagnosis

The clinical picture of anaemia, thrombocytopenia, presence of a cold agglutinin, lymphocytosis, jaundice, hepatosplenomegaly, and lymphadenopathy may indicate any of the 'infectious mononucleoses' (EBV, CMV, HIV, toxoplasmosis or hepatitis B). The biochemistry excludes obstructive jaundice and the clinical picture is not that of Gilbert's syndrome – unconjugated hyperbilirubinaemia in the absence of any sign of liver disease or haemolysis – even though there is a strong familial tendency. He had never been abroad and thus brucellosis is unlikely. Lymphoma and leukaemia must be looked for if the initial infection screen proves to be negative. The presence of a tattoo and several sexual contacts represent risk factors for the hepatitis viruses. The blood film shows atypical lymphocytes that may be seen in EBV, CMV, toxoplasmosis, rubella and lymphoma. EBV is still the most likely diagnosis despite the negative Monospot test. The Monospot test checks for the heterophil antibody, which is absent in up to 15 per cent of cases. EBV remains a diagnosis based on clinical as well as biochemical data.

Answer 16

1 (e)

The CT scan shows a fluid level in the maxillary sinus. She also has ear disease and neuropathy; Wegener's is the likely diagnosis.

Answer 17

1 (e)

The differential diagnosis of a cavitating lesion includes infection, tumour (primary or secondary), granuloma, infarction, or congenital abnormality. Useful distinguishing features include location, single versus multiple, wall thickness and regularity, other pulmonary features. In this case the apical location, thick, smooth wall and surrounding fibrosis suggest tuberculosis.

Answer 18

1 (b)

Be careful in putting together all the unusual information. A 26-year-old who has a normal cranial and peripheral nerve examination, but who has a carer, is highly likely to have learning difficulties. She has had a DVT, and in such a young person you would have to probe deeply as to a cause. You are not given much information in this case. However, she does have a high arch palate and is tall. You may have been tempted to consider Marfan's disease but this is not associated with thrombosis, nor low IQ. The cardiac

murmur is probably an innocent physiological flow murmur – the cardiac defect associated with Marfan's does not cause the patient's murmur.

This patient has homocystinuria. She should be given a trial of pyridoxine, initially at a dose of 150–300 mg/day, to see if the homocystine and methionine levels reduce. In adult patients it is sometimes only possible to achieve this with a low protein diet. As she is at risk of osteoporosis then calcium and vitamin D_3 can be prescribed but this answer is not as favourable as pyridoxine.

Oestrogen and progesterone are used in female Marfan's patients who are prepubertal in an attempt to stop skeletal growth.

Marfan (6 letters)
- Aortic (6) root dilation
- Mitral (6) valve prolapse
- Upward (6) lens dislocation
- Clever (6) – normal IQ

Homocystin (8 letters)
- Clotting (8) abnormal
- Thrombus (8) formation
- Downward (8) lens dislocation
- Retarded (8) – low IQ

Answer 19

1 (b)

Essence

An ECG showing sinus bradycardia with small complexes.

Discussion

The possibilities include hypothermia but the patient is on a long-stay ward, which one can assume is heated adequately. The most likely scenario is of hypothyroidism leading to bradycardia with a pericardial effusion leading to the small complexes.

Answer 20

1 (c)

This characteristic lesion appears as a red-brown patch and slowly enlarges and becomes yellow and atrophic. As almost a half of these patients do not have, or will not develop, diabetes it is reasonable not to use the word 'diabeticorum'.

Answer 21

1 (d)

There are many causes of pubertal delay in adolescents. It is defined as no sign of puberty in a girl of 13 or in a boy of 14. They can be divided into hypogonadism or constitutional. Hypogonadism may be due to hypogonadotrophic failure (where there is a failure of the pituitary to produce LH and FSH) or hypergonadotrophic failure (where there is a failure of the ovary or testis to respond). With constitutional delay there is a delay in bone age and a delay in puberty, whereas in hypogonadism there is a normal bone age and only a delay in puberty. In this case the patient's bone age is still 13, thereby giving indication that he still has growth available to him once he enters

puberty and hence he has constitutional delay. He is on course to be the same height as his parents. As there is no family history of pubertal delay, the likely cause is sporadic.

Answer 22

1 (c)

Essence

A middle-aged woman presents with chronic epigastric pain and weight loss and now with pruritus and cholestatic jaundice.

Differential diagnosis

The combination of cholestatic jaundice, anaemia, high ESR, palpable gallbladder, diabetes and bilirubin in the urine suggests an obstructive jaundice, most likely due to malignancy. The candidate sites are carcinoma of the head of pancreas, bile ducts or secondaries to the porta hepatis. Sixty per cent of pancreatic tumours involve the head of the pancreas, 25 per cent the ampulla, and 15 per cent the tail. Usually enough islet beta cells survive to maintain normoglycaemia, but frank diabetes may occur. It is unlikely that this picture is due to gallstones since a fibrotic reaction is excited by the stones and thus the gallbladder becomes impalpable. Hepatomegaly and diabetes should suggest haemochromatosis; however, she is jaundiced rather than bronzed, has a high ESR and obstructive clinical (palpable gallbladder) and biochemical picture. These latter features are against haemochromatosis.

The highest diagnostic yield will come from an endoscopic retrograde cholangiopancreatogram (ERCP). In practice, patients are likely to have an ultrasound examination first and if the lesion is thought to be hilar, a CT scan of the abdomen also. They will then proceed to ERCP even if the diagnosis has already been made as this allows a stent to be inserted. However, the ultrasound scan may not be diagnostic.

Causes of pubertal delay

Constitutional delay
- Sporadic
- Familial

Hypogonadotrophic hypogonadism
- Chronic diseases
- Malnutrition
- Pituitary disease

Hypergonadotrophic hypogonadism
- Congenital (e.g. Turner's and Klinefelter's)
- Acquired (e.g. post torsion or chemotherapy)

Answer 23

1   (b)

Essence

A young man with self-inflicted eye damage due to obsessive behaviour, foul language and repeated gesturing, presents drunk.

Differential diagnosis

You either do or do not recognize the clinical description. This constellation of obsessive behaviour, often self-destructive, with foul language, tics and gestures are diagnostic of Gilles de la Tourette syndrome. The famous lexicographer Dr Samuel Johnson was said to be a sufferer, and indeed to have lost a job as a schoolteacher because his odd behaviour upset the pupils. The ocular lesion might just sound like severe unilateral chemosis, as occasionally occurs in Graves' disease. However, nothing else is compatible with that diagnosis. Indeed, it is hypothyroidism that is more associated with psychiatric symptoms.

Answer 24

1   (d)

The blood film shows tear-drop poikilocytes which are characteristic of myelofibrosis. They do not qualify as the red cell 'fragments' of microangiopathic haemolytic anaemia. Nor do they look hypochromic or microcytic. The white cells look normal. The presence of nucleated red cells is also characteristic of myelofibrosis. Anisocytosis also occurs, but is not very marked on this particular film. Strictly, bone marrow examination is necessary to confirm the diagnosis.

Answer 25

1   (a), (d)

Explanation

A useful way to interpret arterial blood gases in respiratory disease is to first distinguish acute from chronic hypoxaemia, and then consider the presence or absence of carbon dioxide retention.

- Marked acute hypoxaemia without CO_2 retention is characteristic of pulmonary embolism, asthma, pulmonary oedema, pulmonary haemorrhage and pneumothorax.
- Acute hypoxaemia with CO_2 retention implies a failure of ventilation rather than a problem at the site of gas exchange. Thus there may be failure of the respiratory drive (e.g. respiratory depressants), failure to transmit this drive (e.g. Guillain–Barré syndrome, myasthenia gravis) or mechanical problems of lung expansion (e.g. chest wall injury, severe obstructive defect, stiff lungs due to severe oedema).
- Chronic hypoxaemia without CO_2 retention can develop as a result of any chronic lung disease where ventilation is relatively unimpaired: pulmonary fibrosis, chronic airflow limitation and emphysema and recurrent thromboembolism.
- Chronic hypoxaemia with CO_2 retention will develop as the end stage of chronic hypoxaemia without CO_2 retention, or when a combination of the above develops.
- The acute onset and occupational history are typical clues to suggest pulmonary embolism as a cause of hypoxaemia. The non-invasive investigation to confirm this is a ventilation-perfusion isotope scan (not the shorthand VQ scan). Unfortunately, this may not provide a definitive diagnosis and if the clinical suspicion is high, the next stage will be to perform a CT pulmonary angiogram.
- Massive pulmonary embolism is defined as obstruction of 50 per cent or more of the pulmonary arterial bed on angiography. In the real world, investigations take time and may not be available in the same hospital.

Initiation of therapy may be necessary without definitive diagnosis. If there is systemic hypotension, hypoxia, and evidence of shock in the appropriate clinical context, thrombolytic therapy is warranted; if this is contraindicated, pulmonary embolectomy is the only viable option.

- Smaller pulmonary emboli may cause infarction with or without pleuritic chest pain, with recurrent episodes giving rise to a syndrome of sustained pulmonary hypertension.

Answer 26

1   (d)

As with the classical acute erythematous butterfly rash of SLE, the chronic scarring discoid lesions tend to appear in the malar region, although other sites may be affected. Discoid lesions progress from erythema and oedema to follicular plugging and telangiectasia, and then atrophy with scarring and alteration in pigmentation. They usually have well-defined margins. Discoid lesions are found in about one-fifth of patients with SLE, but only 10 per cent of patients with chronic discoid lesions go on to develop any other feature of lupus. This lesion is rather distinctive clinically. Unusually, sarcoidosis, tuberculosis or lichen planus could produce a similar pattern.

Answer 27

1   (b)

A palliative care question is expected from the RCP guidance on subjects for questions. In this case the patient has obstruction from a compressive lesion. Metoclopramide is a prokinetic agent and would therefore be contraindicated in intestinal obstruction. Ondansetron causes constipation and would therefore make matters worse. Dexamethasone and Nozinan (levomepromazine) are useful second-line agents.

Answer 28

1   (b)

The red cells show microcytosis and hypochromasia. The commonest cause for this anaemia is iron deficiency.

Answer 29

1   (a), (b)

Essence

Sudden-onset severe neck pain and relative hypotension with no physical or ECG signs in a late middle-aged man with a predisposition to atherosclerosis.

Differential diagnosis

Sudden-onset severe pain above the diaphragm does not have a long differential. The most common causes are myocardial infarction, aortic dissection, subarachnoid haemorrhage, pleural disease (including following pulmonary embolism), oesophageal rupture, vertebral collapse (and other fractures), disc prolapse and the neuralgias and neuropathies. The pain of pneumothorax is rarely severe and is usually overshadowed by the dyspnoea. The absence of any other features confines the differential to myocardial infarction and aortic dissection – indeed, there are two predisposing factors for atherosclerosis. (Chronic low back pain is too common to be a valuable pointer to disc prolapse or vertebral collapse.) A normal ECG is entirely compatible with a diagnosis of infarction and normal chest x-ray and peripheral pulses are compatible with aortic dissection. Similarly, the site of the pain, although more typical of a dissection, does not exclude an infarction. Caught in a situation of being unable to differentiate between two or more diagnoses (partly implied by the question, unusually for this examination, by the use of the phrase 'most likely') it is reasonable to choose the more common condition – acute MI. The question allows you to reveal the next most likely diagnosis.

In the event, the patient underwent an urgent angiogram to exclude dissection and was found to have an acute occlusion of his inferior coronary artery. He did very well.

Answer 30

1 (b)

Explanation

Sodium depletion is the major biochemical abnormality resulting from adrenocorticoid hypofunction. When hyponatraemia occurs in the presence of haemoconcentration (raised urea and creatinine) and hypoglycaemia, candidates must think of this diagnosis. Acute adrenal insufficiency is marked by hypotension and shock. Chronic insufficiency often results in postural hypotension. Other symptoms of chronic insufficiency include weight loss, malaise, vomiting, diarrhoea and non-specific abdominal pain.

It is difficult to distinguish primary adrenal insufficiency (Addison's disease) from ACTH deficiency. Pigmentation, which suggests Addison's disease, may be absent in those with autoimmune disease. ACTH deficiency is most commonly the result of exogenous steroid therapy. Otherwise, it occurs as part of generalized pituitary and hypothalamic disease. Spontaneous isolated ACTH deficiency is very rare, as is Sheehan's syndrome (pituitary infarction during pregnancy). Hypoglycaemia (especially fasting) is caused by the absence of glucocorticoids. Other abnormalities include a raised plasma potassium and a metabolic acidosis.

In the West, the commonest form of Addison's is autoimmune. Rarer causes include amyloidosis and disseminated malignancy. However, tuberculosis used to be the most common cause and this must be seriously considered in high-risk individuals, such as the patient in this case. Because of the increased probability of tuberculosis, you would

be awarded more marks for a diagnosis of Addison's than ACTH deficiency.

Answer 31

1 (b)

Despite the presence of a left pleural effusion, there is no doubt about the diagnosis. The whole mediastinum (including the heart) has been pushed across.

Answer 32

1 (b), (d)
2 (d)
3 (e)

You are being asked to understand the principles of electromyography and to recognize a clinical picture. Undamaged normal muscle is electrically quiet at rest; contraction induces large action potentials. If there is muscle loss (myopathy) or 'loss of communication' between nerve and muscle, these action potentials are smaller. If there is denervation (neuropathy, plexopathy, radiculopathy), sensitivity to acetylcholine rises and there are spontaneous discharges (fasciculation and fibrillations), as in this case. Large amplitude motor units reflect sprouting of axons attempting to innervate adjacent muscle. The findings here therefore suggest chronic partial denervation in right supraspinatus, right extensor digitorum communis and right extensor digitorum communis. This is a very typical history for neuralgic amyotrophy, with pain around the shoulder, evidence of patchy denervation (but no generalized polyneuropathy) and then slow recovery. The cause is unknown, it is rarely bilateral or relapsing, and the principal differential is cervical radiculopathy, which might have got some marks. Of course, trapezius is likely to be normal, but you cannot say so on the basis of the available data.

Answer 33

1   (d)

The rash of measles occurs initially on the forehead and then spreads rapidly to involve the rest of the body. At first the rash is discrete but later becomes confluent and patchy. It is dark red initially then fades in a week, leaving a brownish discoloration with desquamation. In rubella a short-lived pink macular rash (if it occurs at all) starts behind the ears and on the forehead and spreads to the face, trunk and limbs. In roseola infantum (also known as exanthem subitum) the rash is pink, more like rubella than measles. The rash in this picture is typical of measles.

Viral causes of maculopapular rash
- Measles (synonym: rubeola)
- Rubella (synonym: German measles)
- Epstein–Barr virus
- Cytomegalovirus
- Adenovirus
- Parvovirus
- Enterovirus
- Hepatitis B

---

important point is that a definitive diagnosis requires muscle biopsy, and that inflammatory and non-inflammatory conditions can be difficult to distinguish.

Insidious symmetrical proximal muscle weakness results from muscle inflammation in dermatomyositis. The disease mainly affects women of between 40 and 50 years. Dysphagia, dysphonia, respiratory weakness, cardiomyopathy, lung collapse and fibrosis may develop. Approximately 25 per cent of patients have a purple skin rash, especially in areas exposed to sunlight, and some may have a 'heliotrope' (a lilac flower) rash around the eyes. Telangiectasia may be found on the face, arms and chest. Diagnosis is by muscle enzymes (CPK and serum aldolase), electromyography and muscle biopsy.

Malignancy is present in approximately 10 per cent of all patients and in over 50 per cent of men presenting over the age of 50 years. The most commonly associated tumours are carcinoma of the lung, prostate, ovary, breast, uterus or large intestine. Treatment or removal of the tumour may result in a remarkable improvement in the muscle disease.

Causes of a raised CPK are given in Exam A, Answer 39.

Answer 34

1   (a), (b)
2   (c)

The picture of muscle weakness with raised muscle enzymes is non-specific and may be found in acute vasculitic neuropathy (both due to acute denervation and involvement of muscle in the vasculitic process, although the CK is not usually this high), muscular dystrophy, myositis and drug-induced myopathies. The use of steroids may have contributed to the telangiectasia but steroid myopathy is not usually associated with raised muscle enzymes. All the investigations are non-specific although all may be helpful and the

Answer 35

1   (a)

These are Leishman–Donovan bodies (amastigotes of *Leishmania donovani*) which can be seen intra- and extracellularly. The amastigotes are ovoid with a large nucleus. The tachyzooites or bradyzooites of *Toxoplasma gondii* have a similar appearance (slightly more elongated than ovoid) but the biopsy material is usually from a fetus or cyst biopsy. If all else fails, go through a list of parasitic causes of hepatomegaly, and having excluded malaria (a purely intracellular parasite, which there is no excuse for missing), leishmaniasis should be your next choice.

Answer 36

1 (e)

The clinical syndrome of erythema nodosum, bihilar lymphadenopathy and ankle ± knee arthritis (Lofgren's syndrome) is sufficiently typical of acute sarcoidosis not to require further investigations. It often requires short courses of prednisolone for adequate anti-inflammatory treatment, but is of benign prognosis (>90 per cent remission). It is prudent to repeat the chest x-ray after a couple of months to ensure regression.

Answer 37

1 (d)

Explanation

This question makes two important points:

*   First, the answer to data interpretation may be in part gleaned from the clinical presentation. Context suggests that you should be looking for a complication of myocardial infarction, and the predominance of signs of right ventricular impairment with no response to diuretics suggests that the right ventricle has infarcted.
*   Second, cardiac pressure questions are easy to answer, even without knowledge of normal values. Basic physiology tells you that left-sided filling pressures should be higher than right-sided; here the end-diastolic or filling pressure of the right ventricle is higher than the end-diastolic pressure in the left ventricle, which is reflected by the left atrial and hence pulmonary wedge pressures.

Right ventricular infarction is usually associated with inferior infarction. The principal differential diagnosis is pulmonary embolism (different presentation, elevated pulmonary artery pressures). Ventricular septal defect would present with dyspnoea and have higher right ventricular

pressures. The answer 'right heart failure following a myocardial infarction' is less precise and might attract fewer marks.

Answer 38

1 (a)

The blood film shows two blast cells each with an Auer rod in the cytoplasm. Auer rods are only seen in myeloid lineage cells and almost always in myeloblasts. In Membership, an Auer rod means AML.

Answer 39

1 (b)

Explanation

The direct cross-match is a test for the presence of pre-existing anti-HLA antibodies, specific for a given donor, in the potential recipient. It is well recognized that the presence of these antibodies may cause devastating hyperacute rejection resulting in the loss of the graft. Thus a positive cross-match is a contraindication to transplantation. It is not to be confused with the cross-match that is done prior to blood transfusion. This is a confusing issue since incompatible ABO blood groups between donor and recipient also constitutes a contraindication for transplantation, but is not the issue being addressed in a direct cross-match test in this context.

Answer 40

1 (c)

Failure of relaxation of the lower oesophageal sphincter and of oesophageal peristalsis causes dysphagia. Solids and liquids are swallowed only slowly and stasis of food with oesophageal expansion occurs. Other pictures of achalasia that may be shown include a chest x-ray with an air/fluid level behind the heart and/or a double right heart border produced by a grossly expanded oesophagus.

Answer 41

1 (e)

There is a nail-fold infarct and proximal interphalangeal joint synovitis.

Answer 42

1 (c)

Essence

A 67-year-old with chronic rheumatoid arthritis, previously on penicillamine and now on steroids and indometacin, has non-specific symptoms, hepatosplenomegaly, proteinuria and renal failure. He bled following a renal biopsy.

Differential diagnosis

There are three 'hard facts' in this case: renal failure, rheumatoid arthritis and hepatosplenomegaly. This triad makes amyloid the only likely explanation. Do not be thrown by the drug history – drugs are not the only cause of problems.

For a discussion of renal disease in rheumatoid arthritis, see Exam C, Answer 84.

Note also that amyloid infiltration can make tissues more prone to haemorrhage and may have predisposed to the haemorrhage post-renal biopsy.

Recently, the serum amyloid P (SAP) scan has been introduced. This is not yet widely available, and there is as yet insufficient experience to advocate its use as the sole diagnostic test. Hence it is reasonable still to require a tissue diagnosis. The diagnostic yield from lip or gingival biopsy is lower than that from rectal biopsy. In this case the full answer of 'deep rectal biopsy with Congo red staining' would have alerted most candidates to the possibility of amyloidosis and hence the

correct answer. The rather nebulous list requires you to know that rectal biopsy is carried out using a rigid sigmoidoscope.

Answer 43

1 (c)
2 (a)

You are being tempted to investigate for myeloma or TB, but the x-rays are typical if subtle. There is periosteal resorption of the radial side of the middle phalanx of the middle and especially index fingers of the left hand (note the convention to show x-rays of hands and feet with right on your right, unlike a chest x-ray), and of the symphysis pubis. Other radiological findings which may be seen are 'basket work' cortical appearance and brown tumours.

Answer 44

1 (b)

The diagnosis is based on the differential of jaundice associated with elevated transaminases (transaminitis) rather than an obstructive picture. In the presence of autoimmune serology, an autoimmune disease is the most likely cause.

Causes of hepatocellular jaundice
Infections
–   Viral
         Hepatitis A, B, C, D, E
         EBV
         CMV
         HIV
         Arboviruses
–   Spirochaetes
         Leptospira
–   Protozoa
         Toxoplasma
         Amoeba

Toxins

Drugs
- Nitrofurantoin
- Halothane
- Isoniazid
- Many others

Inherited disorders
- Wilson's disease
- Galactosaemia

Autoimmune disease/connective tissue disorders
- Chronic active hepatitis
- SLE
- Scleroderma

Answer 45

1 (b)

Using the 'unusual sites' approach, what condition involves pigmentation of the axilla? This question should trigger the answer acanthosis nigricans which typically occurs in the axillae or groin (but also may occur around the anus and involve mucous membranes). In addition to pigmentation, the skin becomes thickened with associated skin tags and warts.

The condition may be benign in the young, but in older patients it is often associated with underlying carcinoma. If all else fails, and nothing springs to mind, then the use of a 'surgical sieve', providing headings of types of pathology, might lead you to an answer.

Answer 46

1 (c)

The radiological diagnosis is easy, especially with the history of loss of pain sensation. The asymmetry in the history is a trick; a syrinx may expand in one direction more than the other. Tonsillar herniation is a frequent association of syringomyelia; it is not clear why the development of syringomyelia occurs so late when some with the malformation develop hydrocephalus in infancy.

Answer 47

1 (b)

Explanation
The differential diagnosis is that of a respiratory alkalosis.

The likely diagnosis in this case is hysterical hyperventilation. Reassurance and rebreathing into a bag is all that is required. Sedation should be used with caution in extreme cases. Remember that hyperventilation can also occur as a result of a metabolic acidosis.

Causes of respiratory alkalosis
- Hysterical overbreathing
- Continuous pain
- Stimulation of respiratory centre by hypoxia
- Pulmonary oedema
- Pneumonia
- Pulmonary collapse or fibrosis
- Pulmonary embolism
- Excessive artificial ventilation
- Brainstem lesions
- Salicylate poisoning/overdose
- Acute liver failure
- Hyperventilation due to metabolic acidosis
- Diabetic ketoacidosis
- Lactic acidosis
- Renal failure
- Renal tubular acidosis
- Transplantation of ureters into colon
- Drugs, e.g. acetazolamide

Answer 48

1   (a)

The blood film shows hypersegmented polymorphonuclear cells characteristic of megaloblastic anaemia. Although folate deficiency and vitamin B_{12} deficiency are the most common causes of this anaemia, it is not possible to ascertain the exact cause from this blood film. Thirty-five is a little young for pernicious anaemia.

Answer 49

1   (c)

This is a reminder to look at the whole chest x-ray. The lung fields are normal and there is no focal bone lesion. The diffuse increase in bone density is due to endosteal new bone, with loss of the corticomedullary distinction. Other causes of increased bone density (metastasis, renal osteodystrophy, fluorosis) tend to be multifocal/patchy rather than diffuse, and with other features, although prostatic metastasis should be considered.

Answer 50

1   (e)
2   (c)

The investigation is coeliac artery angiography showing aneurysms of the hepatic arteries. Obviously an angiogram, this is not recognizable as a coronary, renal, or carotid/cranial study, so this is likely to represent visceral angiography, and, were you asked, this would probably be specific enough. Look hard for aneurysms in such a slide as anything else is unlikely in such a context. For the same diagnosis you might be shown renal

Classification of vasculitides

Vessels involved	Primary	Secondary
Large arteries	Giant cell	Aortitis in RA
	Takayasu	Infection (e.g. treponemal)
	Isolated CNS angiitis	
Medium arteries	Classical PAN	Infection (e.g. hepatitis B)
	Kawasaki disease	
Small vessels and medium arteries	Wegener's granulomatosis	RA/SLE
	Churg–Strauss	Sjögren's
	Microscopic polyarteritis	Drugs
		Infection (e.g. HIV)
Small vessels (leucocytoclastic)	HSP	Drugs
	Essential mixed cryoglobulinaemia	Infection
	Cutaneous leucocytoclastic vasculitis	

Treatment

Vessel involved	Steroids alone	Cyclo+ steroids	Other*
Large	+++	−	+
Medium	+	++	++
Small vessels and medium arteries	+	+++	−
Small	+	−	++

*Includes treatment of underlying disease, plasmapheresis, immunoglobulins, methotrexate, etc.

artery angiography (see figure) with irregular intrarenal vessels which narrow and widen rather than taper.

The diagnosis could be Churg–Strauss or classical polyarteritis; cardiomegaly, ill-health, eosinophilia and late-onset asthma and aneurysms suggest a systemic vasculitis, with features of both Churg–Strauss syndrome and polyarteritis nodosa. The disease classification is primarily to classify patients for trial purposes; in practice, the systemic vasculitides may overlap with each other.

The treatment must be prednisolone **and** cyclophosphamide. Most trials have been performed in Wegener's but similar treatment regimens tend to be used in the other systemic vasculitides. The relative usefulness of cytotoxic versus steroid therapy broadly reflects vessel size.

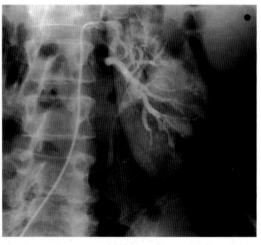

Renal artery angiography in polyarteritis nodosa

Answer 51

1   (e)

An eschar on the finger of a farmer, caused by a bacterial infection, suggests anthrax. (In the UK, the viral infection orf is a more common cause of such an eschar.) Anthrax is caused by *Bacillus anthracis* and transmission is by direct contact with an infected animal. It is seen in farmers, butchers, and wool and hide dealers. The cutaneous form is the most common presentation and is self-limiting in most cases. The lesion is typically erythematous and maculopapular, and eventually forms vesicles and ulcers with a black eschar in the centre. Diagnosis is by demonstration of the organism in smears and culture and by detection of a fourfold rise in antibody titres on ELISA testing of paired sera. Penicillin is the drug of choice although chloramphenicol has also been used successfully. Some vets report incomplete response with tetracyclines.

Answer 52

1   (b)

Explanation

In this case, the differential diagnosis can be centred around causes of hypoalbuminaemia. These are malnutrition (and malignancy), liver

Causes of enteric protein loss

Neoplastic disorders
  Gastric or colonic tumours
  Lymphoma
Inflammatory and infectious disorders
  Ulcerative colitis
  Crohn's disease
  Coeliac disease
  Tropical sprue
  Intestinal infections or infestations
  Post-infective

Lymphatic disorders
  Idiopathic small intestinal lymphangiectasia
  Secondary lymphangiectasia
  Cardiac or pericardial disease
  Abdominal malignancy
  Tuberculous lymphadenitis
Whipple's disease
Giant rugae of stomach (Menetrier's disease)
Villous adenoma of colon
Fistulae and diverticula

failure, renal failure or protein-losing enteropathy. Malnutrition is unlikely, the liver function tests are normal and there is no other evidence to suggest liver failure, and nephrotic syndrome is ruled out by the lack of proteinuria. This leaves a protein-losing enteropathy, causes of which are shown below.

In this case, the key to diagnosis is the lymphopenia and immunoglobulin deficiency, which is characteristic of small intestinal lymphangiectasia. This rare condition may present at any time, but is most common in the first few years of life. The pathological feature is dilatation of lymphatic channels, rupture of which is thought to cause hypoproteinaemia and lymphocyte loss. The condition may be primary, but it has also been described as a secondary condition associated with other disorders such as constrictive pericarditis. The primary abnormality may be associated with lymphatic abnormalities outside of the intestine, but may also be confined to the small bowel.

Clinical presentation may be with diarrhoea or steatorrhoea, hypoproteinaemia and oedema, recurrent infection, or, in childhood, failure to thrive.

Management consists of dietary manipulation to reduce the amount of long-chain fat which is usually absorbed via the small intestinal lymphatics. This in turn reduces pressure in the dilated lymphatics. Surgical resection may be possible if the lesions are localized.

Answer 53

1   (e)

Essence

A middle-aged man presents ill with upper respiratory tract symptoms, confusion, shock, meningism and a petechial rash on his return from North Africa. He had had a splenectomy and his son had just had *Shigella* infection.

Differential diagnosis

The clinical features of this patient are that of an acute bacterial meningitis. This patient does not

have a spleen and, as such, is predisposed to OPSI (overwhelming post-splenectomy infection) with a number of organisms such as *Pneumococcus, Meningococcus, Haemophilus, Capnocytophaga canimorsus* (DF-2), falciparum malaria and *Babesia*, amongst others. The first three of these are recognized causes of meningitis. The early clinical features of acute bacterial meningitis may be very non-specific and, indeed, may be associated with diarrhoea such as to suggest a diagnosis of gastroenteritis. The characteristic skin manifestations of acute meningococcaemia, petechiae and purpura (often appearing first in the conjunctivae and later leading on to skin necrosis and ulceration) are occasionally seen with both *Haemophilus* and pneumococcal meningitis. However, they are so much more common with *Meningococcus* that the presence of the rash in this case makes it the first choice diagnosis. *Shigella* uncommonly produces extra intestinal effects, very rarely seizures, but never meningitis.

Answer 54

1   (a), (b)

The answer to this question should centre on causes of hepatosplenomegaly, as discussed in Exam C, Answer 70.

Although other diagnoses are possible, the nationality of the patient should immediately suggest visceral leishmaniasis. The investigations support this diagnosis.

Kala-azar or visceral leishmaniasis is caused by *Leishmania donovani*. It is transmitted by the bite of a sandfly. The organisms multiply within the macrophages in the reticuloendothelial system and the amastigotes are often seen on liver or bone marrow biopsies or in splenic aspirates. The clinical picture is chronic and non-specific, with intermittent fever, weight loss, lethargy, wasting, epistaxis, cough and diarrhoea, amongst other symptoms. A normochromic normocytic anaemia, neutropenia, thrombocytopenia, hypoalbuminaemia, hypergammaglobulinaemia, massive splenomegaly, lymphadenopathy and hepatomegaly can occur. In HIV-positive patients, the illness is more cryptic and the clinical features are atypical.

Demonstrating the Leishman–Donovan bodies makes the diagnosis. Pentavalent antimony is used in treatment.

Answer 55

1 (d), (g)

Essence

A young man subacutely develops upper motor neurone and sensory signs to T4 and bladder problems after a 1-month history of backache and non-specific symptoms and 3 months after a trip to Kenya.

Differential diagnosis

There are some features of the history that may be misleading (e.g. slipped disc 2 years ago, paracetamol intake). However, the essential feature is that of a spinal cord lesion which, at this age, may have several causes.

The Asian background, raised ESR, raised white count with a lymphocytosis support a diagnosis of Pott's disease of the spine. However, in view of the neurological symptoms and signs compatible with a transverse myelitis and a history of blurred vision, multiple sclerosis must be considered. An epidural abscess is another possibility, as these patients may be surprisingly well. The history is rather rapid to be suggestive of a tumour, and the fact that the patient is not systemically ill makes a pyogenic abscess less likely.

Answer 56

1 (b)

Drugs are by far the commonest cause of this sort of problem. Iatrogenic hepatitis is a regular issue in this situation. It does not undermine the diagnosis of TB at this stage and there is no

---

Causes of weak legs with spasticity

Cord compression
- Disc prolapse at L1–L2 or higher
- Tumours
- Vertebral fractures
- Epidural abscess
- Spinal TB
- Hodgkin's disease
- Myeloma
- Paget's disease
- Schistosomiasis
- Neurocysticercosis
- Hydatid cyst

Myelitis
- Multiple sclerosis
- Transverse myelitis
- SLE
- Infective
    Tuberculous meningitis
    Syphilis
    Mycoplasma
    Mumps
    Measles
    EBV
    HIV
    HTLV-1

- Neurotoxins
- Carcinomatous meningitis
- B_{12} deficiency

Cord infarction
- Vasculitis
    Polyarteritis
    Syphilis

- Anterior spinal artery thrombosis
- Trauma
- Compression
- Dissection of aortic aneurysm

---

reason to search for esoterica, such as a silent myocardial infarction – certainly not as a first step. However, you should not ignore it until the liver damage becomes so severe as to generate jaundice. You may ultimately be forced to stop all this man's drugs. However, this is not a dangerous situation and it is safe to try to identify the culprit by withdrawing drugs one by one. Of all anti-TB drugs, isoniazid most commonly causes this problem.

Answer 57

1   (d)

The shape of an intraocular haemorrhage depends on its site. Preretinal bleeding occurs into a large potential space allowing blood to spread widely, often with a fluid level. Nerve fibre-layer haemorrhages are flame-shaped and obscure the retinal vessels. Intraretinal haemorrhages are confined by the retina as dots, deep to the vessels. Subretinal vessels can spread into a large space but are deep to the vessels. Finally, subchoroidal bleeds are large but appear grey due to overlying pigment.

Answer 58

1   (b)

Explanation
Hyperosmolar non-ketotic diabetic coma presents most frequently in the elderly. These patients have no ketones in the urine or blood, are not acidotic and thus do not hyperventilate. Often there is an insidious onset over weeks. The majority of patients are not comatose, but confused or stuporose. They may present with focal neurological signs. The blood glucose is very high (around 60 mmol/L), resulting in an osmotic diuresis in which large amounts of water, potassium and sodium are lost. Water loss is greatest, so the serum sodium is usually raised. This combination of raised sodium and glucose gives a high serum osmolality. Prerenal uraemia results from fluid depletion.

Answer 59

1   (d)

Following advances in immunochemistry, postmortem studies in the 1980s demonstrated a much higher incidence of Lewy bodies in the neocortex than was previously suspected. What was once thought to be a rare variant of idiopathic Parkinson's disease with dementia has now come to be thought as a common differential of dementia. The distinction between Lewy body and Parkinson's disease is difficult: if the movement disorder presents first then a diagnosis of Parkinson's is often made, and Lewy body disease if the order is reversed. Furthermore, up to 25 per cent of patients previously misdiagnosed with Alzheimer's disease may have Lewy body disease.

Features that suggest Lewy body disease are:

* fluctuations in cognitive function despite being awake
* visual hallucinations
* parkinsonian features that often worsen with antipsychotic medication.

In this question a newly diagnosed dementia patient has developed a movement disorder since the commencement of an antipsychotic agent. He also has visual hallucinations. It may be tempting to counter this with dopamine or a dopamine agonist but either of these may exacerbate the psychiatric symptoms. He is on a very low dose of sulpiride and also reducing the dose will not necessarily relieve the parkinsonian effects which have provoked the referral. Finally donepezil is used in the treatment of Lewy body disease but is associated with dysrhythmia and should not be used in a patient with a recent myocardial infarction.

Answer 60

1   (c), (d)

Essence
A long-standing poorly controlled diabetic with proliferative retinopathy with end-stage renal failure who deteriorates after starting dialysis.

Differential diagnosis
One possible cause of this man's deterioration is a pneumothorax or haemothorax (or both) caused

by the insertion of the subclavian line. This may be a spontaneous event some hours after the insertion of the line, blood may have accumulated gradually, or a bleed may have occurred after the patient was anticoagulated for haemodialysis. Haemothorax is a marginally better answer since a pneumothorax is likely to have been picked up on chest x-ray taken to check the position of the line. Alternatively, he may have pericarditis due to chronic uraemia which, similarly, may be complicated by pericardial haemorrhage as a result of the anticoagulation.

Pulmonary oedema is a less likely explanation of his deterioration. He was fluid overloaded on admission, and certainly had pulmonary oedema; dialysis would, however, make this better, not worse. Indeed, in the clinical situation of fluid overload it is likely that the priority would have been to remove fluid by ultrafiltration before instituting dialysis. On the other hand, he is at risk of ischaemic heart disease and, particularly on dialysis, he might suffer an acute myocardial infarction (often silent in diabetics), which itself could exacerbate the pulmonary oedema.

Pulmonary haemorrhage is a recognized complication of renal failure, but only in certain pathological states (e.g. vasculitis, SLE, Goodpasture's syndrome) and would be very unlikely in this patient.

The treatment of haemo/pneumothorax would be to insert a chest drain. Pericardial haemorrhage might need pericardiectomy, but you may need to insert a pericardial drain initially.

Answer 61

1   (c)

The scan shows a right psoas abscess with ipsilateral hydronephrosis. Tuberculosis is the likeliest cause although inflammatory bowel disease may also cause this combination.

The hydronephrosis is likely to be due to involvement of the ureter by the abscess but may be due to a tubercular stricture.

Answer 62

1   (b)

Essence

A 40-year-old woman with long-standing itching and rheumatoid arthritis treated with paracetamol develops obstructive jaundice.

Differential diagnosis

The history raises the differential diagnosis of pruritus and jaundice. Although pruritus may occur with any liver disease, it is more common with cholestasis. In addition, with the exception of the paracetamol, there is no clue as to an aetiology. The toxicology screen was negative and although this does not rule out a paracetamol overdose, that would be expected to cause a hepatitic picture of abnormalities in the liver function tests. In the absence of any other predisposing feature, the cholestatic picture (alkaline phosphatase raised out of proportion to the transaminases) in a middle-aged female leads to a diagnosis of primary biliary cirrhosis. This is a slowly progressive cholangiohepatitis with destruction of the small interlobular bile ducts. It is thought to have an autoimmune basis and it affects women more than men (90 per cent of patients are females) with a peak incidence of onset at the age of 45 years. Nearly 50 per cent of newly diagnosed patients are symptom-free. Apart from cholestasis and pruritus, other clinical manifestations include hepatosplenomegaly, melanotic pigmentation, clubbing, xanthomata, xanthelesmata, arthralgia, fatigue, osteoporosis, osteomalacia, hirsutism and portal hypertension.

It is not possible to be certain of the diagnosis and the principal differential diagnoses are obstruction by gallstones, cholangiocarcinoma, carcinoma of the head of the pancreas, and sclerosing cholangitis, or, indeed, any cause of obstruction. Gallstones obstruction is less likely without pain and the patient would be young for either malignancy. Sclerosing cholangitis usually occurs in association with ulcerative colitis. Hence, none of these diagnoses is acceptable in this case.

Treatment with several immunosuppressive

agents has been tried but with varying success. Cholestyramine may relieve pruritus and vitamins D, A and K and calcium supplements may be required. End-stage PBC is one of the indications for liver transplantation.

Answer 63

1   (c)

Pattern recognition again. The bilateral symmetrical wasting of the facial and shoulder muscles is striking in this patient.

Answer 64

1   (c)

The best answer would have been lupus anticoagulant levels, but if offered this as a choice most candidates would have been pointed to the diagnosis. The lupus anticoagulant (LA) is an in vitro inhibitor of phospholipid-dependent coagulation assays which was first described in patients with systemic lupus erythematosus. LA activity is believed to be due to an antibody against the phospholipid component of the prothrombinase complex, which cleaves prothrombin to form thrombin. It is associated with high titres of anticardiolipin antibodies and a false-positive test for syphilis.

Individuals with raised anticardiolipin (aCL) antibodies or LA have an increased risk of arterial and venous thrombosis, thrombocytopenia and recurrent abortion. The association of clinical manifestations with raised aCL antibodies or LA has been termed the antiphospholipid syndrome. Thirty to forty per cent of SLE patients have aCL antibodies, but they have also been detected in a number of other disorders, including migraine, malignancy, autoimmune thrombocytopenia, myasthenia gravis and multiple sclerosis. They are also found in patients with vascular disease, e.g. following myocardial infarction or stroke. Patients with cerebral ischaemia associated with aCL antibodies tend to be younger and have recurrent vascular events.

Diagnosis is made on the basis of abnormal coagulation tests and the detection of aCL antibodies. Typically the activated partial thromboplastin time is prolonged and cannot be corrected by mixing with plasma, indicating the presence of an inhibitor rather than the absence of clotting factors. The prothrombin time is usually normal or slightly prolonged. The bleeding time, a measure of platelet function, is normal – in this case it is abnormal because the patient has taken aspirin.

Answer 65

1   (a)

This lesion has the pearly-white edge with a rolled border typical of a basal cell carcinoma (BCC). Any such lesion is to be considered a BCC until biopsy proves otherwise. Keratoacanthoma is sometimes mistaken for a BCC, but BCCs tend to ulcerate in the centre whereas keratoacanthomas, as their name suggests, produce keratin. Squamous cell carcinomas do not have this rolled pearly white margin.

Answer 66

1   (d)

Explanation

The haemolytic-uraemic syndrome (HUS) typically occurs in children shortly after a febrile illness associated with diarrhoea. The commonest culprit is *Escherichia coli* serotype O157:H7, and other *E. coli* serotypes and *Shigella dysenteriae* account for most of the other cases. HUS is a microangiopathic haemolytic anaemia (MAHA), as discussed in Exam C, Answer 13. In this case, the combination of the history, low platelet count, anaemia and renal failure are enough information for the diagnosis. Do not let the age of the patient deceive – the condition can also occur in adults.

The thrombotic microangiopathies are a spectrum of disorders all characterized by intravascular platelet aggregation, resulting in thrombocytopenia and causing mechanical injury to erythrocytes, and hence haemolytic anaemia. The combination of thrombocytopenia, schistocytes (fragmented erythrocytes or helmet cells in the blood film) and elevated lactate dehydrogenase (derived from ischaemic tissue) is usually sufficient to make a diagnosis of TTP. In thrombotic thrombocytopenic purpura the systemic thrombotic features dominate the presentation, classically with the pentad of thrombocytopenia, MAHA, neurological signs, renal failure and fever. If severe renal failure dominates the presentation, HUS is diagnosed.

Pathophysiologically, failure to degrade large multimers of von Willebrand factor causes platelets to aggregate as microvascular thrombi in TTP. They do not contain fibrin, in contrast to thrombi in DIC which do not contain von Willebrand factor. In HUS von Willebrand factor multimers are less prominent in the intrarenal thrombi.

Answer 67

1 (e)

The pelvicalyceal systems are rotated, the kidneys are closer to the midline than normal and a bridge of renal tissue extends across the midline at the lower poles. This is associated with an increased incidence of infection, renal calculi and transitional cell carcinoma.

Answer 68

1 (b)
2 (c)

Explanation
The examiners expect comprehensive knowledge of common medical emergencies. It is important to be aware of basic coronary artery anatomy as this explains both the site of infarction and some of the complications. Supply to the AV node is via the posterior descending artery. In 70 per cent of individuals this is a branch of the right coronary artery, and in 10 per cent this is a branch of the left circumflex artery. In 20 per cent the posterior descending receives supply from both arteries (codominance). The correct answer to question 2 is observation as the patient is asymptomatic. The block is often temporary but normal conduction may not be restored for 2 weeks.

Other important complications of myocardial infarction recognizable on the ECG include:

- AV block in anterior infarction suggests very extensive infarction
- atrial fibrillation
- ventricular tachyarrhythmias
- ventricular aneurysm, more common after anterior than inferior infarction.

Indications for temporary pacing following acute myocardial infarction (MI)
- Only if cardiac output impaired (i.e. low blood pressure, confused)
- Anterior MI
- Complete heart block
- Second-degree heart block
- Alternating left and right bundle branch block
- Right bundle branch block and left axis deviation
- Post-asystolic cardiac arrest

Other indications
- Symptomatic bradycardia or sinus arrest not reversed by atropine
- Complete heart block
- Second-degree heart block if symptomatic
- Pauses with dizziness
- Bradycardia or syncope
- Prior to cardiac surgery
- Prior to general anaesthesia if complete heart block or second-degree heart block
- In selected situations when using anti-arrhythmic drugs

Answer 69

1 (c)

Ultrasound (like echocardiograms) are unusual for Membership. However, the middle two pictures both announce that they are from the liver and two lesions within can be seen clearly in the right-hand picture.

The most common multiple liver lesions, hyper- or hypoechoic on ultrasound, are metastases. Multifocal primary liver cancer can appear similar. Abscesses appear hypoechoic, i.e. dark.

Answer 70

1 (b)
2 (c)

Essence

A young homosexual returning from Zambia develops a febrile illness with a rash, abdominal pain, hepatocellular jaundice, hepatosplenomegaly, and lymphadenopathy.

Differential diagnosis

In this case the number of differential diagnoses is enormous. In every ill traveller returning from the tropics you must exclude malaria, typhoid fever and yellow fever.

Antimalarial prophylaxis does not provide absolute protection, so malaria must be considered in all travellers even if it is an unlikely diagnosis as here. Repeated blood film for malarial parasites is also the most urgent investigation. So here is a situation of the least likely diagnosis still requiring the most urgent investigation. A clinical picture of rigors, macular erythematous rash, and lymphadenopathy (but not the splenomegaly) would be atypical for typhoid. It is difficult to exclude yellow fever clinically, but hepatosplenomegaly (although both organs are involved) and lymphadenopathy are not classical. The patient has had all appropriate immunizations.

Similarly, there are none of the expected features of a viral haemorrhagic fever.

The localizing features – rash, hepatic and splenic involvement, and abdominal pain – are also very common features of many tropical diseases. Hepatitis A is unlikely given a temperature of 39.2, and hepatitis B is also unlikely given the relatively short incubation period. You should

---

Common causes of jaundice in a tropical traveller
- Hepatitis
- Malaria
- Typhoid fever
- G6PD deficiency
- Thalassaemia
- Sickle cell disease

Rarely
- Yellow fever
- Leptospirosis

Causes of hepatosplenomegaly
Common causes
- Kala-azar (visceral leishmaniasis)
- Malaria (tropical splenomegaly syndrome)
- Chronic myeloid leukaemia
- Portal hypertension
- Myelofibrosis

Other causes
- Infections
  - Viral
  - Bacterial (tuberculosis [rarely], typhoid, brucellosis)
  - Helminths (*Schistosoma mansoni* [in natives of endemic areas])

- Malignancies
  - Leukaemia
  - Reticuloendothelial disorders
  - Lymphoma

- Others
  - Sarcoidosis
  - Amyloidosis
  - Glycogen storage disorders
  - Haemochromatosis

also consider the likelihood of acquisition of HIV in East Africa.

Answer 71

1 (a)

Explanation

There are many classical features of hypothyroidism, none of which usually dominates the presentation and all of which occur in other disorders. However, it is difficult to think of another condition which includes a myopathy with only mildly elevated muscle enzymes, hyponatraemia and macrocytosis.

Hyponatraemia in hypothyroidism is due to inappropiate secretion of antidiuretic hormone. The macrocytosis is probably related to increased lipid deposition in the red cell membrane. The muscle enzymes are insufficiently raised for there to be significant myositis. She might be on a statin but you are given no hint of this.

The thyroid antibodies usually measured are antimicrosomal and antithyroglobulin antibodies. Both are present in signficant titre in Hashimoto's thyroiditis. A more likely aetiology in a woman of this age is spontaneous atrophic non-goitrous hypothyroidism. This is also an organ-specific autoimmune disease with lymphoid infiltration of

---

The aetiology of primary hypothyroidism can be classified as follows:

- Non-goitrous
  - Spontaneous atrophic
- Goitrous
  - Hashimoto's thyroiditis
  - Drug-induced (lithium, amiodarone)
  - Iodine deficiency
  - Dyshormonogenesis (e.g. Pendred's syndrome)
  - Post-ablative (postoperative or radiodine
    - often transient if develops within 6 months of therapy)

---

the thyroid and TSH receptor blocking antibodies (cf. receptor stimulating antibodies in Graves' disease). These antibodies are not useful clinically.

Treatment of primary hypothyroidism is aimed at keeping the TSH within the low normal range in conjunction with clinical findings.

Answer 72

1 (c)

Essence

A patient develops anaphylactic shock and becomes cyanosed.

Management

This is one of the few cases in which you will be expected to know doses of drugs. The first drug to be given is adrenaline. It can be given intramuscularly or subcutaneously, but not intravenously. You should give 0.5–1.0 mL of a 1:1000 dilution.

Answer 73

1 (b)

Diverticula are frequently found in the colon in 50 per cent of patients over the age of 50 years. Diverticulitis is inflammation of these diverticula. Diverticular disease is asymptomatic in 90 per cent of cases. In the rest it may present as constipation, pain in the left iliac fossa and frequent passage of loose stools. Diagnosis is made on barium enema, as in this case.

Complications of diverticular disease
- Diverticulitis
- Abscess formation
- Perforation
- Fistula formation
- Intestinal obstruction
- Rectal bleeding
- Iron deficiency anaemia

Diagnoses often missed on barium enemas

- Pneumatosis cystoides intestinalis
  - Multiple gas-filled cysts in the submucosa of the colon
- Ischaemic colitis
  - 'Thumb printing' and strictures
- Polyps
  - Solitary polyp
  - Familial colonic polyposis
  - Gardener's syndrome
- Intussusception
  - Ileocaecal
- Normal barium enema but incidental finding of
  - Bamboo spine
  - Pancreatic calcification
  - Dense vertebra
- Silhouette of *Ascaris lumbricoides*

Antineutrophil cytoplasmic antibodies (ANCA)

Since 1985, ANCA has been useful in the diagnosis of the systemic vasculitides. It produces two different patterns of immuno-fluorescence on staining ethanol-fixed neutrophils:

- cytoplasmic staining (described as cANCA) is probably synonymous with the presence of an antibody to proteinase 3
- perinuclear ANCA (pANCA) represents a variety of antibody specificities, including one to myeloperoxidase (MPO).

cANCA is a highly sensitive marker of systemic Wegener's granulomatosis (WG) and is found at lower frequencies in diseases with incomplete forms and variants of WG. Anti-MPO antibodies are found in pANCA-positive patients with idiopathic or vasculitis-associated necrotizing crescentic glomer-ulonephritis, particularly if they are also negative for cANCA, and in diseases not associated with granulomatous involvement of the respiratory tract. Anti-MPO is also found in anti-GBM disease and, possibly, also in SLE (at low titre). However, pANCA, but not anti-MPO, is present in some patients with other autoimmune diseases, such as ulcerative colitis, autoimmune liver disease, and rheumatoid arthritis.

Answer 74

1 (d)

Another one you either know or you don't!

Occurrence of pANCA in other conditions

Disease	Prevalence of pANCA (per cent)
Ulcerative colitis	60–70
Crohn's disease	10–20
Autoimmune chronic active hepatitis	60–70
Primary biliary cirrhosis	30–40
Primary sclerosing cholangitis	60–85
Rheumatoid arthritis	
with Felty's syndrome	90–100
with vasculitis	50–75
uncomplicated	20–40

Disease	Sensitivity (per cent) cANCA/anti-proteinase 3	Anti-MPO
Wegener's granulomatosis (all)	80	20
Systemic Wegener's granulomatosis[a]	>90	
Limited Wegener's granulomatosis[b]	75	
Idiopathic crescentic glomerulonephritis	30	70
Microscopic polyarteritis	50	50
Classical polyarteritis nodosa	10	20
Churg–Strauss syndrome	10	70

[a]Respiratory tract granulomata, crescentic nephritis and systemic vasculitis.

[b]Without renal involvement.

Answer 75

1   (a)

The lesion shown is an eschar. In some rickettsial infections parasites invade endothelial cells where they multiply and cause a derma-epidermal necrosis called an eschar. A similar appearance is also seen in cutaneous anthrax or aspergillus (both of which have a black centre) and the chancre of African trypanosomiasis. American trypanosomiasis is also associated with a skin lesion at the entry point but this chagoma does not usually ulcerate. A tarantula bite may, despite Hollywood appearances to the contrary, rarely cause problems with neurotoxicity leading to muscle spasm. Spiders of the genus *Loxosceles* may cause an eschar, but the tarantula is not from this genus. Typhoid infection is associated with rose spots that do not ulcerate to give an eschar.

Answer 76

1   (c)
2   (a), (d)

Essence

A cachectic elderly lady presents with an acute febrile illness associated with haemoptysis and chronic diarrhoea, tricuspid regurgitation, opacities on chest x-ray and hepatic ultrasound, anaemia and leucocytosis.

Differential diagnosis

Given the cachexia, this is clearly an acute-on-chronic problem. The only other chronic feature described is the diarrhoea. Most other abnormalities (except the hepatic lesions) point above the diaphragm. The heavy smoking could predispose her to malignancy, but there are no other clues as to the site of a primary; the multiple opacities in the lungs and liver could represent metastases, but these tend to be uniform and well defined, with a predilection for the periphery and lower lobes. There are no specific features of Wegener's granulomatosis (ENT disease or suggestion of renal involvement) other than haemoptysis associated with pulmonary nodules. The pulmonary nodules in Wegener's are usually well-defined (0.5–10 cm in size) and often cavitate.

The acute lesion is likely to be infective and the opacities in the lung are likely to be the source of the haemoptysis and purulent sputum. This suggests either that underlying lesions have become infected or that they are pulmonary abscesses. The radiographic features are more in keeping with the latter, being poorly defined and of varying size; abscesses often cavitate. The tricuspid regurgitation could be secondary to an underlying pulmonary problem. However, right-heart strain tends to result from a pathological process that affects the lung fields globally. Multiple isolated lesions are less likely to do so. In this case the cardiac lesion is likely to be primary. If we postulate an underlying right-sided endocarditis, then all the acute findings follow on from that. Although right-heart endocarditis is more common in drug abusers, it also occurs on the background of general debility, and this may account for at least part of the chronic component of the illness but there is not enough information to hypothesize further. The hepatic lesions are probably due to mycotic embolic originating in the lungs and which have traversed to the left side of the heart.

Another lesion that has been suggested for this case is carcinoid syndrome. However, diarrhoea is the only other feature supporting this. A patient with carcinoid of sufficiently advanced stage to affect the right heart would be more generally symptomatic.

Yet another explanation offered is of a *Streptococcus bovis* endocarditis associated with colonic carcinoma and causing also hepatic and pulmonary abscesses. However, the signs of right-heart disease mean you would have to postulate an uncommon complication occurring in an uncommon site. With a primary diagnosis of right-heart endocarditis, everything else follows on.

> The major difficulty with this case is untangling all the strands, deciding what to disregard (diarrhoea) and establishing causes and effects. Isolate one finding (preferably the least common or the best defined, such as tricuspid regurgitation) and analyse it separately. How do the other features of the case relate to it? If this approach does not work for the first feature chosen, choose a second, then a third.

Answer 77

1 (b)

Haemoglobin H is a tetramer of normal haemoglobin β-chains. It is produced when there is marked reduction in α-chain synthesis, most commonly when an individual inherits α^0-thalassaemia from one parent and α^+-thalassaemia from the other. Affected patients may survive to adult life and have less severe bone changes or growth retardation than patients with homozygous β-thalassaemia. The degree of anaemia and splenomegaly is variable. The numerous inclusion bodies which make the red cells look like golf balls are generated by the precipitation of HbH under the redox action of the dye. Note also several reticulocytes; individuals usually have a haemoglobin of 7–10 g/dL and a moderate reticulocytosis.

Answer 78

1 (d)
2 (b)

Explanation

The combination of systemic hypotension with low left- and low right-heart pressures means either hypovolaemia or septic shock (or a combination of both, which is often the case in clinical practice). In this case, the key to the correct diagnosis is the cardiac output (or cardiac index, which is the cardiac output/m^2 of body surface area). When this increases and the blood pressure falls, as here, then systemic vascular resistance must have fallen (as cardiac output = blood pressure/systemic vascular resistance). This is the predominant situation during the vasodilatation of septicaemic shock. In hypovolaemia, systemic vascular resistance should rise as a result of vasoconstriction.

Note, however, that septic shock and hypovolaemia often occur together and that the immediate management of septic shock usually involves fluid replacement.

Septic shock leads to a metabolic acidosis because of poor tissue perfusion. The respiratory centre will respond with hyperventilation in order to lower blood Pa_{CO_2}.

Answer 79

1 (b), (e)

Essence
An elderly man develops intermittent confusion and weakness of his left leg, with documented fluctuations in signs.

Differential diagnosis
Confusion and weakness are compatible with cerebrovascular disease. Although it is common for signs of dementia to fluctuate, it is unusual for motor signs to come and go rapidly. Although the motor features could be due to recurrent TIAs, the association with confusion is less likely, unless one postulates pre-existing permanent damage on which the TIAs are superimposed. Fluctuating signs are a feature of certain space-occupying lesions, of which chronic subdural haematoma is the most likely in this age group, and is a better answer than TIAs. The lack of a history of trauma does not detract from the likelihood of that diagnosis. Glioma would be less likely in this age group.

Answer 80

1 (b), (c), (i)

Management
The patient is cyanosed – she needs oxygen. Give her 35 per cent. Do not forget to include it – even although the nurse will probably have the mask on the patient long before you get there. The second agent to be given is an antihistamine – you are interested in H_1 rather than H_2 blockade. Chlorpheniramine is particularly popular. Given that she is shocked, your final answer should be to set up central venous access and administer fluid.
  Any other management measure is 'second line', e.g. aminophylline infusion or starting a course of hydrocortisone. Other measures, such as intubation and artificial ventilation or use of an inotrope, would only be justified after the above measures failed.

Answer 81

1 (a)

  Diabetic eye disease
There are three classes of changes to the eye in diabetes mellitus:

* cataracts (six times as common as in an age-matched non-diabetic population)
* rubeosis iridis, with its complications such as secondary glaucoma
* retinopathy.

Retinopathy
Background ('simple') retinopathy
– Microaneurysms or dot haemorrhages
– Hard exudates (acuity normal)

Maculopathy (macular exudative retinopathy)
– Hard exudates and oedema near macula (acuity impaired)

Pre-proliferative retinopathy
– Cotton wool spots
– Flame and blot haemorrhages
– Tortuous arteries
– Irregular calibre veins (indication for pan-peripheral photocoagulation of the retina)

Proliferative retinopathy
– New vessels
– Pre-retinal/vitreous haemorrhage (e.g. subhyoloid)
– Fibrous overgrown/retinitis proliferans
– Retinal detachment

Answer 82

1 (e)

Explanation

This is a difficult question in which all but two of the data are abnormal. There is a clearly discernible pattern of results which, taken with the history, suggests chronic renal failure. However, this alone cannot explain the grossly depressed MCV of 58 fL. The logical approach is to consider the differential diagnosis of a microcytic anaemia.

The most common cause of a microcytic anaemia is iron deficiency. This diagnosis can be confirmed by a low serum iron, low serum ferritin and a high total iron binding capacity (TIBC) or transferrin. The reticulocyte count is appropriately low for the degree of anaemia.

The anaemia of chronic disease is usually normocytic or mildly microcytic. Both serum iron and TIBC are low and ferritin normal or raised.

In thalassaemia traits, the MCV is always very low for the degree of anaemia, which is often mild or absent. Serum iron and ferritin are normal.

Sideroblastic anaemias are characterized by ring sideroblasts in the bone marrow. The disorder may be congenital or acquired: the MCV is often very low in the former but often raised in the latter. Serum iron and ferritin are both raised.

The anaemia of aluminium toxicity is seen exclusively in patients with long-standing dialysis-dependent renal failure who have either used dialysates containing high levels of aluminium or who have received large amounts of aluminium-containing phosphate binders.

The patient in this question has chronic renal failure and a severe microcytic anaemia. The anaemia of chronic disease (associated in this case with renal failure) undoubtedly contributes to her anaemia, but does not explain the low MCV. The normal ferritin makes iron deficiency and congenital sideroblastic anaemia unlikely. The history suggests that the patient has not yet received renal replacement therapy (i.e. dialysis), so aluminium toxicity is unlikely. Thalassaemia trait could be clinically silent and still cause this degree of microcytosis. This should be confirmed by haemoglobin electrophoresis.

Causes of microcytic anaemia
- Iron deficiency
- Anaemia of chronic disease
- Thalassaemia
- Sideroblastic anaemia
- Aluminium toxicity

Answer 83

1 (c)

The differential is of multifocal intracranial calcification. The distribution in the region of the basal ganglia makes hypo (or pseudo- or pseudopseudo-) most likely, with chronic carbon monoxide poisoning next. Other diagnoses on the list are congenital toxoplasmosis/CMV/rubella (which tend to be periventricular), cysticercosis, tuberous sclerosis and lead poisoning.

Answer 84

1 (b)
2 (f), (h)

Essence

A 74-year-old lady with rheumatoid arthritis develops acute GI upset and a rash and presents with hypertension, evidence of renal inflammation without infection, renal failure and hyperkalaemia.

Differential diagnosis

Your approach to this question should centre on the differential diagnosis of renal disease in a patient with rheumatoid arthritis.

Dealing first with the non-drug-related disorders, renal amyloid is the most common. Patients present with the nephrotic syndrome and progressive renal failure. A sudden decline in renal function might suggest renal vein thrombosis, as thromboses are a common complication of the nephrotic state. As there are no other features of systemic amyloidosis, this is unlikely. By contrast, glomerulonephritis and renal vasculitis are rarely a clinical problem in rheumatoid arthritis.

Drugs are a more common cause of renal problems in rheumatoid arthritis. Gold and penicillamine may cause proteinuria which usually resolves once the drug is discontinued. The renal lesion in these cases is usually membranous glomerulonephritis. Non-steroidal anti-inflammatory drugs can cause renal impairment by a variety of means, including reduction of glomerular filtration rate (GFR). This may be worse in patients with renovascular disease. Alternatively, interstitial nephritis may occur. Chronic analgesic abuse, particularly with combination analgesics, may cause 'analgesic nephropathy'.

In this question, an important clue lies in the data obtained by urinalysis – white cell casts in the absence of infection suggest an interstitial inflammatory infiltrate, i.e. interstitial nephritis, or a glomerulonephritis. The likeliest cause in this patient are the NSAIDs, of which we are told she has had several. The rash which preceded her illness is also typical of an acute allergic disease.

Management

The immediate management must be to correct her hyperkalaemia. Examination reveals she is already fluid overloaded. But the level of overload described is not so severe that it should be considered life-threatening. The hyperkalaemia is – hence it takes priority. Calcium ions protect the myocardium from the effects of hyperkalaemia. Intravenous dextrose and insulin and intravenous bicarbonate sequester potassium in the intracellular compartment, thus protecting the heart temporarily. Both these techniques (and of course dialysis) will lower the potassium in a few hours. Calcium Resonium will take up to a day and is therefore too slow for a life-threatening situation. Reports have shown that intravenous salbutamol is an effective hypokalaemic agent. Intravenous

bicarbonate is an inferior answer because it contains a heavy sodium load that carries the risk of precipitating pulmonary oedema.

At least one of your management measures must address the hyperkalaemia, although it would be reasonable to nominate two lines of management to deal with it. Calcium ions only represent a holding measure, so a calcium infusion as the only response to the hyperkalaemia is inadequate. Prescribing dialysis will deal with the hyperkalaemia. However, the patient is probably not ill enough to demand urgent dialysis, which is why that represents an inferior answer. You would want to attempt to establish a diuresis. However, you would not get away with a fluid challenge in someone as fluid overloaded, and in the real world infusions of high-dose furosemide are rarely effective. This patient has been oliguric for too long for dopamine to be considered. Because of the level of fluid overload, it would be reasonable to require a central line to manage this patient, but not before dealing with the life threatening hyperkalaemia – the insertion of a central line may induce an arrhythmia that can be impossible to terminate with coexisting severe hyperkalaemia.

Answer 85

1 (b)

The hands are classically 'spade like'. Everything about them is big. Relative to their length, the circumference of the fingers is particularly large.

Answer 86

1 (b)

Explanation

There are a number of multiple endocrine diseases, and MEN 1 and MEN 2 are particular favourites. MEN 1 consists of the three 'P' tumours: anterior pituitary adenomata, parathyroid adenomata causing hypercalcaemia, and pancreatic tumours of diverse types (most commonly insulinomas or gastrinomas). Any of these may dominate the clinical presentation. Other occasional features include thyroid disease, carcinoid tumours and multiple lipomata. The gene for MEN 1 has been mapped to chromosome 11q13 but the function of the nuclear protein for which it codes is not known. MEN 1 gene screening is used in presymptomatic diagnosis.

MEN 2, often inherited, consists of medullary carcinoma of the thyroid, phaeochromocytoma and, frequently, parathyroid hyperplasia. Medullary carcinoma of the thyroid comprises only a small proportion of thyroid neoplasms, and usually presents either as goitre or is found incidentally when screening patients suspected of having MEN 2. Even in the absence of other endocrine disease defining MEN 2, the tumour is often familial. The C cells of the thyroid produce calcitonin, and serum levels can be used for screening family and to determine adequacy of surgical clearance, but the calcitonin appears to have no significant effect on calcium metabolism. Treatment is total thyroidectomy as the tumour is often multifocal.

Medullary carcinoma of the thyroid (MTC) is associated with phaeochromocytoma in MEN 2a and with mucosal neuromas in MEN 2b, but may be inherited in isolation. Mutations in a proto-oncogene on chromosome 10q11 have been found in all three clinical variants and can be used to assess risk and the need for prophylactic surgery.

Phaeochromocytoma

As in this patient, it may be part of MEN 2 (and patients should have calcitonin levels measured) but is also associated with neurofibromatosis. The clinical manifestations and stage at which the tumour presents depend in part on how far the catecholamines are metabolized prior to their release into the circulation. Thus, if adrenaline, with predominant β-receptor affinity, is the major metabolite, the hypertension may be predominantly systolic. Clues which the examiners may leave to suggest the diagnosis of phaeochromocytoma in the appropriate context include:

- sustained rather than paroxysmal hypertension, in 50 per cent

- postural hypotension due to reduction in intravascular volume
- anxiety, fear and sweating with or after paroxysms
- palpitations
- paroxysms after particular movements, or after micturition in patients with bladder wall tumours
- impaired glucose tolerance – adrenaline inhibits the hepatic uptake of glucose.

Diagnostic tests are confounded by the large number of drugs and foods which interfere with catecholamine metabolism (methyldopa, tetracyclines, phenothiazines, banana, tea, coffee, vanilla, etc.) and by their variable metabolism within the tumours themselves. The initial test for urinary catecholamine metabolites (vanillylmandelic acid, metanephrines) has in most centres been replaced by the ability to test directly for urine catecholamines, with careful attention to diet and drugs. Plasma catecholamines can be measured by high-pressure liquid chromatography but will be elevated by stress and exercise.

Most tumours occur in the adrenal glands and most will be visualized by CT scanning. [^{131}I]metaiodobenzylguanadine (MIBG) binds to the tumour and is being increasingly used to visualize it. If selective venous sampling is performed, α-blockade and then β-blockade is essential prior to the procedure which may provoke paroxysms. β-Blockade protects against arrhythmias. Similar precautions are necessary before surgery.

A popular question concerns those drugs which you would want on the anaesthetic trolley at surgery for a phaeochromocytoma. They are:

- phentolamine and nitroprusside for control of blood pressure
- propranolol to protect the heart from the arrhythmogenic catecholamines
- isoprenaline and noradrenaline in case of excessive α-blockade.

It is clearly a better answer to recognize that these two tumours comprise a syndrome rather than naming them individually. Having made the diagnosis, serum calcitonin is the definitive investigation.

Answer 87

1 (a)

She has developed a unilateral Horner's syndrome following attempted stellate ganglion block, as a form of sympathectomy to improve peripheral circulation. The upper cervical chain has been damaged, resulting in a Horner's syndrome.

Answer 88

1 (a)
2 (a)

The British Thoracic Society (BTS) has produced guidelines that outline severe features in community-acquired pneumonia. They include the

- core 'CURB' adverse prognostic features
  - Confusion: new onset of mental confusion with an MTS of 8 or less
  - Urea: renal failure with a urea of greater than 7 mmol/L
  - Respiratory rate: tachypnoea with a RR of greater than 30
  - Blood pressure: a systolic of less than 90 or a diastolic of less than 60
- Pre-existing adverse prognostic features
  - age over 50
  - previous medical illness
- Additional clinical adverse prognostic features
  - O_2 sats of less than 92 per cent regardless of F_{iO_2}
  - bilateral or multilobar involvement.

The BTS guidelines suggest that where a patient has no adverse prognostic features then community management or early hospital discharge may be indicated.

In this question then, the adverse prognostic features are potentially the age over 50 but this patient is only just over 50 and is otherwise well.

As with all testing scores your use of them needs to be accurate as others will perform the same test later and should therefore use the same questions. The mental test score asks for the date of the first world war and so strictly speaking he would lose no marks for failing to know 1914–18. In addition, to be confused under the C of CURB he needs an MTS of less than 8 out of 10, but in being told that he is otherwise well you cannot make that assumption.

As with all guidelines, they do not supplant clinical decision making but act as a guide – the patient can go home. In patients with non-severe CAP the guidelines suggest that oral amoxicillin should be the first-line treatment.

Detailed knowledge of guidelines for rare conditions is not expected, but this is a clinical situation that you deal with daily, and therefore detailed knowledge can be expected.

Answer 89

1 (d)

This purple papular lesion appears to be made up of numerous coalescing small lesions. Not visible here, a close-up would show arborizing white lines (Wickham's striae) on the surface of the lesions. Scratch marks are often also seen because it is very itchy.

Answer 90

1 (b), (d)

Essence

A young man develops over several years two episodes of a 'flu-like' illness, nodular shadows on chest x-ray, negative Kveim and Mantoux tests and later has a seizure.

Differential diagnosis

The important point about this question is to understand the limitations of special investigations. The negative Kveim test is of no help since it does not exclude sarcoidosis. Similarly, the negative bronchoscopy and transbronchial biopsy are of no help. We know from the radiography that there is an abnormality. The failure to respond to a reducing course of steroids is a rather useless piece of information; it is only of diagnostic value if you know how much was given for how long and the nature of the follow-up.

Kveim testing is now no longer used owing to the potential infectious risk to the patient from nvCJD with little diagnostic yield in most cases.

Of more interest is the negative Mantoux test. If he had tuberculosis, one would expect this man to be much worse in order to be anergic to PPD. Similarly, one would expect most British people to be positive to a Mantoux of 1:1000. This fact, coupled with relatively asymptomatic pulmonary disease, and subsequent CNS involvement produces a syndrome that is really only compatible with sarcoidosis.

The two investigations of choice would be an MRI or CT scan to identify the CNS lesions, and a repeat transbronchial biopsy to try and obtain a tissue diagnosis. It would be inappropriately invasive to proceed to an open lung biopsy before trying another bronchoscopy, and it would be unreasonable, in the face of such a striking clinical syndrome, to subject him to an open operation for the purpose of obtaining tissue from what is probably now rather a chronic scarred lesion.

Answer 91

1 (d)

While allergic reactions to antituberculous drugs are common, the time frame is against that as a cause. The emergence of resistance is unlikely to present in this way. The killing of mycobacteria is a slow process and unlike that causing the Jarisch–Herxheimer reaction with treponemal disease. The diagnosis is fairly sound, so (c) is an

unlikely diagnosis. However, it is well recognized in urinary tuberculosis that the ureteric orifices may become scarred in the healing process and precipitate ureteric obstruction.

Answer 92

1 (a)

The blood film shows fragmented red cells characteristic of a microangiopathic haemolytic anaemia (MAHA). However, given the history, the likely diagnosis is the haemolytic-uraemic syndrome (HUS).

MAHA is discussed further in the answer to Exam C, Question 13.

Answer 93

1 (d)

Explanation

Protein-losing enteropathy in general and small intestinal lymphangiectasia in particular have been discussed in Exam B, Answer 90 and Exam C, Answer 52. A firm diagnosis is made by establishing lymphatic abnormalities on small intestinal biopsy; however, lesions may be intermittent along the course of the bowel and thus a negative biopsy may not necessarily exclude the diagnosis. Barium studies typically show coarse mucosal folds. Radioisotopic techniques may demonstrate abnormal enteric loss of protein; intravenous $^{51}CrCl_3$ is most commonly used.

Answer 94

1 (d)

Unequal fingers in a patient born with normal sized fingers in the absence of trauma is most likely due to repeated episodes of inflammation and joint destruction or to infarction. The fact that the patient is black makes the diagnosis of sickle cell anaemia more likely.

Answer 95

1 (b)

Explanation

The differential diagnosis must centre around causes of lymphocytosis in the CSF. The history is most suggestive of tuberculous meningitis. Investigations should be aimed at confirming this as quickly as possible.

> **Causes of lymphocytosis in the cerebrospinal fluid**
> - Tuberculous meningitis
> - Viral meningitis
> - Fungal meningitis
> - Meningovascular syphilis
> - Cerebral abscess
> - Cerebral toxoplasmosis
> - Sarcoidosis
> - CNS lymphoma/leukaemia

Answer 96

1 (b)

These are the Gottron's papules of dermatomyositis.

Answer 97

1 (d)
2 (b), (d)

Explanation

Primary biliary cirrhosis (PBC) characteristically occurs in middle-aged women. Itching is a common feature and is caused by retention of bile salts. Anti-mitochondrial antibodies directed against the inner casing of mitochondria are found in 90 per cent of patients. Liver biopsy usually shows piecemeal necrosis, prominent septa and infiltration with lymphocytes and plasma cells. Inflammation and resulting fibrosis around the bile ductules result in cholestasis with consequent pruritus, hypercholesterolaemia, and malabsorption of fat.

Low-titre positive ANAs are common in women, and more so in the context of autoimmune disease. The history of hypertension and hence possible drug-induced lupus might tempt you to pursue that avenue of investigation further but there are no other specific lupus features and the ANA is likely to be non-specific. Paracetamol analgesia may cause acute liver disease in excess, and non-steroidal analgesia can cause a usually hepatitic picture. Nevertheless, the picture of PBC is fairly typical.

Answer 98

1 (d)

The ECG was caught at a very opportune moment as the patient switches from right bundle branch block to sinus rhythm at the mid-recording point of the chest leads. The appearance in the chest leads looks like a partial bundle branch block in that the ECG shows broad complexes in leads V1–V3 but then narrow complexes in leads V4–V6. The complexes in leads V1–V3 look like a right bundle branch block and hence the answer of partial RBBB. However, the patient also has left axis deviation and therefore left anterior hemiblock would be a better answer. Nevertheless trumping this, is examination of the rhythm strip for V1 – whose complexes also become narrow at the point in time that the chest leads record V4–V6, indicating a change from bundle block to sinus rhythm.

Answer 99

1 (b)

The sardonic smile of tetanus (risus sardonicus) due to tonic muscle spasm of the facial and neck muscles is illustrated. This is evidence of end stage of the disease and there will be considerable difficulty in swallowing and breathing capacity. Tonic muscle spasm remains between reflex convulsions and this distinguishes it from strychnine poisoning.

Answer 100

1 (c)

The history fits with the development of constipation following the prescription of presumably codeine based medication. There is however little faecal material visible on the film. There is a collection of what appears to be teeth in the region of the iliac fossa. This is most likely to be a collection of ectodermal, mesodermal and endodermal tissue that in most cases also contains cystic material and is called a dermoid cyst. The majority are benign, but should be removed in order to prevent growth and to exclude malignancy.

Appendices

Appendix A – normal ranges

There are a few very basic investigations for which you will not be provided normal ranges in the MRCP examination. You will have to memorize these in advance if you have not already absorbed them by osmosis. We think the following lists include the only cases in which this will apply.

Haematology

	Male adult	Female adult
Hb (g/dL)	13.0–18.0	11.5–16.5
MCV (fL)	80–96	80–96
MCH (pg)	28–32	28–32
MCHC (g/dL)	32–35	32–35
WBC ($\times10^9$/L)	4–11	4–11
Platelets ($\times10^9$/L)	150–400	150–400

	Percentage	Absolute count
Neutrophils ($\times10^9$/L)	40–75	1.5–7
Eosinophils ($\times10^9$/L)	1–6	0.04–0.4
Basophils ($\times10^9$/L)	0–1	0–0.1
Monocytes ($\times10^9$/L)	0–8	0–0.8
Lymphocytes ($\times10^9$/L)	20–45	1.5–4
ESR (male, age <50 years)		<15 mm in first hour
ESR (female, age <50 years)		<20 mm in first hour

Biochemistry

Plasma sodium	137–144 mmol/L
Plasma potassium	3.5–4.9 mmol/L
Plasma urea	2.5–7.5 mmol/L
Plasma creatinine	60–110 µmol/L
Plasma bicarbonate	20–28 mmol/L
Plasma chloride	95–107 mmol/L
Plasma albumin	37–49 g/L
Plasma total protein	61–76 g/L
Plasma glucose (fasting)	3.0–6.0 mmol/L
Plasma bilirubin	1–22 µmol/L
Plasma calcium (total)	2.2–2.6 mmol/L
Plasma phosphate (inorganic)/inorganic phosphorus	0.8–1.4 mmol/L

Arterial blood gases

pH	7.36–7.44 kPa
$Pa\text{CO}_2$	4.7–6.0 kPa
$Pa\text{O}_2$	11.3–12.6 kPa

Cerebrospinal fluid analysis

Opening pressure	50–180 mmH$_2$O
Protein	0.15–0.45 g/L
Glucose	3.3–4.4 mmol/L

Appendix B – approach to a 12-lead ECG in the MRCP Part 2 written paper

Checklist

- Sensitivity marker
- Rate
- Mean frontal axis
- P wave
    height
    width
    shape
    relationship to QRS complexes

- PR interval
    length
    consistency

- Rhythm
    origin
    activation sequence

- QRS complex
    Q waves
    height/depth of QRS
    width of QRS
    pattern

- QT interval
- ST segments
    displacement
    gradient
    morphology

- T waves
    inverted or upright
    morphology

Sensitivity marker

Convention
The standard sensitivity marker (1 mV) measures 10 mm at full sensitivity, and 5 mm at half sensitivity. It may have been necessary to set the ECG machine at half sensitivity to fit in particularly large QRS complexes, e.g. in left ventricular hypertrophy. All the figures provided in this appendix assume that the ECG machine has been calibrated at standard sensitivity and speed.

Rate

Normal range: 55–100/min

Mean frontal axis

Normal range: −30° to +90°

Calculating the mean frontal axis, usually referred to simply as 'the axis', has been endowed with much mystery and needless misery. The underlying idea is simple: that the heart is assessed in a single two-dimensional coronal plan. An analogy might help: imagine you are looking down on an area of land from an aeroplane. You will only see movements in two dimensions. If there were a hot air balloon coming straight up it would not appear to be moving until it got close, and even then you would only assume it was moving from the fact that it appeared to be getting bigger. In terms of your two-dimensional plane, it would not be moving at all.

The mean frontal axis is the sum of all the movements of the wave of depolarization in that two-dimensional coronal plane over the whole period of depolarization. Let us go back to the aeroplane: imagine that a group of people are standing in the top left-hand corner of a field and over a few minutes they drift towards the bottom right-hand corner (Figure 1a). You are too far away to be able to count every movement and add them up, but you can get a general impression that the movements are happening rapidly and simultaneously. Figure 1(b) represents the sum of the movements of these individuals; by analogy, the ECG represents the sum of the 'electrical movements'.

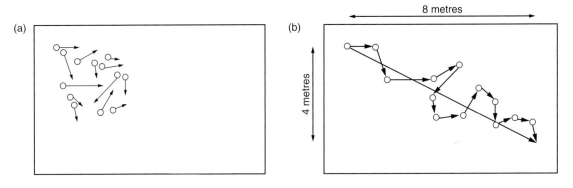

Figure 1   The movements (a) and the summation of all the movements (b) of 13 people in a field.

In an ECG, this 'sum of the electrical movements' is assessed by measuring the amplitudes of the QRS complexes in the limb leads. Standard lead I has an orientation of left to right (by convention labelled 0°; Figure 2). It is the equivalent of looking at our field from its north side. In one-dimensional terms, the total movement of our group of people with respect to the north side of the field is 8 metres. Standard lead aVF has the orientation north to south (by convention labelled 90°; Figure 2). It is the equivalent of looking at our field from its west side. In one-dimensional terms, the total movement of our group of people with respect to the west side of the field is 4 metres. These two vectors can be added together nose to tail to estimate the direction of the mass movement (Figure 3).

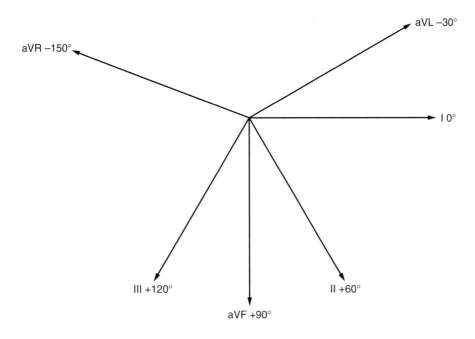

Figure 2   Conventional orientation of limb leads.

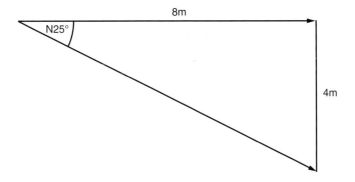

Figure 3   Resultant vector of movements in figure 1.

Using the extent of deflection of the ECG as a measure of movement of the wave of depolarization and repolarization, an identical process can be performed to calculate the mean frontal axis. However, the precision of measurement of the deflection is such that it is meaningless to report the angle to less than the nearest 5°.

Here are two worked examples:

Example 1

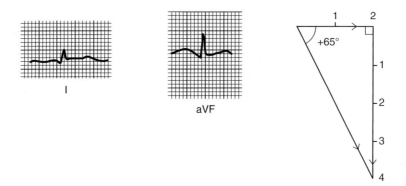

I

aVF

1   In lead I, the net sum of forces in the QRS complex is +2 mm (3 mm positive deflection from which subtract 1 mm negative deflection).
2   In lead aVF, it is +4 mm (5 mm positive, 1 mm negative).
3   Add the vectors of these two leads together in a nose-to-tail manner; both are positive, thus they are oriented in the direction of the lead.
4   The mean frontal axis is the resultant vector, approximately +65°. This is normal.

Example 2

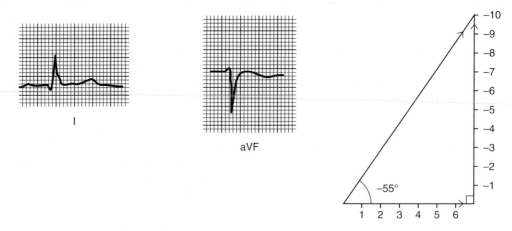

I

aVF

1   In lead I, the net sum of forces is +7 mm (8 mm positive deflection, 1 mm negative deflection).
2   In lead aVF, it is −10 mm (1 mm positive, and 11 mm negative).
3   Add these vectors nose-to-tail, taking into account the fact that aVF is negative, and thus goes away from the direction of the normal vector of aVF (i.e. −90° rather than +90°).
4   The mean frontal axis is thus approximately −55°. This is left axis deviation.

In a short period of time, you should be able to calculate axes in your head. For most clinical purposes, it is enough to be no more precise than ±30°. The only real exception to this is when you are trying to compare the QRS axis with the T axis.

Some rules of thumb

- If the complexes in I and II are both predominantly positive, the axis is normal.
- The axis lies at 90° to an isoelectric complex, i.e. positive and negative deflections are equal in size.

Note: While it is usually effective to use leads I and aVF to calculate the mean frontal axis, occasionally it seems that all leads seem to have an isoelectric complex and no axis can be calculated. This is presumably because the true axis is nearly perpendicular to the coronal plane.

P wave

Normal dimensions: height, 0.25 mV (0.5 mm); width, 0.12 s (3 mm).
Leads to view: the lead with the large P waves should be used. Leads II and V1 are usually the best.

Height

P waves more than 0.25 mV tall (2.5 mm) in the limb leads imply right atrial enlargement.

Width

P waves more than 0.12 s wide (3 mm) in the limb leads imply left atrial enlargement.

Shape

In right atrial enlargement, the P waves are tall, in left atrial enlargement, they are broad and bifid. Also in left atrial enlargement, in V1 the P wave is biphasic with a negative component that is at least one small square in area and larger than the area of the positive component.

If the P waves look unusual, e.g. prominent in leads in which they are usually poorly seen, or predominantly negative, they may not be originating from the sinus node. They may be ectopic within the atria, or be originating from the atrioventricular node or junction and be being retrogradely conducted. In the latter case, they tend to be predominantly negative. Alternatively, they may in fact be the F or f waves of atrial flutter or fibrillation, respectively. Suspect atrial flutter if the ventricular rate is approximately 150/min (i.e. 2:1 AV block: the atrial rate is 300/min). Suspect atrial fibrillation if the ventricular rhythm is irregular.

Note for the perverse

Beloved of examiners is the ECG in which the baseline clearly looks like atrial fibrillation but the ventricular rate is strictly regular. The catch is that there is also complete heart block. There are therefore two independent foci of electrical activation: the fibrillating atria and the isolated ventricles.

Relationship with QRS complexes

The presence of true P waves implies sinus rhythm. Check that each is followed by a QRS complex. If not, then there is at, least second degree heart block.

PR interval

The PR interval stretches from the **beginning** of the P wave to the **beginning** of the QRS complex.
Normal range: 0.12–0.20 s (3–5 mm).

Leads to view: use the lead in which the P wave is best seen (usually II and V1) and accept the longest measurement of the PR interval.

Length
If it is longer than 0.02 s, there is some degree of heart block. If it is shorter than 0.12 s, this implies either (a) that there is an accessory pathway with rapid conduction between the atria and ventricles (Wolff–Parkinson–White, Lown–Ganong–Levine syndrome, etc.) or (b) that the P wave is not originating from the sinoatrial node. Atrial ectopic foci may be associated with a short PR interval, as are beats originating from the AVN. If the pacemaker is distal in the junctional tissue, the wavefront may depolarize the ventricles before the atria, in which case there is a consistent relationship between the QRS complex and a P wave which is seen **after** it. In the intermediate situation of a pacemaker in the centre of the junctional tissue, P wave and QRS complex coincide and the former may not be seen.

Consistency
Make sure the relationship between P waves and QRS complex is seen in all, or nearly all, leads. If the relationship is not consistent, consider second- or third-degree heart block.

Rhythm
The term rhythm, refers to two things:

1   the origin of the wave of depolarization
2   the sequence in which it proceeds, the 'activation sequence'.

You have gathered all the necessary information to determine both by examining the P waves and the PR interval.

The origin of the wave of depolarization
In normal rhythm the sequence begins at the sinoatrial node, producing sinus rhythm. However, it may begin anywhere else in the heart. Other sources within the conduction system include the atrioventricular node (AVN). It is this 'node' which is referred to in the term 'nodal rhythm'. The term 'junctional rhythm' is less anatomically specific and implies a rhythm originating from the junction of the atria and ventricles. This includes the AVN and also the specialized conduction tissue distal to it, the bundle of His. If the sequence is triggered from a point anywhere else in the myocardium, it is an ectopic rhythm. These may take over control of cardiac depolarization for a single beat, a run, or for prolonged periods, and may be atrial or ventricular. Any such non-sinus supraventricular origin of the rhythm may produce an atypical P wave, which in turn may be conducted anterogradely and/or retrogradely.

In certain circumstances, there is continuous electrical activity in parts of the heart, most commonly **atrial flutter** and **fibrillation**. When these exist, they stimulate depolarization of the ventricles and are the origin of the activation sequence.

Finally, it is possible to have more than one source of depolarization operating at the same time. Most commonly, one or more ectopic foci and the sinoatrial node are firing simultaneously. Which is responsible for a particular cardiac beat depends entirely on the timing of each with respect to adjacent refractory periods, and the source may change from moment to moment. Occasionally, they share responsibility for a single beat, with their respective waves of depolarization meeting half-way. This is the origin of the fusion beat. In complete heart block, the atria and ventricles are electrically isolated from each other and each has a separate source of depolarization.

Appendix: B

The activation sequence

In normal beats the wave of depolarization originating in the sinoatrial node passes through the atria to the AVN, bundle of His, the specialized conducting tissue in the ventricles and from these through the ventricular myocardium. This can be interrupted or slowed at any point. If there is a delay or blockage in the area of the AVN or bundle of His, then this is a form of heart block. More distal blocks may produce left and right bundle branch blocks and hemiblocks.

QRS complex

Examine all QRS complexes in sequence. Bear in mind the sequence of orientation (see Figure 2). We suggest looking at the limb leads first in the order: aVL, I, II, aVF, III, and aVR and then at the chest leads in order V1–V6. Consider each of the following points:

1   Are there any Q waves and are they pathological? Q waves may be found in any lead of a normal ECG except V2. To be pathological, however, they must be at least 0.04 s in duration (one small square) and in the vertical axis be more than 25 per cent of the height of the ensuing R wave. Even then, what appears to be a pathological Q wave may actually be a prominent S wave which has completely obliterated the R wave. Since it is then the first deflection of the QRS complex and is negative it conforms to the definition of a Q wave. These waves are called QS waves and may be seen in aVL, III and V1. A QS wave (or apparently pathological Q wave) is normal in aVL if the axis is >+60° and normal in III if the axis is <+30°.

2   The height/depth of QRS complexes: at least one R wave in the precordial leads must be greater than 8 mm. Otherwise, the QRS complexes may be said to be pathologically small. The definition of pathologically tall/deep QRS complexes is complex. The size of the R wave in aVL must not exceed 13 mm and in aVF, 20 mm. In the chest leads, the tallest R wave should not exceed 27 mm and the deepest S/QS wave should not exceed 30 mm. The sum of the tallest R wave and the deepest S/QS should not exceed 40 mm. If any of these dimensions is exceeded, the ECG cannot be declared unequivocally normal. However, it is harder to assert that a particular chamber is hypertrophied without accompanying ST/T wave abnormalities, particularly in young people.

3   The width of QRS complexes: no QRS complex should exceed 0.12 s (three small squares). If it does, this implies an intraventricular conduction defect. This may be due to ventricular hypertrophy or a defect in the conduction system. Look at the height of the complexes and their morphology for further clues.

4   Pattern: normally, R waves become progressively taller across the chest, but it is a normal variant for them to decrease in size from V4 to V5. Conversely, S waves should become progressively smaller across the chest, although V1 may be smaller than V2. Finally, the morphology of broadened complexes may characterize a pattern of conduction defects.

QT interval

Prolonged QT intervals may be due to metabolic abnormalities (e.g. hypocalcaemia) or drugs (e.g. amiodarone, quinidine, disopyrimide), or be a congenital abnormality (e.g. Romano–Ward syndrome). It may be associated with significant dysrhythmias, but it is difficult to assess since it is rate related. (So is the PR interval, but it varies rather less.) The QT interval may be corrected using the formula $QTc=QT/\sqrt{(R\text{-}R\ interval)}$. This produces the range of 0.35–0.43 s. However, rather than calculate this on each occasion, some find it easier to note a few specific values:

Rate (per min)	Upper limit of QT interval (seconds)	
	Male	Female
150	0.25	0.28
100	0.31	0.34
75	0.36	0.39
60	0.40	0.44
50	0.44	0.48

ST segments

The ST segment runs from the J point, the end of the S wave, to the beginning of the T wave.

Displacement from the isoelectric line

The ST segment must not deviate from the isoelectric line by more than 1 mm either upwards or downwards. However, it often slopes, causing much angst in quantifying the degree of deviation. In exercise ECG testing, the crucial place at which deviation is assessed is taken to be 0.06 s (1.5 small squares) along the ST segment from the J point.

Gradient

A downsloping ST segment is much more likely to imply significant ischaemic heart disease than an upsloping one, even if both are 1 mm depressed 0.06 s from the J point. However, it can only finally be interpreted in the light of the clinical scenario.

Morphology

Pericarditis is associated with saddle-shaped ST elevation in many leads of the ECG. Some apparent ST elevation is often shrugged off as an abnormally 'high take-off' and of no clinical significance, and may be a normal racial variant. This is usually seen in the right precordial leads. It can be difficult to assert what is significant ST segment elevation in leads V1–V3. Again, the apparent abnormality must be interpreted in the clinical context, and mild to moderate (<2 mm) ST elevation in V1–V3 with no other ECG abnormality is unlikely to be significant unless accompanied by clinical features of right ventricular infarction.

T waves

Inverted or upright

Inverted T waves can only be said to be unequivocally abnormal if they are found in I, II, or V4–V6. They may or may not be pathological if found in other leads. Of more value is the assertion that a T wave should be upright if the QRS complex in that lead is predominantly positive, and inverted if the QRS is predominantly negative. There can be a small amount of deviation from this rule, but almost never in more than one lead. The T-wave axis (calculated in the same way as the QRS axis) should not differ from the mean frontal axis by more than 45°. The one exception to this rule is in inferior infarction, when inverted T waves are abnormal findings (part of the ECG findings of MI) despite having a similar axis to the QRS complexes.

Morphology

Peaked or flattened T waves are found in metabolic abnormalities, e.g. peaked in hyperkalaemia and flattened (with ensuing U waves) in hypokalaemia. Size should be assessed in leads V3–V6. The T wave should be no more than 2/3 and no less than 1/8 of the height of the preceding R wave.

Index